Commemorative Issue: 15 Years of the Sleep Medicine Clinics - Part 1: Sleep and Sleep Disorders

Editors

ANA C. KRIEGER
TEOFILO LEE-CHIONG Jr

SLEEP MEDICINE CLINICS

www.sleep.theclinics.com

June 2022 • Volume 17 • Number 2

ELSEVIER

1600 John F. Kennedy Boulevard • Suite 1800 • Philadelphia, Pennsylvania, 19103-2899

http://www.theclinics.com

SLEEP MEDICINE CLINICS Volume 17, Number 2
June 2022, ISSN 1556-407X, ISBN-13: 978-0-323-96163-9

Editor: Joanna Collett
Developmental Editor: Axell Ivan Jade M. Purificacion

Sleep Medicine Clinics (ISSN 1556-407X) is published quarterly by Elsevier Inc., 360 Park Avenue South, New York, NY 10010-1710. Months of issue are March, June, September and December. Business and Editorial Offices: 1600 John F. Kennedy Blvd., Ste. 1800, Philadelphia, PA 19103-2899. Customer Service Office: 3251 Riverport Lane, Maryland Heights, MO 63043. Periodicals postage paid at New York, NY and additional mailing offices. Subscription prices are $234.00 per year (US individuals), $100.00 (US and Canadian students), $653.00 (US institutions), $272.00 (Canadian individuals), $267.00 (international individuals) $135.00 (International students), $682.00 (Canadian and International institutions). Foreign air speed delivery is included in all *Clinics* subscription prices. All prices are subject to change without notice. **POSTMASTER:** Send change of address to *Sleep Medicine Clinics*, Elsevier Health Sciences Division, Subscription Customer Service, 3251 Riverport Lane, Maryland Heights, MO 63043. Customer Service: **Tel: 1-800-654-2452 (U.S. and Canada); 314-447-8871 (outside U.S. and Canada). Fax: 314-447-8029. E-mail: journalscustomerservice-usa@elsevier.com (for print support); journalsonline-support-usa@elsevier.com (for online support).**

Reprints. For copies of 100 or more of articles in this publication, please contact the Commercial Reprints Department, Elsevier Inc., 360 Park Avenue South, New York, NY 10010-1710. Tel.: 212-633-3874; Fax: 212-633-3820; E-mail: reprints@elsevier.com.

Sleep Medicine Clinics is covered in *MEDLINE/PubMed (Index Medicus)*.

SLEEP MEDICINE CLINICS

FORTHCOMING ISSUES

September 2022
Commemorative Issue: 15 years of the Sleep Medicine Clinics, Part 2: Medication and treatment effect on sleep disorders
Ana C. Krieger and Teofilo Lee-Chiong, *Editors*

December 2022
A review of PAP therapy for the treatment of OSA
Matthew R. Ebben, *Editor*

March 2023
Adjunct Interventions to Cognitive Behavioral Therapy for Insomnia
Joshua Hyong-Jin Cho, *Editor*

RECENT ISSUES

March 2022
Causes of Sleep Complaints
Keith Romeo A. Aguilera, and Agnes T. Remulla, *Editor*

December 2021
Measuring Sleep
Erna Sif Arnardottir, *Editor*

September 2021
Sleep Medicine: Current Challenges and its Future
Barbara Gnidovec Stražišar, *Editor*

SERIES OF RELATED INTEREST

Neurologic Clinics
Available at: https://www.neurologic.theclinics.com/

Contributors

CONSULTING EDITORS

TEOFILO LEE-CHIONG Jr, MD
Professor of Medicine, National Jewish Health, Professor of Medicine, University of Colorado, Denver, Colorado, USA; Chief Medical Liaison, Philips Respironics, Pennsylvania, USA

ANA C. KRIEGER, MD, MD, MPH, FCCP, FAASM
Chief, Division of Sleep Neurology Medical Director, Weill Cornell Center for Sleep Medicine, New York, Professor of Clinical Medicine, Professor of Medicine in Neurology and Genetic Medicine,Weill Cornell Medical College, Cornell University, New York, New York, USA

EDITORS

ANA C. KRIEGER, MD, MPH, FCCP, FAASM
Chief, Division of Sleep Neurology, Medical Director, Weill Cornell Center for Sleep Medicine, Professor of Clinical Medicine, Professor of Medicine in Neurology and Genetic Medicine, Weill Cornell Medical College, Cornell University, New York, New York, USA

TEOFILO LEE-CHIONG Jr, MD
Professor of Medicine, National Jewish Health, Professor of Medicine, University of Colorado, Denver, Colorado, USA; Chief Medical Liaison, Philips Respironics, Murrysville, Pennsylvania, USA

AUTHORS

RITA AOUAD, MD
Division of Pulmonary, Critical Care, and Sleep Medicine, Department of Internal Medicine, The Ohio State University, Columbus, Ohio, USA

VINEET M. ARORA, MD, MAPP
Herbert T Abelson Professor of Medicine Dean, Pritzker School of Medicine, Department of Medicine, University of Chicago, Chicago, Illinois, USA

FIONA C. BAKER, PhD
Human Sleep Research Program, SRI International, Menlo Park, California, USA; Brain Function Research Group, School of Physiology, University of the Witwatersrand, Johannesburg, South Africa

GLENNA S. BREWSTER, PhD, RN, FNP-BC
Assistant Professor, Nell Hodgson Woodruff School of Nursing, Emory University, Atlanta Georgia, USA

JONATHAN CHAREST, PhD
Department of Kinesiology, University of Calgary, Calgary, Alberta, Canada; Centre for Sleep & Human Performance, Department of Psychology, Universite Laval, Quebec City, Quebec, Canada

NATALIE DAUTOVICH, PhD
Department of Psychology, Virginia Commonwealth University, Richmond, Virginia, USA

JEANNE F. DUFFY, MBA, PhD
Division of Sleep and Circadian Disorders, Department of Medicine, Brigham and Women's Hospital, Division of Sleep Medicine, Harvard Medical School, Boston, Massachusetts, USA

JOSEPH M. DZIERZEWSKI, PhD
Department of Psychology, Virginia Commonwealth University, Richmond, Virginia, USA

ALEXANDRIA R. ELKHADEM
Division of Sleep and Circadian Disorders, Department of Medicine, Brigham and Women's Hospital, Boston, Massachusetts, USA

PHILIP R. GEHRMAN, PhD, CBSM, FAASM
Associate Professor of Clinical Psychology in Psychiatry, Hospital of the University of Pennsylvania, Philadelphia, Pennsylvania, USA

NALAKA S. GOONERATNE, MD, MSc
Associate Professor, Geriatrics Division, Perelman School of Medicine, University of Pennsylvania, Center for Sleep and Circadian Neurobiology, Philadelphia, Pennsylvania, USA

MICHAEL A. GRANDNER, PhD, MTR, CBSM
Department of Psychiatry, College of Medicine, University of Arizona, Tucson, Arizona, USA

SEBASTIAN C. HOLST, PhD
Neuroscience and Rare Diseases Discovery and Translational Area, Roche Pharmaceutical Research and Early Development, Roche Innovation Center Basel, Basel, Switzerland

ALEX IRANZO, MD, PhD
Neurology Service, Hospital Clinic de Barcelona, Barcelona, Spain

DENISE C. JARRIN, PhD
School of Psychology and Centre de Recherche CERVO, Université Laval, Quebéc, Canada

ILIA N. KARATSOREOS, PhD
Department of Psychological and Brain Sciences, Neuroscience and Behavior Program, University of Massachusetts Amherst, Amherst, Massachusetts, USA

MEENA S. KHAN, MD
Division of Pulmonary, Critical Care, and Sleep Medicine, Departments of Internal Medicine and Neurology, The Ohio State University, Columbus, Ohio, USA

JEE HYUN KIM, MD, PhD
Department of Neurology, Ewha Womans University Seoul Hospital, Ewha Womans University College of Medicine, Gangseo-gu, Seoul, Republic of Korea

HANS-PETER LANDOLT, PhD
Institute of Pharmacology and Toxicology, Zürich Center for Interdisciplinary Sleep Research (ZiS), University of Zürich, Zürich, Switzerland

KATHRYN ALDRICH LEE RN, PHD, CBSM
Department of Family Health Care Nursing, UCSF School of Nursing, University of California, San Francisco, San Francisco, California, USA

JUNXIN LI, PhD
Assistant Professor, Johns Hopkins University, School of Nursing, Baltimore, Maryland, USA

RAMAN K. MALHOTRA, MD
Professor of Neurology, Washington University Sleep Medicine Center, Department of Neurology, Washington University in St. Louis School of Medicine, St Louis, Missouri, USA

BRUCE S. MCEWEN, PhD
Harold and Margaret Milliken Hatch Laboratory of Neuroendocrinology, The Rockefeller University, New York, New York, USA

CHARLES M. MORIN, PhD
School of Psychology and Centre de Recherche CERVO, Université Laval, Quebéc, Canada

ELLIOTTNELL PEREZ, MS
Department of Psychology, Virginia Commonwealth University, Richmond, Virginia, USA

SCOTT G. RAVYTS, MS
Department of Psychology, Virginia Commonwealth University, Richmond, Virginia, USA

BARBARA RIEGEL, PhD, RN, FAAN, FAHA
Professor, School of Nursing, Perelman School of Medicine, University of Pennsylvania, Philadelphia, Pennsylvania, USA

ALAN M. ROSENWASSER, PhD
Department of Psychology, School of Biology and Ecology, Graduate School of Biomedical Science and Engineering, University of Maine, Orono, Maine, USA

NANCY H. STEWART, DO, MS
Assistant Professor of Medicine, Department of Medicine, University of Kansas Medical Center, Kansas City, Kansas, USA

FRED W. TUREK, PhD
Department of Neurobiology, Center for Sleep and Circadian Biology, Northwestern University, Evanston, Illinois, USA

MICHAEL V. VITIELLO, PhD
Professor, Department of Psychiatry and Behavioral Sciences, University of Washington, Seattle, Washington, USA

Contents

Insufficient sleep and sleep disorders are highly prevalent in the population and are associated with significant morbidity and mortality. Adverse outcomes of insufficient sleep and/or sleep disorders are weight gain and obesity, cardiovascular disease, diabetes, accidents and injuries, stress, pain, neurocognitive dysfunction, psychiatric symptoms, and mortality. Exposure to sleep difficulties varies by age, sex, race/ethnicity, and socioeconomic status; significant sleep health disparities exist in the population. Societal influences, such as globalization, technology, and public policy, affect sleep at a population level.

In this review, we provide a summary of the field of mammalian circadian neurobiology circa 2015. While many additional details have emerged in the intervening seven years, understanding of the fundamental structure and function of this critical neural system remains intact. Thus, the present review continues to provide a valuable introduction for those seeking an integrative multilevel overview of the circadian system. In brief, the circadian system comprises a coupled network of molecular/cellular- and tissue-level oscillators, hierarchically coordinated by the hypothalamic suprachiasmatic nuclear circadian pacemaker, and entrained by both photic and nonphotic signals.

Behavioral states naturally alternate between wakefulness and the sleep phases rapid eye movement and nonrapid eye movement sleep. Waking and sleep states are complex processes that are elegantly orchestrated by spatially fine-tuned neurochemical changes of neurotransmitters and neuromodulators including glutamate, acetylcholine, γ-aminobutyric acid, norepinephrine, dopamine, serotonin, histamine, hypocretin, melanin concentrating hormone, adenosine, and melatonin. However, as highlighted in this brief overview, no single neurotransmitter or neuromodulator, but rather their complex interactions within organized neuronal ensembles, regulate waking and sleep states. The neurochemical pathways presented here are aimed to provide a conceptual framework for the understanding of the effects of currently used sleep medications.

Sleep is a key determinant of healthy and cognitive aging. Sleep patterns change with aging, independent of other factors, and include advanced sleep timing, shortened nocturnal sleep duration, increased frequency of daytime naps, increased number of nocturnal awakenings and time spent awake during the night, and decreased slow-wave sleep. The sleep-related hormone secretion changes with aging. Most changes seem to occur between young and middle adulthood; sleep parameters remain largely unchanged among healthy older adults. The circadian system and sleep homeostatic mechanisms become less robust with normal aging. The causes of sleep disturbances in older adults are multifactorial.

associated with worse health outcomes, including; cardio-metabolic derangements and increased risk of delirium. Because older patients are at risk of; polypharmacy and medication side effects, a variety of nonpharmacological interventions are recommended first to improve sleep loss for hospitalized older adults.

speed, and other aspects of physical performance. Sleep issues can also increase risk of concussions and other injuries and impair recovery after injury. Cognitive performance is also impacted in several domains, including vigilance, learning and memory, decision making, and creativity.

Sleep and circadian rhythms are altered in association with the hormonal changes in the menstrual cycle and in the presence of menstrual-associated disorders. The magnitude of the effect varies, particularly for self-reported sleep quality, which worsens in some, but not all, women when premenstrual symptoms emerge. Importantly, women with polycystic ovary syndrome (PCOS) have an increased risk for sleep-disordered breathing (SDB), which should be treated to mitigate health impacts. Potential menstrual cycle variability in sleep quality, as well as upper airway resistance, should be considered when evaluating reproductive-age women. For research purposes, the impact of the menstrual cycle phase should be kept in mind when data are collected and, ideally, the phase should be documented. When comparing women with men, women of reproductive age should be studied in the early-mid follicular phase before there is potential influence from ovarian hormones.

Sleep paralysis is rare in the elderly but may occur particularly in families suffering from this phenomenon. In a minority of patients with disorders of arousal, the episodes persist until the age of 70. Zolpidem and other medications may induce sleepwalking and sleep eating-related syndrome. Most patients with idiopathic REM sleep behavior disorder (RBD) eventually develop Parkinson disease and dementia with Lewy bodies. Anti-IgLON5 disease includes abnormal behaviors in both non-rapid eye movement sleep and rapid eye movement sleep (REM) sleep. Restless legs syndrome prevalence increases with age until the sixth decade. A severe form of periodic limb movements in sleep may clinically mimic REM sleep behavior disorder (RBD).

Patients suffering from neurodegenerative conditions frequently report sleep complaints, such as insomnia and excessive daytime sleepiness. These symptoms are likely multifactorial, caused by their underlying neurologic disorder and also by medications and other comorbidities associated with the progressive condition. A detailed history, sleep logs, actigraphy, or polysomnography may be necessary to properly diagnosis and manage these patients. Improvement in sleep may result in improvement in neurologic symptoms and quality of life in this population. There is growing evidence that disrupted sleep may lead to acceleration in the progression of the neurodegenerative disorder and may play a role in the pathogenesis.

Preface
Sleep Medicine: Its Imperfect Past

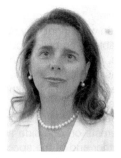 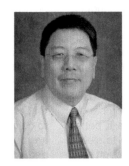

Ana C. Krieger, MD, MPH, FCCP, FAASM   Teofilo Lee-Chiong Jr, MD

Editors

It could be said that the past of Sleep Medicine is forgettable: as with life in general, it is sometimes easy to forget what brought us to today and simply ignore the past. It would be a mistake not to learn from the past journey, as it took a lot of courage, dedication, and determination from many scientists and clinicians to help develop this eclectic field and bring Sleep Medicine to what it is today. Unfortunately, much of the past of Sleep Medicine has already been forgotten or has never really been learned by the new generation of professionals working in or joining the field. Even more concerning is the fact that remembering the past is often tinted by today's knowledge unfettered by the sobering perspective of hindsight.

Sleep medicine is a field that is still growing and in conflict with itself. It is easy to recall with contempt those dreadful, large, and uncomfortable early CPAP masks, painful and untested surgical approaches, and dangerous medications prescribed many decades ago, without conceding that those were the best approaches available at that time. From looking at challenging conditions, such as insomnia, broken down to at least a dozen different potential causes, over time, however, were clumped into two categories; we appreciate the practicality of the current classification but yearn for the pathophysiologic insights gained from the earlier divisions. We edge idiopathic hypersomnia closer to narcolepsy but at the same time try to move the latter further away from the former: this tug-and-pull continues today with no clarifying pathophysiology, clinical feature, biomarker, or diagnostic test in sight for

hypersomnia. Each day, we treat more patients with parasomnias, either primary or secondary, and yet recognize that we know very little about these conditions and their true cause. Many circadian rhythm sleep disorders are increasingly becoming a lifestyle choice, as is chronic sleep deprivation, despite its public health hazards; we are powerless in the midst of this societal shift. There are more articles about sleep disorders, nightmares, and sleepwalking in the lay media than there are in our science journals, and personal opinions are often used to make recommendations instead of sound clinical research.

We learn that sleep is "of, by, and for" the brain and relearn that sleep predates the brain; how many textbook chapters, presentations, and mindsets must be revised! We venture into sleep's microarchitecture searching for the origins of cognition, memory, and emotion, and attempt to manipulate its hertzes, spindles, and waves to augment, replace, or regulate them, and fail. It is peculiar to realize that the "microtuning" of sleep waves that is sought by the lay public and media has no real scientific basis. Superficial discussions about having more of an X or Y stage of sleep are often presented, as if someone could easily manipulate the electrical activity of the brain. This shows the lack of understanding of what sleep truly is, a complex chemical process, orchestrated by yet unknown factors with intended results.

As a field, Sleep Medicine has its share of rules, policies, guidelines, best-practices, and coverage determinations for service and care, which have a clear impact but do not necessarily bring value; we

Sleep Med Clin 17 (2022) xiii–xiv
https://doi.org/10.1016/j.jsmc.2022.03.007
1556-407X/22/© 2022 Published by Elsevier Inc.

trust the need for regulation but not always their purpose. The most embarrassing and inexcusable of all is our "4-hour, 70% of nights PAP use" rule, which, for many, has become a quasi-religion. Indeed, so much of Sleep Medicine was, and still is, a magic show, with all of us willingly or forcefully participating but none of us fully comprehending. One can only imagine if such rules would be expanded to other fields; imagine access to anticoagulants or antihypertensive medications being denied to patients if they are not used more than 70% of the time!

Finally, our clinical recommendations have become platitudes that are often incompatible with the realities of contemporary life. Is it better to tell our patients what is the ideal way to sleep, or to help them sleep better as they go through their lives in the modern world? Is it more important to develop devices to detect sleepiness among drivers, or to invent technology to always ensure safe driving for everyone? Is it more effective to limit work hours among health care workers in order to reduce medical errors, or to create algorithms and systems to prevent errors by anyone at any time? Do we modify school times, or should we help change the methods of teaching? Perhaps both approaches should be considered, and if so, which one should be prioritized?

The march of science is slow and tedious. We increasingly expect science to eventually give us the (a) knowledge, (b) understanding, and (c) solution for everything in Sleep Medicine. However, many of us value facts over methods, choose confirmation rather than discovery, favor standardization to heterogeneity, and try to find solutions and not answers. But this isn't science, and misinterpreting what science is can be threateningly dangerous or annoyingly frustrating. How can science help us standardize approaches and still personalize care? Understanding and coping with these disparities is a major challenge, and looking to our past may help guide us.

The biggest danger of the past of Sleep Medicine is mistrust. In a "temporary society," the next best thing is always just around the corner. In an "information society," there are multiple versions of the truth. When we cannot fully remember our history, we are liable to embellish our failures and distort our errors, both of which can magnify the mistrust of our past choices, actions, and science. It is, therefore, essential to acknowledge that, even in an imperfect past, each of us tried to do our best in the field and remember that there are opinions and interests on one side and facts and science on the other end of the spectrum. At a societal level, our role is to help these two ends meet in order to implement a healthier and improved sleep for all.

Ana C. Krieger, MD, MPH, FCCP, FAASM
Division of Sleep Neurology
Weill Cornell Center for Sleep Medicine
Weill Cornell Medical College
Cornell University
New York, NY 10065, USA

Teofilo Lee-Chiong Jr, MD
National Jewish Health
University of Colorado
Denver, CO 80206, USA

Philips Respironics
Murrysville, PA 15668, USA

E-mail addresses:
ack2003@med.cornell.edu (A.C. Krieger)
lee-chiongT@njc.org (T. Lee-Chiong)

Sleep, Health, and Society

Michael A. Grandner, PhD, MTR, CBSM

KEYWORDS

• Sleep • Sleep disorders • Epidemiology • Social factors • Health • Disparities • Society

KEY POINTS

- Insufficient sleep and sleep disorders are highly prevalent in the population and are associated with significant morbidity and mortality.
- Adverse outcomes of insufficient sleep and/or sleep disorders are weight gain and obesity, cardiovascular disease, diabetes, accidents and injuries, stress, pain, neurocognitive dysfunction, psychiatric symptoms, and mortality.
- Exposure to sleep difficulties varies by age, sex, race/ethnicity, and socioeconomic status; significant sleep health disparities exist in the population.
- Societal influences, such as globalization, technology, and public policy, affect sleep at a population level.

CONCEPTUALIZING SLEEP IN A SOCIAL CONTEXT

Sleep represents an emergent set of many physiologic processes under primarily neurobiological regulation that impact many physiologic systems. As such, many advances have been made over the past several decades that have shed light on these neurobiologic mechanisms of sleep-wake,[1–4] with especially exciting work in the area of functional genetics/genomics[5,6] and molecular mechanisms of sleep-related regulation.[7–9] Still, the phenomenon of sleep exists outside the nucleus and the cell membrane: sleep is experienced phenomenologically. Sleep is a biological requirement for human life, alongside food, water, and air. Like consumption of food and unlike breathing air, achieving this biological need requires the individual to engage in volitional behaviors. Although many of these behaviors are genetically and intrapersonally driven (eg, it is not a coincidence that most people prefer to sleep at night, and that most humans sleep in a stereotypical posturally recumbent manner), there is still much variability in sleep behaviors and practices. Because of this, sleep is also socially driven, dictated by the environment, and subject to interpersonal and societal factors.

Sleep in most humans occupies between 20% and 40% of the day. Even prehistoric evidence suggests the importance of sleep in human life[10]; this is consistent with archaeological and historical accounts of sleep having a prominent and important role in even early human society. Sleep was a universal phenomenon that was inescapable and thus was incorporated in social structures. In this way, sleep became not just a set of physiologic processes, but one represented in sociocultural structures. Thus, the timing, environment, and constraints surrounding sleep across human societies began to differ between rich and poor, powerful and powerless, rural and urban, and so forth. As sociologist Simon Williams writes, "Where we sleep, when we sleep, and with whom we sleep are all important markers or indicators of social status, privilege, and prevailing power relations."[11]

CONCEPTUALIZING DOWNSTREAM CONSEQUENCES

The downstream consequences of insufficient sleep duration and/or inadequate sleep quality (including sleep disorders and circadian misalignment of sleep) are varied and impact many physiologic systems. Conceptualizing these is therefore

This article previously appeared in *Sleep Med Clin* 12 (2017) 1–22.

Department of Psychiatry, College of Medicine, University of Arizona, 1501 North Campbell Avenue, PO Box 245002, BUMC Suite 7326, Tucson, AZ 85724-5002, USA

E-mail address: grandner@email.arizona.edu

Sleep Med Clin 17 (2022) 117–139

https://doi.org/10.1016/j.jsmc.2022.03.001

difficult. One way to do so is to acknowledge domains of outcomes and recognize the overlaps and relationships among those domains. The recent position statement from the American Academy of Sleep Medicine and Sleep Research Society[12–15] broadly categorizes effects of insufficient sleep as pertaining to the following categories: general health, cardiovascular health, metabolic health, mental health, immunologic health, human performance, cancer, pain, and mortality.

CONCEPTUALIZING UPSTREAM INFLUENCES: SOCIAL-ECOLOGICAL MODELS

Upstream social and environmental influences on sleep are also complex and overlapping and implicate many potential pathways. With this in mind, a social-ecological framework may be best suited to describe this relationship. The social-ecological model was originally developed to describe the complex ways that an individual's behavior related to their health is a product of influences at the individual level, but that the individual operates in the context of social structures that they are a member of, but these structures exist outside of the individual.[16] For example, an individual has genetic, psychological, and other reasons for consuming a healthy diet, but social structures that they are a part of but exist outside of that individual (like their neighborhood, which may have healthy food; their job, which may or may not have a cafeteria; their family, which may have other food restrictions, and so forth) play a role in that individual's behavior.

This model also may be appropriate for understanding sleep. At the individual level, factors that influence a person's sleep include that person's genetics, knowledge, beliefs, and attitudes about sleep, their overall health, and so forth. The individual level is embedded, though, within a social level, which includes the home (family, bedroom, and so forth), neighborhood, work/school, socioeconomics, religion, culture, race/ethnicity, and other factors. All of these factors influence sleep through the individual. Still, this social level is embedded within a societal level, which includes social forces that exist outside of things like work, family, and neighborhood, including globalization, geography, technology, public policy. These factors, at this high of a level, filter through the social structures that eventually come to bear on the individual. For example, as society embraced the Internet, it caused changes in jobs and families, which led to individual changes that play a role in sleep (such as social networking in bed or browsing the Internet late at night). **Fig. 1** displays a social-ecological model of sleep, illustrating that sleep duration and quality are influenced by factors at the individual level, which is embedded within a social level, which itself is embedded within a societal level. **Fig. 2** brings these models together, with sleep as the fulcrum (shown in **Fig. 1**) at the interface of upstream social-environmental influences (shown in more detail in **Fig. 3**) and downstream health and functional outcomes (shown in more detail in **Fig. 2**). This model brings all of these concepts together to describe how sleep is influenced by these societal factors and how those influences, through sleep, may play a role in health. The first version of this model was published in 2010,[17] and it has appeared in several other publications since then.[14,18–20] It may serve as a useful framework for conceptualizing the physiologic processes of sleep in a social context.

POPULATION PREVALENCE OF SLEEP DURATION AND SLEEP DISTURBANCES
Sleep Duration

Population estimates of habitual sleep duration are variable, because few studies used identical methods to derive estimates. The best population-level estimates come from 1 of 3 sources: (1) self-reported time use data, (2) self-reported typical weeknight/work-night sleep, and (3) self-reported average sleep within 24 hours. For US-based data, the primary sources of these estimates come from the American Time Use Survey (ATUS) for time use data, the National Health Interview Survey or National Health and Nutrition Examination Survey (NHANES) for weeknight sleep, and the Behavioral Risk Factor Surveillance System (BRFSS) for 24-hour sleep.

Longitudinal analysis of time use diaries by Knutson and colleagues[21] found that the proportion of Americans reporting short (<6 hours) sleep was 7.6% in 1975 and 9.3% in 2006. Bin and colleagues[22] examined similar time use data from several countries and showed that, in the United States, sleep duration has generally declined since the 1960s, if only by a small amount. The most comprehensive analysis of time use data related to sleep was recently undertaken by Basner and colleagues.[23] They report that the age group that receives the most sleep is young adults (8.86 hours on weeknights and 10.02 hours on weekends) and that those aged 25 to 64 report about 0.70 to 0.99 fewer hours on weeknights and 0.62 to 1.16 fewer hours on weekends. Prevalence of sleep duration by hour is not reported, though.

Regarding weekday sleep duration, Grandner and colleagues[24] reported census-weighted

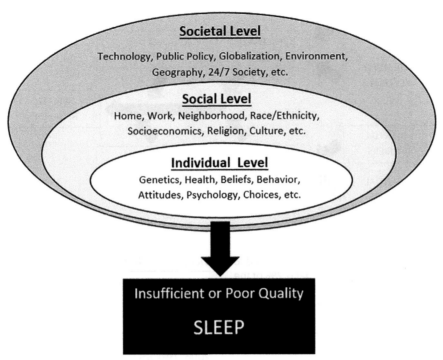

Fig. 1. Social-ecological model of sleep.

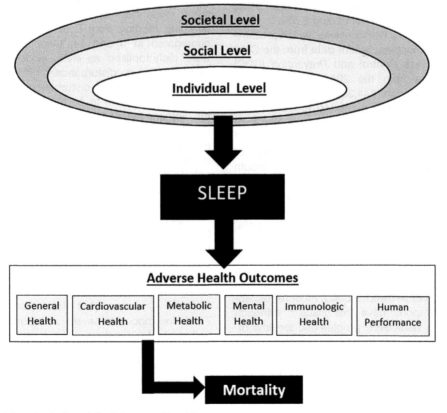

Fig. 2. Social-ecological model of sleep and health.

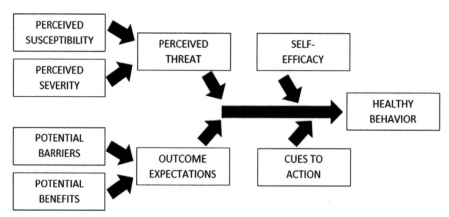

Fig. 3. Health belief model.

estimates of sleep duration using the 2007 to 2008 wave of the NHANES. They report that 6.2% of the population reports less than 5 hours of sleep, 33.78% reports 5 to 6 hours of sleep, 52.68% report 7 to 8 hours of sleep, and 7.38% report at least 9 hours of sleep per typical weeknight. These values from NHANES is similar to values reported from Krueger and Friedman,[25] who assessed similar data from the National Health Interview Survey using data from 2004 to 2007. They report prevalence of 5 hours or less being 7.8%, 6 hours being 20.5%, 7 hours being 30.8%, 8 hours being 32.5%, and 9 or more hours being 8.5%.

Regarding typical 24-hour sleep, which presumably includes napping, recent data from the Centers for Disease Control and Prevention (CDC) released data from the 2014 BRFSS, which included data from 444,306 American adults. Based on the recently published guidelines,[12,15] the CDC calculated the prevalence of less than 7 hours of sleep duration across all 50 states.[26] The median prevalence of less than 7 hours of sleep was 35.1%, with a range of 28.4% (South Dakota) to 43.9% (Hawaii). This report also documents that the prevalence of 5 hours or less was 11.8%, with prevalence of 6, 7, 8, 9, and 10 or more hours being 23.0%, 29.5%, 27.7%, 4.4%, and 3.6%, respectively.

Taken together, the time diaries generally show more sleep than other retrospective reports, perhaps because they may better capture time in bed but not actual sleep. Indeed, most retrospective sleep reports have this issue,[27] although perhaps it is particularly problematic for time diaries. In general, though, at least one-third of the population seems to be reporting habitual sleep of 6 hours or less. The proportion of those with 6 hours or less is salient, given the risk factors associated with sleep duration described in more detail in later discussion.

Sleep Disturbances

Sleep disturbances are difficult to measure at the population level. Often, population-level assessments of general sleep disturbances subsume insufficient sleep duration and/or sleep disorders that may not expressly fit into this category. The 2006 BRFSS asked the following question to more than 150,000 residents of 36 US states/territories: "Over the last 2 weeks, how many days have you had trouble falling asleep or staying asleep or sleeping too much?" In an analysis of these responses, values were coded in whole numbers ranging from 0 to 14, but responses aggregated at 0 and 14; therefore, responses were dichotomized as either endorsing or not endorsing "sleep disturbance."[28,29] For men, the prevalence of sleep disturbance ranged from 13.7% (ages 70–74) to 18.1% (ages 18–24), and for women, the prevalence ranged from 17.7% (ages 80 or older) to 25.1% (ages 18–24).[29] Interestingly, reports of sleep disturbance generally declined with age. This finding was recently replicated using data from the 2009 BRFSS, which showed a similar pattern of declining self-report of insufficient sleep with age.[30]

Regarding sleep symptoms, data from the 2007 to 2008 NHANES were examined with regard to prevalence of various sleep symptoms.[31] Long sleep latency (more than 30 minutes) was reported by 18.8% of Americans. Self-reported difficulty falling asleep was reported at a rate of 11.71% for mild symptoms (1–3 times per week) and 7.7% for moderate-severe symptoms (at least half of nights). Similarly, sleep maintenance difficulties were reported by 13.21% endorsing mild and 7.7% endorsing moderate-severe symptoms, and early morning awakenings were reported at a rate of 10.7% for mild and 5.8% for moderate-severe symptoms. Daytime sleepiness and nonrestorative sleep were reported at a rate of 13.0% and 17.8% for mild symptoms, respectively, and 5.8% and 10.9% for moderate-severe symptoms, respectively. Frequent snoring was reported by 31.5% of adults and snorting/gasping during sleep was reported by 6.6% "occasionally" and 5.8% "frequently."

SLEEP EFFECTS ON HEALTH AND LONGEVITY

Because sleep is involved with many physiologic systems, insufficient sleep duration and poor sleep quality have been associated with several adverse health outcomes. Separate literature texts have emerged describing some of the negative effects of insufficient sleep duration, sleep apnea, and insomnia.

Mortality

The first report documenting the relationship between sleep duration and mortality risk was published more than 50 years ago.[32] This first study, an analysis of data from the American Cancer Society's first Cancer Prevention Study of more than 1 million US adults, found that increased mortality risk was associated with both short (6 hours or less) and long (9 hours or more) sleep duration. Since that time, many other studies have been published, from both large and small cohorts, covering both short and long follow-up periods, from 6 continents. Taken together, this overall pattern of findings, that both short and long sleep are associated with mortality risk, has generally remained consistent across studies, although not all studies found this pattern.[17] Two meta-analyses have been published, using slightly different methods and controls.[33,34] Still, their findings were highly consistent, indicating a 10% to 12% increased risk for short sleep and a 30% to 38% increased risk associated with long sleep duration. Much controversy remains, though, regarding this issue. For example, the precision of measurement of sleep in these studies is often poor.[17,27,35] Self-reported sleep time may better approximate time in bed, and although an actigraphic study found a similar pattern,[36] the cutoffs for short and long sleep indicated an overestimate among self-reports. Also, there is still a lack of clarity on the biological plausibility of the long sleep relationship, although some ideas have been proposed.[37,38] For this reason, most of the attention has been focused on risks associated with short sleep duration, which may be far more prevalent.

Weight Gain and Obesity

Many studies have found associations between sleep duration and adiposity and obesity.[39–41] Although most of these studies are cross-sectional, precluding causality, several other studies have longitudinally examined this relationship, demonstrating that short sleep duration is associated with increased weight gain over time.[42–46] These studies include individuals with otherwise low obesity risk, diverse community samples, and samples in which effectiveness of weight loss interventions was mitigated by sleep and circadian factors. Several important caveats seem to be present in this relationship. First, this relationship is dependent on age, with the strongest relationships among younger adults and U-shaped relationships more common in middle-aged adults.[47] Also, this relationship may be moderated by race/ethnicity, with stronger relationships between sleep and obesity among non-Hispanic White and Black/African American adults.[24]

Diabetes and Metabolism

Several studies have documented a cross-sectional relationship between insufficient sleep and diabetes risk.[40,48–51] A recent meta-analysis showed that insufficient sleep is associated with a 33% increased risk of incident diabetes.[52] These studies are supported by laboratory findings that show that physiologic sleep loss is associated with diabetes risk factors, including insulin resistance,[53–56] and other diabetes risk factors, such as increased consumption of unhealthy foods.[57–59] Physiologic studies also show that sleep loss can influence metabolism through changes in metabolic hormones,[60,61] adipocyte function,[62] and beta-cell function.[63]

Inflammation

Laboratory studies have shown that physiologic sleep restriction is associated with a proinflammatory state, including elevations in inflammatory cytokines, such as interleukin (IL)-1B,[64,65] IL-6,[64,66–68] IL-17,[64–69] tumor necrosis factor-α,[64,68,70–72] and C-reactive protein.[64,69,73–76] Findings at the population level have been more difficult to assess,[64] but similar relationships were found. A recent meta-analysis found no consistent relationship between sleep duration and inflammation,[77] but this may be because it did not include some studies that were more generalizable and with larger samples (eg, Ref.[76]). Also, it is plausible that population-level samples did not optimally measure these markers, because relationships with sleep vary across 24 hours and single time-point blood draws may miss the window of difference.[68]

Cardiovascular Disease

In addition to increased likelihood of obesity, diabetes, and inflammation, insufficient sleep is associated with increased risk of cardiovascular disease. Many studies have found that short sleep duration is associated with hypertension.[24,78–80] Although directionality is difficult to ascertain, several of these studies were longitudinal in nature. A meta-analysis of these longitudinal studies indicated that habitual short sleep duration is associated with a 20% increased likelihood of hypertension, relative to normal sleep duration.[81] Other studies have supported this association, showing increased 24-hour blood pressure in short sleepers.[82] Other studies have also shown short sleep to be associated with hypercholesterolemia[24,79] and atherosclerosis risk.[83] Regarding cardiovascular endpoints, there is some evidence that habitual short sleep increases the likelihood of cardiovascular events,[84] although meta-analyses do not generally show short sleep to be associated with increased cardiovascular mortality.[33,34,85]

Neurocognitive Functioning

Many studies have examined the relationship between laboratory-induced sleep loss and neurocognitive function. The domain that is most often studied is vigilant attention,[86,87] most often operationalized with the psychomotor vigilance task.[87,88] These studies show that as sleep time declines, attentional lapses increase in a somewhat dose-dependent manner.[86,89] Furthermore, these impairments often become cumulative over time[90] and do not seem to level off even after weeks in a laboratory. Other domains of neurocognitive function have also been assessed. For example, reduced sleep duration has been shown to cause impairments in working memory,[91] executive function,[92] processing speed,[93–95] and cognitive throughput.[96] Although some of these effects may be rescued with stimulants such as caffeine, the effects on executive function particularly do not seem to be rescued.[92] Although studies of this phenomenon in the general population are scarce, some studies show that reduced sleep time is associated with drowsy driving[97] and occupational accidents.[98–100]

Mental Health

Many studies have shown that short sleep duration is associated with poor mental health. Sleep disruptions are a common diagnostic feature of many mental health disorders.[101] Patients with mood disorders and anxiety disorders frequently experience short sleep duration. Sleep duration also has been identified as a suicide risk factor.[102] In the general population, overall mental health has been identified as the leading predictor of self-reported insufficient sleep.[30]

BELIEFS AND ATTITUDES ABOUT SLEEP

Real-world sleep may be driven by many of the same factors that drive other health-related behaviors, such as diet and exercise. With this in mind, previous literature from health behavior researchers has identified several models that explain healthy behavior, identifying the roles of beliefs and attitudes.

The Health Belief Model and Application to Sleep

The Health Belief Model was originally developed in the 1960s,[103,104] but has since been used in the study of many health-related behaviors. See **Fig. 3** for a schematic of this model. This model can be applied to sleep behaviors. For example, a person will engage in healthy sleep behaviors (eg, making time for sufficient sleep or adhering to treatment) if they (1) believe that they are susceptible to the adverse effects of insufficient/poor sleep, (2) believe that the adverse effects are severe enough to warrant action, (3) believe that the action will mitigate the adverse effects, (4) believe that barriers to performing the action are sufficiently reduced, (5) are reminded to engage in the action, and (6) believe that performing the action is under their control. According to the Health Belief Model, all of these are required for action. Therefore, just educating patients about the severity of outcomes of inaction, for example, is not sufficient to motivate behavior.

The Integrated Behavioral Model and Application to Sleep

The Integrated Behavioral Model arose from the Theory of Planned Behavior and Theory of Reasoned Action[105] to describe why people engage in behaviors. A schematic for this model is presented in **Fig. 4**. According to this model, attitudes, norms, and agency need to be addressed. Regarding attitudes, this would involve leading individuals to not only endorse helpful beliefs and attitudes about healthy sleep but also associate healthy sleep with positive feelings. Regarding norms, more research is needed to understand how the sleep of a person's (perceived) peers

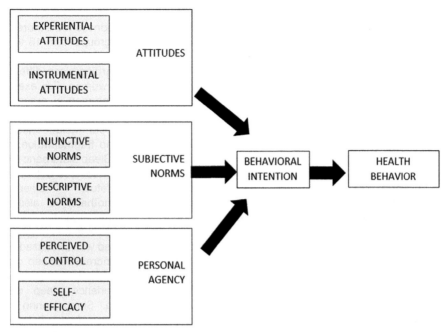

Fig. 4. Integrated behavior model.

and those to whom that individual wishes to conform influences individual sleep behaviors.

Beliefs and Attitudes About Sleep

Across segments of society, sleep practices and beliefs can vary to a great extent. For example, bed-sharing with infants and other family members differentially exists across cultures.[106–111] The cultural impact of dreaming also varies widely across cultures.[112] As globalization and technology penetrate society, sleep-related beliefs and practices can change, including the provision of longer working hours,[113–120] shift work,[121–124] and discouraging otherwise culturally appropriate naps.[125–127] There have been a few studies that examined beliefs and attitudes about sleep. In a sample from Brooklyn, New York, Black/African American individuals who were at high risk of obstructive sleep apnea had higher scores on the Dysfunctional Beliefs and Attitudes about Sleep scale, compared with those who were not at high risk.[128] In a study in the Philadelphia area among older Black and White women,[129] participants were administered a questionnaire to evaluate sleep-related beliefs and practices. Black women were more likely to endorse incorrect and unhelpful statements. Sell and colleagues[130] examined sleep knowledge among Mexican American individuals in San Diego. Non-Hispanic White individuals were more likely than Mexican American individuals to know what sleep apnea was, but

when describing the symptoms, both groups had similar knowledge that such a problem existed. Taken together, the role of sleep and health in society is driven by healthy behavior choices. These behavioral decisions, as described in the preceding models, are largely influenced by beliefs and attitudes about sleep. These beliefs and attitudes, though, are differentially endorsed by racial/ethnic groups, which may underlie sleep difficulties in those populations.

GENDER AND AGE IMPACTS SLEEP IN THE POPULATION
Sleep Changes with Normal Aging in the Population

Physiologic changes in sleep have been well-documented. In a landmark meta-analysis by Ohayon and colleagues,[131] polysomnographic sleep characteristics across the lifespan were examined across 65 studies spanning more than 40 years. This analysis found that with age, polysomnographic total sleep time, sleep efficiency, slow-wave sleep, rapid eye movement (REM) sleep, and REM latency decline, whereas sleep latency, wake after sleep onset, stage 1 sleep, and stage 2 sleep increase. This finding suggests a phenomenon of more disturbed and lighter sleep. In addition to these changes, melatonin secretion declines with age, which may also impact sleep consolidation in older adults.[132] Risk for many sleep disorders also increases with age.[133–135] In particular, sleep disorders, such as insomnia,[136] restless legs syndrome,[137,138] sleep apnea,[139] and REM behavior disorder,[140] include older age as a risk factor. However, a paradox exists, which was highlighted in a large, international cohort study by Soldatos and colleagues.[141] In this study, older adults were more likely to report difficulties initiating and maintaining sleep; however, they did not endorse a greater level of dissatisfaction with their sleep. A lack of dissatisfaction is similar to results reported in Italy by Zilli and colleagues,[142] who found that younger adults were more likely to report dissatisfaction with sleep than older adults. In the US population, general dissatisfaction with sleep associated with age was examined using the 2006 BRFSS. In a study of more than 150,000 US adults, general sleep disturbance (general difficulties with sleep) was most frequently reported in young adults, and rates generally declined with age.[29] In controlled analyses, no age groups were statistically less likely to report sleep disturbances than the oldest adults, aged 80 or older, although many of the younger groups reported higher levels. These results were replicated using the 2009 BRFSS, which examined self-reported perceived insufficient sleep among more than 350,000 US adults and found a decline in general sleep insufficiency associated with age.[30] Thus, it appears that sleep objectively worsens with age, but that subjective dissatisfaction with sleep is not associated with normal aging. In fact, this may be a sign of illness or depression.[143]

Population-level Differences in Sleep between Men and Women

Differences in sleep between men and women have been widely reported in the literature for decades.[144–149] Overall, in the general population, women report shorter sleep duration,[150] more sleep symptoms,[31] greater rates of insomnia,[151] and lower rates of sleep apnea.[152] In an analysis of sleep disturbances reported in the 2006 BRFSS, it was found that women reported more nighttime sleep disturbances and daytime tiredness than men. Across all age groups, sleep disturbance was reported by between 13.7% and 18.1% of men, depending on age group, and between 17.7% and 25.1% of women.[29] Similarly, for daytime tiredness, rates were 16.4% to 22.9% of men and 20.5% to 29.9% of women, depending on age. In all age groups, women reported nominally more disturbances than men. Statistically, after adjusting for demographics, socioeconomics, health variables, and depression, rates of sleep disturbances were more prevalent among women

for all age groups between 25 and 69 years old and rates of daytime tiredness were more common in women for all age groups from 18 to 59 and 75 to 79.

Other issues regarding sleep differences exist between men and women. For example, sleep disturbances are common in pregnancy,[153–155] especially the first and third trimesters. These sleep disturbances can include insomnia, short sleep duration, sleep fragmentation, and gestational sleep apnea. Sleep disturbance in pregnant women can result in adverse outcomes for both the mother and the fetus.[156,157] Sleep in new parents (especially mothers) is also frequently disturbed,[158,159] especially in the first few months after birth. Sleep disturbances among parents of infants are associated with increased postpartum depression,[160–162] increased sleep disturbances among infants, and other adverse outcomes. Women also experience sleep disturbances around menopause. Sleep during the menopausal transition is often characterized by insomnia symptoms and increased sleep fragmentation.[163] Hot flashes are also a common source of sleep disturbance around the menopausal transition.[164]

Some sleep disturbances are disproportionately experienced by men. For example, men are more likely to have obstructive sleep apnea,[139] are more likely to have difficulty adhering to sleep apnea treatment,[165,166] and are more likely to die as a result of complications or consequences of sleep apnea.[167] In addition, men are more likely to be diagnosed with REM behavior disorder, which is typically diagnosed among older adults and likely predates neurodegenerative disorders.[168] During the aging process, men are also more likely to demonstrate a steeper decline in slow-wave sleep generation,[131] with lower amounts of slow-wave sleep among older man versus older women.

RACE, ETHNICITY, AND CULTURE ASSOCIATED WITH SLEEP
Insufficient Sleep Associated with Race/ Ethnicity

Many studies have documented a "sleep disparity" in the population,[19,39] such that racial/ ethnic minorities, especially in the context of socioeconomic disadvantage, achieve less quality sleep. Most studies in this area have shown that, overall, Black/African American individuals are more likely to experience short sleep duration compared with non-Hispanic White individuals.[19,39] One nationally representative study found that this pattern is robust even after adjustment for a large number of other demographic and socioeconomic covariates, such that the rate of very short sleep (<4 hours) was 2.5 times those of non-Hispanic White individuals and the rate of short (5–6 hours) sleep was about twice as high.[150] A similar pattern was seen for Asian individuals/others, who reported very short sleep at a rate of 4 times that seen in non-Hispanic White individuals and a short sleep about twice as frequently. Among Hispanic/Latino individuals, there is less clear evidence of habitual short sleep, especially among Mexican American individuals. In addition to epidemiologic studies, some laboratory studies have also examined this issue. For example, Blacks/African American individuals have been shown to sleep less in the laboratory.[169–171] Also, this group has been shown to demonstrate less slow-wave sleep, compensated by increased stage 2 sleep. Other studies have shown similar patterns for sleep duration in other samples that included minority groups,[172,173] and this topic was the subject of multiple recent reviews.[19,174,175]

Sleep Disturbances Associated with Race/Ethnicity in the Population

Less work has been done to characterize rates of sleep disturbances in racial/ethnic minorities. One previous study showed that racial/ethnic minorities demonstrated a lower sleep efficiency based on actigraphy.[176] A study in the Philadelphia area found that race differences in poor sleep quality largely depended on socioeconomic status.[177] A nationally representative study found that Black/African American individuals were 60% more likely than non-Hispanic White individuals to report sleep latency more than 30 minutes, although they (along with Hispanic/Latino individuals) were less likely to report "difficulty falling asleep."[31] This discrepancy between self-reported "problems" and computed long sleep latency suggests that symptom reports may vary based on the question asked. Overall, minority groups were less likely to report insomnia symptoms, nonrestorative sleep, and daytime sleepiness, although non-Mexican Hispanic/Latino individuals were more likely to endorse sleep apnea symptoms such as snoring.

Several studies have examined the role of racial discrimination as a unique stressor that impacts sleep. A study of residents in Michigan and Wisconsin found that exposure to racial discrimination was associated with sleep disturbances, above the effects of race, sociodemographics, and even depressed mood.[178] This finding, that sleep disturbance is associated with exposure to racism is consistent with other findings that

showed that exposure to discrimination was associated with shorter sleep and more sleep difficulties[179] and that these findings are also seen in objective sleep assessments.[169,170] Interestingly, polysomnography differences in slow-wave sleep between Black/African American and non-Hispanic White individuals (ie, reduced slow-wave sleep) were mediated by exposure to discrimination.

Sleep, Acculturation, and Immigration

Few studies have examined sleep related to acculturation. Sell and colleagues[130] found that Mexican American individuals who were more acculturated to American lifestyle were more familiar with information about sleep disorders. Also, in a nationally representative sample, speaking only Spanish at home was associated with a decreased likelihood of sleep duration in the short (5–6 hours) and very short (<4 hours) categories compared with 7 to 8 hours. In this same sample, being born in Mexico (but not any other country) was associated with decreased likelihood of both short and very short sleep duration, but these effects were not significant after adjusting for other demographic and socioeconomic factors, which likely explain this finding.[129]

EMPLOYMENT, NEIGHBORHOOD, AND SOCIOECONOMICS

Although sleep is an important factor in overall health, society has incentivized insufficient sleep. Many of these incentives involve finances and employment. Because of this, there is evidence that one of the strongest societal determinants of sleep is work. The relationship between work and sleep is especially important for safety-sensitive occupations that not only incentivize insufficient sleep but also for which the associated fatigue also jeopardizes the public safety.

Trading Sleep for Work Hours

Replicating and extending prior work in this area, Basner and colleagues[23] examined data from more than 100,000 Americans over a 9-year period who participated in the ATUS, which is performed annually by the US Bureau of Labor Statistics and uses time diaries to determine work and other activities across 24 hours.[180] In a recent report, Basner and colleagues[23] show that work time, including actual work and other related activities (such as commuting), was the primary determinant of sleep duration. In addition, later start times of school and work were associated with longer sleep, such that each hour of delayed work or training start time was associated with 20 more minutes of sleep. Also, those holding multiple jobs were at greater risk for short sleep duration compared with those only working one job at a time. Although work is a strong determinant of sleep duration, other studies show that employed individuals report the lowest rates of self-reported sleep disturbance.[28] Unemployment, on the other hand, is associated with more sleep problems.[28,30]

Sleep Deprivation and Sleep Disorders in Occupational Settings

Recognition of the role of sleep disorders and sleep deprivation in occupational settings is gaining increased attention. Rosekind and colleagues[181] showed that the typical well-rested worker costs an employer approximately $1300 per year in lost sleep-related productivity, and this number increases to approximately $3000 for those with insomnia or insufficient sleep. Furthermore, the loss to productivity permeates many areas of functioning, including time management, mental and interpersonal demands, output demands, and physical job demands. Hui and Grandner[182] show that not only is self-reported poor sleep quality associated with decreased work performance, but also worsening sleep longitudinally predicts worsening performance over time. In addition, difficulty sleeping is associated with increased health care costs. Those with difficulty sleeping "often" or "always" were associated with additional health care costs of $3600 to $5200 per person per year more than those who "never" have sleep problems, and these costs increased over time if sleep became worse. Additional analyses from this dataset also showed that poor sleep may motivate employees to make healthy changes as part of a workplace wellness program, but it may also limit those employees' ability to maintain healthy change.[183]

Regarding safety-sensitive occupations, such as medicine, law enforcement, and transportation, sleep plays a critical role in safety. For example, sleep apnea occurs at high rates among commercial drivers[184–186] and impairs their ability to drive safely. Accordingly, workplace programs to increase screening and treatment of sleep apnea may have financial benefits for companies.[184] Similar efforts may show effectiveness in rail workers as well.[187,188] Airline pilots face similar challenges, in addition to challenges presented by crossing many time zones. To address these concerns, sleep disorders screening in addition to circadian approaches and scheduled napping have shown effectiveness in improving safety.[189–197] Among law enforcement and first responders, several studies have shown that sleep disturbances are common among police officers[198–203] and firefighters.[204,205] In particular, issues such as sleep apnea, insomnia, and shift work are the most common problems.[206] In a landmark study by Rajaratnam and colleagues,[198] police officers who were at greatest risk of sleep disorders were also more likely to be at risk for job-related problems, such as falling asleep at meetings and using unnecessary violence against citizens. Studies have shown that sleep disturbances in police officers and firefighters are associated with reduced ability to maintain job performance and safety.[198,203,207]

Several studies have been conducted among medical residents and nurses. For nurses, shift work and long work hours have been shown to be related to adverse health outcomes and indicators of reduced functioning.[208–217] Among medical residents, long work hours and shift work have been shown to lead to insufficient sleep duration.[218–221] Furthermore, longer work hours in medical residents have been associated with markers of reduced work performance, although impacts on actual work performance are more inconsistent.[115,222] In a landmark study that compared 2 groups of residency programs, those that gave more time off for sleep did not show measurable changes in work performance.[223] Paradoxically, residents given more time to sleep were more worried about decreases in their quality of work as a result of working less, yet they were more satisfied with the quality of their life and social functioning.

Sleep, Poverty, and Neighborhood Factors

Several studies have shown that poverty is associated with both shorter sleep duration and worse sleep quality.[30] However, once the benefits of income are accounted for (by statistically covarying education, access to health care, and so forth), associations with income are often nonexistent and may go in the opposite direction. For example, in an analysis of data from more than 350,000 US adults, insufficient sleep was associated with poverty before adjusting for covariates, but after adjustment, the opposite relationship was seen.[30] A positive relationship between income and insufficient sleep after adjusting for covariates suggests that money may not buy sleep, but many of the benefits of income may contribute to healthy sleep. One aspect of this relationship is neighborhood quality. Several studies have investigated the role of the neighborhood in an individual's sleep quality, showing that neighborhoods that are crime-ridden, not socially cohesive, and dirty, are associated with worse sleep quality.[224-227] Furthermore, sleep quality may partially mediate the relationship between neighborhood quality and both mental[227] and physical[225] health. One way that a neighborhood may directly influence sleep would be via the physical environment. There is substantial literature showing that environmental noise[228,229] and light[230-233] can adversely impact sleep and that neighborhoods that are active at night may directly impact sleep through these.

INFLUENCES OF HOME, FAMILY, AND SCHOOL ENVIRONMENT

The home, family, and school environments also likely play important roles in an individual's sleep. For example, household size is negatively associated with sleep, such that more crowded homes are more likely to foster insufficient sleep.[30] Also, as mentioned previously, the physical sleep environment can also play a role. Bedrooms that have levels of light, noise, and temperature that are not conducive to sleep may contribute to insufficient sleep.[234-236] Although data on beds and other sleeping surfaces are relatively scarce, an uncomfortable sleeping environment may also reduce sleep ability.[237-239]

Another key issue of the home and family environment on sleep regards the marital relationship. Although most sleep research is performed on individuals sleeping alone in a laboratory, most adults do not sleep alone most nights.[240,241] With this in mind, several studies have explored the important role of marital and relationship quality in sleep quality and how this relates to health. For example, relationship quality has been shown to be an important predictor of sleep health, especially among women, and relationship quality may be an important moderator between sleep quality and health.[241-244]

TECHNOLOGY IN AND OUT OF THE BEDROOM

In 2011, the National Sleep Foundation polled Americans regarding their use of technology in the bedroom. In a report of the findings of this survey, Gradisar and colleagues[245] note that 90% of Americans use some sort of electronic device in the hour before bed. Also, more than two-thirds of adolescents and young adults used a Smartphone in the hour before bed, compared with approximately one-third of middle-aged adults and approximately one-fifth of older adults. Furthermore, the more engaging the technology

application, the more the electronic device use was associated with difficulties falling asleep and nonrestorative sleep. This finding is supported by other work that shows that not only is electronic media use near bedtime prevalent[246] but also the light emitted by the devices[247] as well as the mental engagement[248] can interfere with sleep. Growing awareness of the influence of mobile electronic device use on sleep is a key example of a societal-level change (use of technology) impacting an individual's sleep.

GLOBALIZATION AND 24/7 SOCIETY

Another societal-level factor that impacts sleep is the advent of globalization and a 24/7 society. In the past, social interactions, commercial activities, and work responsibilities were dictated by more local factors. Now, though, the advent of globalization and 24/7 operations often impinge on sleep. Regarding globalization, individuals and organizations are connected across the globe. In combination with a society that institutes shift work and 24-hour operations, entire segments of the population are awake across all hours of the 24-hour day, and access to individuals across time zones is easier than ever. Because of this, social interactions (such as interactions with friends, family, and even online groups), commercial activities (such as eCommerce and availability of entertainment around the clock on demand), and work responsibilities (such as e-mails outside of business hours and business conducted across the globe) can impinge on sleep. The influence of globalization and 24/7 society on sleep behaviors is particularly relevant, because shift work has been repeatedly shown in both laboratory and field studies to be related to adverse health outcomes.

PUBLIC SAFETY AND PUBLIC POLICY

As mentioned previously, many safety-sensitive occupations, such as those in transportation, law enforcement, and medicine, require healthy sleep for optimal performance. The problem is that these professions often institute policies that make healthy sleep difficult. As a result, the sleep of an individual in one of those occupations may have ramifications for others in the public. For example, when a large commercial truck crashes, it causes more damage and a greater likelihood of fatal injury.[249,250] For this reason, several policy approaches to sleep and public safety have been proposed. The Accreditation Council for Graduate Medical Education has already instituted duty hour restrictions on medical residents, based on results from a report by the Institute of Medicine.[218] These restrictions, although controversial,[115,251–253] are likely resulting in increased sleep among medical residents.[222] In the transportation industry, recommendations by the National Highway Transportation and Safety Administration address the need for sleep disorders screening and fatigue mitigation among commercial drivers,[250] although formal regulations have not yet been passed. The Federal Aviation Administration also recently issued guidelines to address sleep issues in pilots.[254] More work is needed in this area, and although regulations to ensure public safety have been proposed, they still have not yet been passed.

Another domain of public safety is drowsy driving. Even among noncommercial drivers, drowsy driving is an important public safety issue. Drowsy driving is prevalent, reported among approximately 5% of the US population over a 6-month period.[255] Population-level data suggest that short sleep duration is an independent risk factor for drowsy driving, even if respondents believe that they are completely well rested.[97]

Another area of public policy related to sleep involves school start times. Existing evidence suggests that most US schools, especially high schools, start too early for most adolescents.[256–259] Earlier start times not only promote shorter sleep duration among adolescents (who need more sleep than adults) but also do not take into account natural circadian delays that occur in adolescence.[260] It has been proposed that delaying school start times can improve academic performance, improve mental health, and improve overall health in students.[261–266]

Other public policy initiatives have addressed the issue of environmental light and noise in neighborhoods. There are several policies in place, and more being proposed, that limit the brightness of street lights in neighborhoods, increase "quiet time" regulations at night, direct airplanes to avoid some residential areas at night, reduce traffic and train noise at night, and so forth. These approaches are usually regional, and many efforts are ongoing.

One more public policy implication relevant to sleep would be health policy legislation. For example, improving mental health parity laws will do much to intervene on perhaps the most important determinant of sleep health at the population level[30] and will facilitate treatment of insomnia with the most well supported therapy.[267] In addition, health equity legislation may help to address some of the disparities seen in sleep in the population.[20]

These and other future approaches may better promote healthy sleep from a policy standpoint.

IMPORTANT LIMITATIONS OF THE EXISTING LITERATURE

There are several important limitations to the existing literature, which constrain interpretations and generalizations of the data. The most important limitation is that there is a lack of consistency in sleep assessment methods across studies, and this is a problem for several reasons. First, retrospective self-report (eg, survey), prospective self-report (eg, diary), laboratory-based objective (eg, polysomnography), and field-based objective (eg, actigraphy) estimates of sleep tend to disagree with each other, because they capture different elements of sleep well. It is likely that physiologic sleep is substantially less than that which is self-reported.[27] Even among survey methods, there seems to be systematic variation.[35] Second, because there is still no nationally representative dataset that includes any well-validated estimate of sleep duration or quality, generalizability from one dataset to the next is limited. Third, cutoffs and categories used to describe sleep are often inconsistent across studies; for example, the cutoff for the shortest sleep duration category can be as low as 4 hours or less or as high as 7 hours.

Another important limitation is a general lack of physiologic sleep measures at the societal level. Because these measures are typically more expensive and require more infrastructure to implement, they are often infeasible for large studies that require assessment of thousands of people. Until sleep assessment becomes more of a priority, otherwise rich datasets will continue to have just a few nonvalidated survey items measuring sleep. Suboptimal measurement of sleep will make data interpretation difficult, because it is unclear the degree to which associations are referring to physiologic sleep or other factors that become subsumed in self-reported sleep experience.

A third important limitation regards the complexity of social environments. As shown in the Social-Ecological Model, the influences that may play a role in sleep are many, varied, and exist at several levels. Still, most studies do not address the complex nature of social-environmental influences on health. Also, future studies that will examine epigenetic effects will need to better account for gene-environment interactions, and this will require a better operationalization of environmental variables in many cases. An example of one study that brought these methodologies together is cited by Watson and colleagues,[268] who combined geospatial neighborhood analyses with sleep genetic information to characterize a social-environmental influence on sleep duration.

A fourth important limitation to the existing literature is a lack of interventional studies. If, for example, sleep represents a modifiable factor in health disparities, it is plausible that improvements in sleep at the community level could reduce effects of health disparities. However, there is a lack of interventional studies that can demonstrate this; rather, the best examples of investigations in this area use mediational analysis to show that changes in sleep account for changes in health outcomes across groups, such as blood pressure.[269] More sleep interventions at the community level are going to be needed to understand the causal role of sleep in these outcomes. Also, there is a general lack of empirically supported interventions for sleep health. Although many interventions exist to promote healthy diet, physical activity, and substance cessation, a lack of standardized sleep health interventions limits knowledge in this area.

FUTURE RESEARCH DIRECTIONS

Several potential future research directions may help advance knowledge in this area. First, expanded epigenetic studies are needed to explore gene-environment interactions. As the science of human sleep genetics develops, more research into how genetic vulnerabilities interact with environmental influences is needed. For example, although it is unlikely that genetics explains racial disparities in sleep, it is plausible that some genetic adaptations to one geographic region may confer risk in another region (eg, less sunlight, different food availability). Also, it may be possible that certain genetic vulnerabilities (eg, airway collapse) may differentially affect groups because body mass indexes increase in the presence of increasing obesity rates due to westernized diets.

Another important direction in research will be to clarify the sleep phenotypes and endophenotypes. Currently, typing of sleep at the community and population level is frequently based on broad sleep duration groups (eg, "short sleepers") or sleep symptoms ("difficulty falling asleep"), although these groups can be highly heterogeneous. Genetic studies are limited by this limited clarity in sleep phenotypes. Short sleepers, for example, may comprise individuals who are "true" short sleepers and need less sleep, those who need more sleep but are able to tolerate less sleep for an extended period ("resilient"), and those who are insufficient sleepers. Still, insufficient sleepers may belong to groups that demonstrate neurocognitive and metabolic impairments at variable rates (eg, some individuals may demonstrate more metabolic impairments and some more cognitive). Perhaps more clarity regarding phenotypes will help move forward an agenda of better human sleep genetics.

More intervention studies are also needed at the laboratory, clinical, and community levels that address real-world sleep concerns. As mentioned previously, there is a lack of healthy sleep interventions, relative to healthy diet or physical activity recommendations. Without these data, it is difficult to make recommendations in addition to just stating a problem. Also, interventions need to address issues that have generally been ignored yet carry real-world significance For example, despite many adults sleeping between 6 and 7 hours per night, this sleep duration is almost never included in the literature, either because epidemiologic studies categorize at the hour (including them in either 6-hour or 7-hour groups) or because laboratory studies try to maximize difference between groups (usually comparing 8–6, 5, or 4 hours but not between 6 and 7).[14] These and other real-world issues need to be better captured in intervention studies.

Finally, intervention studies are needed that identify real-world approaches to increasing sleep time among chronically sleep-deprived individuals. Unlike traditional intervention study designs, where changing sleep is the intervention and some health marker is the outcome (which would address the question of whether changing sleep impacts health), study designs are needed whereby changing sleep itself is the outcome. For example, it is known that smoking cessation can positively impact health. However, how does one quit smoking? Just recommending that someone quit is not enough, and literature has emerged that proposes novel ways to achieve this difficult behavioral change. Likewise, changing sleep duration in a real-world setting (with home, work, and other societal pressures) may be difficult, and useful strategies besides simply making recommendations need to be explored.

CLINICS CARE POINTS

- Patients presenting to the sleep clinic may also be experiencing a wide range of potential comorbidities, including conditions reflecting impaired cardiovascular, metabolic, immune, behavioral, cognitive, and mental health. It is important to screen for these issues and refer to other providers when appropriate.

- Sleep is impacted by many social, behavioral, and environmental factors, in addition to individual-level factors such as genetics, beliefs and attitudes, etc. These factors may be useful to identify for the purpose of case conceptualization, as well as treatment optimization.

- Individuals from racial/ethnic minority backgrounds, socioeconomically disadvantaged contexts, and other marginalized groups, may be more likely to be at risk for sleep problems and disorders and may have morre difficulties receiving adequate treatment.

- Behavior change is complex, and requires a number of conditions to be met, including understanding barriers and facilitators, self-efficacy, and behavioral intentions.

DISCLOSURE

Dr M.A. Grandner is supported by National Heart, Lung, and Blood Institute (K23HL110216).

REFERENCES

1. Cajochen C, Chellappa S, Schmidt C. What keeps us awake?-the role of clocks and hourglasses, light, and melatonin. Int Rev Neurobiol 2010;93: 57–90.

2. Fuller PM, Lu J. Neurobiology of sleep. In: Amlaner CJ, Fuller PM, editors. Basics of sleep guide. 2nd edition. Westchester (IL): Sleep Research Society; 2009. p. 53–62.

3. Mackiewicz M, Naidoo N, Zimmerman JE, et al. Molecular mechanisms of sleep and wakefulness. Ann N Y Acad Sci 2008;1129:335–49.

4. Schwartz JR, Roth T. Neurophysiology of sleep and wakefulness: basic science and clinical implications. Curr Neuropharmacol 2008;6(4):367–78.

5. Franken P. A role for clock genes in sleep homeostasis. Curr Opin Neurobiol 2013;23(5):864–72.

6. Feng D, Lazar MA. Clocks, metabolism, and the epigenome. Mol Cell 2012;47(2):158–67.

7. Gerstner JR, Lenz O, Vanderheyden WM, et al. Amyloid-beta induces sleep fragmentation that is rescued by fatty acid binding proteins in Drosophila. J Neurosci Res 2016. [Epub ahead of print].

8. Xu M, Chung S, Zhang S, et al. Basal forebrain circuit for sleep-wake control. Nat Neurosci 2015; 18(11):1641–7.

9. Cox J, Pinto L, Dan Y. Calcium imaging of sleep-wake related neuronal activity in the dorsal pons. Nat Commun 2016;7:10763.

10. Park DA. The fire within the eye: a historical essay on the nature and meaning of light. Princeton (NJ): Princeton University Press; 1997.

11. Williams S. Sleep and society: sociological ventures into the (Un)known. London: Taylor & Francis; 2005.

12. Watson NF, Badr MS, Belenky G, et al. Recommended amount of sleep for a healthy adult: a joint consensus statement of the American Academy of Sleep Medicine and Sleep Research Society. Sleep 2015;38(6):843–4.

13. Consensus Conference Panel, Watson NF, Badr MS, et al. Joint consensus statement of the American Academy of Sleep Medicine and Sleep Research Society on the recommended amount of sleep for a healthy adult: methodology and discussion. J Clin Sleep Med 2015;11(8):931–52.

14. Consensus Conference Panel, Watson NF, Badr MS, et al. Joint consensus statement of the American Academy of Sleep Medicine and Sleep Research Society on the recommended amount of sleep for a healthy adult: methodology and discussion. Sleep 2015;38(8):1161–83.

15. Consensus Conference Panel, Watson NF, Badr MS, et al. Recommended amount of sleep for a healthy adult: a joint consensus statement of the American Academy of Sleep Medicine and Sleep Research Society. J Clin Sleep Med 2015; 11(6):591–2.

16. Bronfenbrenner U. Toward an experimental ecology of human development. Am Psychol 1977;32: 513–31.

17. Grandner MA, Patel NP, Hale L, et al. Mortality associated with sleep duration: the evidence, the possible mechanisms, and the future. Sleep Med Rev 2010;14:191–203.

18. Grandner MA. Addressing sleep disturbances: an opportunity to prevent cardiometabolic disease? Int Rev Psychiatry 2014;26(2):155–76.

19. Grandner MA, Williams NJ, Knutson KL, et al. Sleep disparity, race/ethnicity, and socioeconomic position. Sleep Med 2016;18:7–18.

20. Grandner MA. Sleep disparities in the American population: prevalence, potential causes, relationships to cardiometabolic health disparities, and future directions for research and policy. In: Kelly R, editor. Health disparities in America. Wash ington, DC: US Congress; 2015. p. 126–32.

21. Knutson KL, Van Cauter E, Rathouz PJ, et al. Trends in the prevalence of short sleepers in the USA: 1975-2006. Sleep 2010;33(1):37–45.

22. Bin YS, Marshall NS, Glozier N. Secular trends in adult sleep duration: a systematic review. Sleep Med Rev 2012;16(3):223–30.

23. Basner M, Spaeth AM, Dinges DF. Sociodemographic characteristics and waking activities and their role in the timing and duration of sleep. Sleep 2014;37(12):1889–906.

24. Grandner MA, Chakravorty S, Perlis ML, et al. Habitual sleep duration associated with self-reported and objectively determined cardiometabolic risk factors. Sleep Med 2014;15(1):42–50.

25. Krueger PM, Friedman EM. Sleep duration in the United States: a cross-sectional population-based study. Am J Epidemiol 2009;169(9):1052–63.

26. Liu Y, Wheaton AG, Chapman DP, et al. Prevalence of healthy sleep duration among adults -United States, 2014. MMWR Morb Mortal Wkly Rep 2016;65(6):137–41.

27. Kurina LM, McClintock MK, Chen JH, et al. Sleep duration and all-cause mortality: a critical review of measurement and associations. Ann Epidemiol 2013;23(6):361–70.

28. Grandner MA, Patel NP, Gehrman PR, et al. Who gets the best sleep? Ethnic and socioeconomic factors related to sleep disturbance. Sleep Med 2010;11:470–9.

29. Grandner MA, Martin JL, Patel NP, et al. Age and sleep disturbances among American men and women: data from the U.S. Behavioral Risk Factor Surveillance System. Sleep 2012;35(3):395–406.

30. Grandner MA, Jackson NJ, Izci-Balserak B, et al. Social and behavioral determinants of perceived insufficient sleep. Front Neurol 2015;6:112.

31. Grandner MA, Petrov MER, Rattanaumpawan P, et al. Sleep symptoms, race/ethnicity, and socio-economic position. J Clin Sleep Med 2013;9(9): 897–905, 905A-D.

32. Hammond EC. Some preliminary findings on physical complaints from a prospective study of 1,064,004 men and women. Am J Public Health Nations Health 1964;54:11–23.

33. Gallicchio L, Kalesan B. Sleep duration and mortality: a systematic review and meta-analysis. J Sleep Res 2009;18(2):148–58.

34. Cappuccio FP, D'Elia L, Strazzullo P, et al. Sleep duration and all-cause mortality: a systematic review and meta-analysis of prospective studies. Sleep 2010;33(5):585–92.

35. Grandner MA, Patel NP, Gehrman PR, et al. Problems associated with short sleep: bridging the gap between laboratory and epidemiological studies. Sleep Med Rev 2010;14:239–47.

36. Kripke DF, Langer RD, Elliott JA, et al. Mortality related to actigraphic long and short sleep. Sleep Med 2011;12(1):28–33.

37. Youngstedt SD, Kripke DF. Long sleep and mortality: rationale for sleep restriction. Sleep Med Rev 2004;8(3):159–74.

38. Grandner MA, Drummond SP. Who are the long sleepers? Towards an understanding of the mortality relationship. Sleep Med Rev 2007;11(5): 341–60.

39. Adenekan B, Pandey A, McKenzie S, et al. Sleep in America: role of racial/ethnic differences. Sleep Med Rev 2013;17(4):255–62.

40. Morselli LL, Guyon A, Spiegel K. Sleep and metabolic function. Pflugers Arch 2012;463(1):139–60.

41. Knutson KL. Does inadequate sleep play a role invulnerability to obesity? Am J Hum Biol 2012; 24(3):361–71.

42. Watanabe M, Kikuchi H, Tanaka K, et al. Association of short sleep duration with weight gain and obesity at 1-year follow-up: a large-scale prospective study. Sleep 2010;33(2):161–7.

43. Chaput JP, Bouchard C, Tremblay A. Change in sleep duration and visceral fat accumulation over 6 years in adults. Obesity (Silver Spring) 2014; 22(5):E9–12.

44. Chaput JP, Despres JP, Bouchard C, et al. The association between sleep duration and weight gain in adults: a 6-year prospective study from the Quebec Family Study. Sleep 2008;31(4):517–23.

45. Baron KG, Reid KJ, Kern AS, et al. Role of sleep timing in caloric intake and BMI. Obesity (Silver Spring) 2011;19(7):1374–81.

46. Shechter A, Grandner MA, St-Onge MP. The role of sleep in the control of food intake. Am J Lifestyle Med 2014;8(6):371–4.

47. Grandner MA, Schopfer EA, Sands-Lincoln M, et al. Relationship between sleep duration and body mass index depends on age. Obesity (Silver Spring) 2015;23(12):2491–8.

48. Barone MT, Menna-Barreto L. Diabetes and sleep: a complex cause-and-effect relationship. Diabetes Res Clin Pract 2011;91(2):129–37.

49. Aldabal L, Bahammam AS. Metabolic, endocrine, and immune consequences of sleep deprivation. Open Respir Med J 2011;5:31–43.

50. Bopparaju S, Surani S. Sleep and diabetes. Int J Endocrinol 2010;2010:759509.

51. Zizi F, Jean-Louis G, Brown CD, et al. Sleep duration and the risk of diabetes mellitus: epidemiologic evidence and pathophysiologic insights. Curr Diab Rep 2010;10(1):43–7.

52. Shan Z, Ma H, Xie M, et al. Sleep duration and risk of type 2 diabetes: a meta-analysis of prospective studies. Diabetes Care 2015;38(3):529–37.

53. Buxton OM, Pavlova M, Reid EW, et al. Sleep restriction for 1 week reduces insulin sensitivity in healthy men. Diabetes 2010;59(9):2126–33.

54. Morselli L, Leproult R, Balbo M, et al. Role of sleep duration in the regulation of glucose metabolism and appetite. Best Pract Res Clin Endocrinol Metab 2010;24(5):687–702.

55. Tasali E, Leproult R, Spiegel K. Reduced sleep duration or quality: relationships with insulin resistance and type 2 diabetes. Prog Cardiovasc Dis 2009;51(5):381–91.

56. Spiegel K, Knutson K, Leproult R, et al. Sleep loss: a novel risk factor for insulin resistance and Type 2 diabetes. J Appl Physiol 2005;99(5):2008–19.

57. Spaeth AM, Dinges DF, Goel N. Sex and race differences in caloric intake during sleep restriction

in healthy adults. Am J Clin Nutr 2014;100(2):559–66.

58. Kim S, Deroo LA, Sandler DP. Eating patterns and nutritional characteristics associated with sleep duration. Public Health Nutr 2011;14(5):889–95.

59. Nedeltcheva AV, Kilkus JM, Imperial J, et al. Sleep curtailment is accompanied by increased intake of calories from snacks. Am J Clin Nutr 2009;89(1):126–33.

60. Van Cauter E, Spiegel K, Tasali E, et al. Metabolic consequences of sleep and sleep loss. Sleep Med 2008;9(Suppl 1):S23–8.

61. Spiegel K, Tasali E, Penev P, et al. Brief communication: sleep curtailment in healthy young men is associated with decreased leptin levels, elevated ghrelin levels, and increased hunger and appetite. Ann Intern Med 2004;141(11):846–50.

62. Hayes AL, Xu F, Babineau D, et al. Sleep duration and circulating adipokine levels. Sleep 2011;34(2):147–52.

63. Perelis M, Ramsey KM, Marcheva B, et al. Circadian transcription from beta cell function to diabetes pathophysiology. J Biol Rhythms 2016;31(4):323–36.

64. Grandner MA, Sands-Lincoln MR, PakVM etal. Sleep duration, cardiovascular disease, and proinflammatory biomarkers. Nat Sci Sleep 2013;5:93–107.

65. Frey DJ, Fleshner M, Wright KP Jr. The effects of 40 hours of total sleep deprivation on inflammatory markers in healthy young adults. Brain Behav Immun 2007;21(8):1050–7.

66. Ferrie JE, Kivimaki M, Akbaraly TN, et al. Associations between change in sleep duration and inflammation: findings on C-reactive protein and interleukin 6 in the Whitehall II Study. Am J Epidemiol 2013;178(6):956–61.

67. Rohleder N, Aringer M, Boentert M. Role of interleukin-6 in stress, sleep, and fatigue. Ann N Y Acad Sci 2012;1261:88–96.

68. Vgontzas AN, Zoumakis E, Bixler EO, et al. Adverse effects of modest sleep restriction on sleepiness, performance, and inflammatory cytokines. J Clin Endocrinol Metab 2004;89(5):2119–26.

69. van Leeuwen WM, Lehto M, Karisola P, et al. Sleep restriction increases the risk of developing cardiovascular diseases by augmenting proinflammatory responses through IL-17 and CRP. PLoS One 2009;4(2):e4589.

70. Chennaoui M, Sauvet F, Drogou C, et al. Effect of one night of sleep loss on changes in tumor necrosis factor alpha (TNF-alpha) levels in healthy men. Cytokine 2011;56(2):318–24.

71. Shearer WT, Reuben JM, Mullington JM, et al. Soluble TNF-alpha receptor 1 and IL-6 plasma levels in humans subjected to the sleep deprivation model of spaceflight. J Allergy Clin Immunol 2001;107(1):165–70.

72. Patel SR, Zhu X, Storfer-Isser A, et al. Sleep duration and biomarkers of inflammation. Sleep 2009;32(2):200–4.

73. Meier-Ewert HK, Ridker PM, Rifai N, et al. Effect of sleep loss on C-reactive protein, an inflammatory marker of cardiovascular risk. J Am Coll Cardiol 2004;43(4):678–83.

74. Miller MA, Kandala NB, Kivimaki M, et al. Gender differences in the cross-sectional relationships between sleep duration and markers of inflammation: Whitehall II study. Sleep 2009;32(7):857–64.

75. Matthews KA, Zheng H, Kravitz HM, et al. Are inflammatory and coagulation biomarkers related to sleep characteristics in mid-life women? Study of Women's Health across the Nation sleep study. Sleep 2010;33(12):1649–55.

76. Grandner MA, Buxton OM, Jackson N, et al. Extreme sleep durations and increased C-reactive protein: effects of sex and ethnoracial group. Sleep 2013;36(5):769–779E.

77. Irwin MR, Olmstead R, Carroll JE. Sleep disturbance, sleep duration, and inflammation: a systematic review and meta-analysis of cohort studies and experimental sleep deprivation. Biol Psychiatry 2016;80(1):40–52.

78. von Ruesten A, Weikert C, Fietze I, et al. Association of sleep duration with chronic diseases in the European Prospective Investigation into Cancer and Nutrition (EPIC)-Potsdam study. PLoS One 2012;7(1):e30972.

79. Altman NG, Izci-Balserak B, Schopfer E, et al. Sleep duration versus sleep insufficiency as predictors of cardiometabolic health outcomes. Sleep Med 2012;13(10):1261–70.

80. Wang Q, Xi B, Liu M, et al. Short sleep duration is associated with hypertension risk among adults: asystematic review and meta-analysis. HypertensRes 2012;35(10):1012–8.

81. Meng L, Zheng Y, Hui R. The relationship of sleep duration and insomnia to risk of hypertension incidence: a meta-analysis of prospective cohort studies. Hypertens Res 2013;36(11):985–95.

82. Mezick EJ, Hall M, Matthews KA. Sleep duration and ambulatory blood pressure in black and white adolescents. Hypertension 2012;59(3):747–52.

83. King CR, Knutson KL, Rathouz PJ, et al. Short sleep duration and incident coronary artery calcification. JAMA 2008;300(24):2859–66.

84. Amagai Y, Ishikawa S, Gotoh T, et al. Sleep duration and incidence of cardiovascular events in a Japanese population: the Jichi Medical School cohort study. J Epidemiol 2010;20(2):106–10.

85. Cappuccio FP, Cooper D, D'Elia L, et al. Sleep duration predicts cardiovascular outcomes: a

systematic review and meta-analysis of prospective studies. Eur Heart J 2011;32(12):1484–92.

86. Goel N, Rao H, Durmer JS, et al. Neurocognitive consequences of sleep deprivation. Semin Neurol 2009;29(4):320–39.

87. Lim J, Dinges DF. Sleep deprivation and vigilant attention. Ann N Y Acad Sci 2008;1129:305–22.

88. Dinges DF, Powell JW. Microcomputer analyses of performance on a portable, simple visual RT task during sustained operations. Beh Res Meth Instrcomp 1985;17:652–5.

89. Banks S, Dinges DF. Behavioral and physiological consequences of sleep restriction. J Clin Sleep Med 2007;3(5):519–28.

90. Van Dongen HP, Baynard MD, Maislin G, et al. Systematic interindividual differences in neurobehavioral impairment from sleep loss: evidence of trait-like differential vulnerability. Sleep 2004;27(3): 423–33.

91. Verweij IM, Romeijn N, Smit DJ, et al. Sleep deprivation leads to a loss of functional connectivity in frontal brain regions. BMC Neurosci 2014;15:88.

92. Killgore WD, Grugle NL, Balkin TJ. Gambling when sleep deprived: don't bet on stimulants. Chronobiollnt 2012;29(1):43–54.

93. Jackson ML, Croft RJ, Kennedy GA, et al. Cognitive components of simulated driving performance: sleep loss effects and predictors. Accid Anal Prev 2013;50:438–44.

94. Saint Martin M, Sforza E, Barthelemy JC, et al. Does subjective sleep affect cognitive function in healthy elderly subjects? The Proof cohort. Sleep Med 2012;13(9):1146–52.

95. Rupp TL, Wesensten NJ, Balkin TJ. Trait-like vulnerability to total and partial sleep loss. Sleep 2012; 35(8):1163–72.

96. Banks S, Van Dongen HP, Maislin G, et al. Neurobehavioral dynamics following chronic sleep restriction: dose-response effects of one night for recovery. Sleep 2010;33(8):1013–26.

97. Maia Q, Grandner MA, Findley J, et al. Short and long sleep duration and risk of drowsy driving and the role of subjective sleep insufficiency. Accid Anal Prev 2013;59:618–22.

98. Chiu HY, Tsai PS. The impact of various work schedules on sleep complaints and minor accidents during work or leisure time: evidence from a national survey. J Occup Environ Med 2013; 55(3):325–30.

99. Lilley R, Day L, Koehncke N, et al. The relationship between fatigue-related factors and work-relatedinjuries in the Saskatchewan Farm Injury Cohort Study. Am J Ind Med 2012;55(4):367–75.

100. Kucharczyk ER, Morgan K, Hall AP. The occupational impact of sleep quality and insomnia symptoms. Sleep Med Rev 2012;16(6):547–59.

101. American Psychiatric Association. Diagnostic and statistical manual of mental disorders. 5th edition. Washington, DC: American Psychiatric Association; 2003. DSM-5.

102. Chakravorty S, Siu HY, Lalley-Chareczko L, et al. Sleep duration and insomnia symptoms as risk fac-tors for suicidal ideation in a nationally representative sample. Prim Care Companion CNS Disord 2015;17(6).

103. Rosenstock IM. Why people use health services. Milbank Mem Fund Q 1966;44(3 Suppl):94–127.

104. Champion VL, Skinner CS. The health belief model. In: Glanz K, Rimer BK, Viswanath K, editors. Health behavior and health education: theory, research, and practice. San Francisco (CA): Jossey-Bass; 2008. p. 45–65.

105. Montano DE, Kasprzyk D. Theory of reasoned action, theory of planned behavior, and the integrated behavioral model. In: Glanz K, Rimer BK, Viswanath K, editors. Health behavior and health education: theory, research, and practice. San Francisco (CA): Jossey-Bass; 2008. p. 68–96.

106. Hooker E, Ball HL, Kelly PJ. Sleeping like a baby: attitudes and experiences of bedsharing in northeast England. Med Anthropol 2001;19(3):203–22.

107. Thoman EB. Co-sleeping, an ancient practice: issues of the past and present, and possibilities forthe future. Sleep Med Rev 2006;10(6):407–17.

108. Mindell JA, Sadeh A, Wiegand B, et al. Cross-cultural differences in infant and toddler sleep. Sleep Med 2010;11(3):274–80.

109. Norton PJ, Grellner KW. A retrospective study on infant bed-sharing in a clinical practice population. Matern Child Health J 2011;15(4):507–13.

110. Gettler LT, McKenna JJ. Evolutionary perspectives on mother-infant sleep proximity and breastfeedingin a laboratory setting. Am J Phys Anthropol 2011; 144(3):454–62.

111. Jain S, Romack R, Jain R. Bed sharing in school-age children-clinical and social implications. J Child Adolesc Psychiatr Nurs 2011;24(3): 185–9.

112. Shulman D, Strousma GG. Dream cultures: explorations in the comparative history of dreaming. Oxford (United Kingdom): Oxford University Press; 1999.

113. Spurgeon A, Harrington JM, Cooper CL. Health and safety problems associated with long working hours: a review of the current position. Occup Environ Med 1997;54(6):367–75.

114. Goto A, YasumuraS, Nishise Y, et al. Association of health behavior and social role with total mortality among Japanese elders in Okinawa, Japan. Aging Clin Exp Res 2003;15(6):443–50.

115. Lockley SW, Landrigan CP, Barger LK, et al. When policy meets physiology: the challenge of reducing

resident work hours. Clin Orthop Relat Res 2006; 449:116–27.

116. Ko GT, Chan JC, Chan AW, et al. Association between sleeping hours, working hours and obesity in Hong Kong Chinese: the 'better health for better Hong Kong' health promotion campaign. Int Jobes (Lond) 2007;31(2):254–60.

117. Basner M, Dinges DF. Dubious bargain: trading sleep for Leno and Letterman. Sleep 2009;32(6): 747–52.

118. Gangwisch JE. All work and no play makes Jack lose sleep. commentary on Virtanen et al. Long working hours and sleep disturbances: the Whitehall II prospective cohort study. Sleep 2009;32: 737–45.

119. Virtanen M, Ferrie JE, Gimeno D, et al. Long working hours and sleep disturbances: the Whitehall II prospective cohort study. Sleep 2009;32(6): 737–45.

120. Nakata A. Effects of long work hours and poor sleep characteristics on workplace injury among full-time male employees of small- and medium-scale businesses. J Sleep Res 2011;20(4):576–84.

121. Mahan RP, Carvalhais AB, Queen SE. Sleep reduction in night-shift workers: is it sleep deprivation or a sleep disturbance disorder? Percept Mot Skills 1990;70(3 Pt 1):723–30.

122. Rajaratnam SM, Arendt J. Health in a 24-h society. Lancet 2001;358(9286):999–1005.

123. Nag PK, Nag A. Shiftwork in the hot environment. J Hum Ergol (Tokyo) 2001;30(1–2):161–6.

124. Costa G. Shift work and health: current problems and preventive actions. Saf Health Work 2010; 1(2):112–23.

125. Owens J. Sleep in children: cross-cultural perspectives. Sleep Biol Rhythms 2004;2:165–73.

126. Milner CE, Cote KA. Benefits of napping in healthy adults: impact of nap length, time of day, age, and experience with napping. J Sleep Res 2009;18(2): 272–81.

127. Worthman CM, Brown RA. Sleep budgets in a globalizing world: biocultural interactions influence sleep sufficiency among Egyptian families. Soc Sci Med 2013;79:31–9.

128. Pandey A, Gekhman D, Gousse Y, et al. Short sleep and dysfunctional beliefs and attitudes toward sleep among black men. Sleep 2011; 34(Abstract Suppl):261–2.

129. Grandner MA, Patel NP, Jean-Louis G, et al. Sleep-related behaviors and beliefs associated with race/ethnicity in women. J Natl Med Assoc 2013;105(1): 4–15.

130. Sell RE, Bardwell W, Palinkas L, et al. Ethnic differences in sleep-health knowledge. Sleep 2009; 32(Abstract Supplement):A392.

131. Ohayon MM, Carskadon MA, Guilleminault C, et al. Meta-analysis of quantitative sleep parameters from childhood to old age in healthy individuals: developing normative sleep values across the human lifespan. Sleep 2004;27(7):1255–73.

132. Hardeland R. Melatonin in aging and disease-multiple consequences of reduced secretion, options and limits of treatment. Aging Dis 2012;3(2): 194–225.

133. Neikrug AB, Ancoli-Israel S. Sleep disorders in the older adult - a mini-review. Gerontology 2010;56(2): 181–9.

134. Roepke SK, Ancoli-Israel S. Sleep disorders in the elderly. Indian J Med Res 2010;131:302–10.

135. Martin J, Shochat T, Gehrman PR, et al. Sleep in the elderly. Respir Care Clin N Am 1999;5(3):461–72, ix.

136. Ruiter ME, VanderWal GS, Lichstein KL. Insomnia in the elderly. In: Pandi-Perumal SR, Monti JR, Monjan AA, editors. Principles and practice of geriatric sleep medicine. Cambridge (United Kingdom): Cambridge; 2010. p. 271–9.

137. Yeh P, Walters AS, Tsuang JW. Restless legs syndrome: a comprehensive overview on its epidemiology, risk factors, and treatment. Sleep Breath 2012;16(4):987–1007.

138. Spiegelhalder K, Hornyak M. Movement disorders in the elderly. In: Pandi-Perumal SR, Monti JR, Monjan AA, editors. Principles and practice of geriatric sleep medicine. Cambridge (United Kingdom): Cambridge; 2010. p. 233–40.

139. Peppard PE, Young T, Barnet JH, et al. Increased prevalence of sleep-disordered breathing in adults. Am J Epidemiol 2013;177(9):1006–14.

140. Ferini Strambi L. REM sleep behavior disorder in the elderly. In: Pandi-Perumal SR, Monti JR, Monjan AA, editors. Principles and practice of geriatric sleep medicine. Cambridge (United Kingdom): Cambridge; 2010. p. 241–7.

141. Soldatos CR, Allaert FA, Ohta T, et al. How do individuals sleep around the world? Results from a single-day survey in ten countries. Sleep Med 2005;6(1):5–13.

142. Zilli I, Ficca G, Salzarulo P. Factors involved in sleep satisfaction in the elderly. Sleep Med 2009; 10(2):233–9.

143. Grandner MA, Patel NP, Gooneratne NS. Difficulties sleeping: a natural part of growing older? Aging Health 2012;8(3):219–21.

144. Roehrs T, Kapke A, Roth T, et al. Sex differences in the polysomnographic sleep of young adults: a community-based study. Sleep Med 2006;7(1): 49–53.

145. Kimura M. Minireview: gender-specific sleep regulation. Sleep Biol Rhythms 2005;3:75–9.

146. Vitiello MV, Larsen LH, Moe KE. Age-related sleep change: gender and estrogen effects on the subjective-objective sleep quality relationships of healthy, noncomplaining older men and women. J Psychosom Res 2004;56(5):503–10.

147. Voderholzer U, Al-Shajlawi A, Weske G, et al. Are there gender differences in objective and subjective sleep measures? A study of insomniacs and healthy controls. Depress Anxiety 2003;17(3): 162–72.

148. Mohsenin V. Gender differences in the expression of sleep-disordered breathing: role of upper airway dimensions. Chest 2001;120(5):1442–7.

149. Armitage R, Hudson A, Trivedi M, et al. Sex differences in the distribution of EEG frequencies during sleep: unipolar depressed outpatients. J Affect Disord 1995;34(2):121–9.

150. Whinnery J, Jackson N, Rattanaumpawan P, et al. Short and long sleep duration associated with race/ethnicity, sociodemographics, and socioeconomic position. Sleep 2014;37(3):601–11.

151. Green MJ, Espie CA, Hunt K, et al. The longitudinal course of insomnia symptoms: inequalities by sex and occupational class among two different age cohorts followed for 20 years in the west of Scotland. Sleep 2012;35(6):815–23.

152. Ye L, Pien GW, Weaver TE. Gender differences in the clinical manifestation of obstructive sleep apnea. Sleep Med 2009;10(10):1075–84.

153. Del Campo F, Zamarron C. Sleep apnea and pregnancy. an association worthy of study. Sleep Breath 2013;17(2):463–4.

154. Ibrahim S, Foldvary-Schaefer N. Sleep disorders in pregnancy: implications, evaluation, and treatment. Neurol Clin 2012;30(3):925–36.

155. Facco FL, Kramer J, Ho KH, et al. Sleep disturbances in pregnancy. Obstet Gynecol 2010; 115(1):77–83.

156. Chen YH, Kang JH, Lin CC, et al. Obstructive sleep apnea and the risk of adverse pregnancy outcomes. Am J Obstet Gynecol 2012;206(2):136. e1–5.

157. Okun ML, Luther JF, Wisniewski SR, et al. Disturbed sleep, a novel risk factor for preterm birth? J Womens Health (Larchmt) 2012;21(1): 54–60.

158. Moore M, Meltzer LJ, Mindell JA. Bedtime problems and night wakings in children. Sleep Med Clin 2007;2:377–85.

159. Mindell JA, Kuhn B, Lewin DS, et al. Behavioral treatment of bedtime problems and night wakings in infants and young children. Sleep 2006;29(10): 1263–76.

160. Okun ML, Luther J, Prather AA, et al. Changes in sleep quality, but not hormones predict time to postpartum depression recurrence. J Affect Disord 2011;130(3):378–84.

161. Chang JJ, Pien GW, Duntley SP, et al. Sleep deprivation during pregnancy and maternal and fetal outcomes: is there a relationship? Sleep Med Rev 2010;14(2):107–14.

162. Pires GN, Andersen ML, Giovenardi M, et al. Sleep impairment during pregnancy: possible implications on mother-infant relationship. Med Hypotheses 2010;75(6):578–82.

163. Ameratunga D, Goldin J, Hickey M. Sleep disturbance in menopause. Intern Med J 2012;42(7): 742–7.

164. Regestein QR. Do hot flashes disturb sleep? Menopause 2012;19(7):715–8.

165. Baron KG, Smith TW, Berg CA, et al. Spousal involvement in CPAP adherence among patients with obstructive sleep apnea. Sleep Breath 2011; 15(3):525–34.

166. McDowell A. Spousal involvement and CPAP adherence: a two-way street? Sleep Breath 2011; 15(3):269–70.

167. Punjabi NM, Caffo BS, Goodwin JL, et al. Sleep-disordered breathing and mortality: a prospective cohort study. PLoS Med 2009;6(8):e1000132.

168. Mahowald MW, Schenck CH. REM sleep behaviour disorder: a marker of synucleinopathy. Lancet Neurol 2013;12(5):417–9.

169. Tomfohr L, Pung MA, Edwards KM, et al. Racial differences in sleep architecture: the role of ethnic discrimination. Biol Psychol 2012;89(1):34–8.

170. Thomas KS, Bardwell WA, Ancoli-Israel S, et al. The toll of ethnic discrimination on sleep architecture and fatigue. Health Psychol 2006;25(5):635–42.

171. Profant J, Ancoli-Israel S, Dimsdale JE. Are there ethnic differences in sleep architecture? Am J Hum Biol 2002;14(3):321–6.

172. Ruiter ME, Decoster J, Jacobs L, et al. Normal sleep in African-Americans and Caucasian-Americans: a meta-analysis. Sleep Med 2011; 12(3):209–14.

173. Ruiter ME, DeCoster J, Jacobs L, et al. Sleep disorders in African Americans and Caucasian Americans: a meta-analysis. Behav Sleep Med 2010; 8(4):246–59.

174. Grandner MA, Knutson KL, Troxel W, et al. Implications of sleep and energy drink use for health disparities. Nutr Rev 2014;72(Suppl 1):14–22.

175. Knutson KL. Sociodemographic and cultural determinants of sleep deficiency: implications for cardio-metabolic disease risk. Soc Sci Med 2013; 79:7–15.

176. Mezick EJ, Matthews KA, Hall M, et al. Influence of race and socioeconomic status on sleep: Pittsburgh Sleep SCORE project. Psychosom Med 2008;70(4):410–6.

177. Patel NP, Grandner MA, Xie D, et al. Sleep disparity" in the population: poor sleep quality is strongly associated with poverty and ethnicity. BMC Public Health 2010;10(1):475.

178. Grandner MA, Hale L, Jackson N, et al. Perceived racial discrimination as an independent predictor

of sleep disturbance and daytime fatigue. Behav Sleep Med 2012;10(4):235–49.

179. Slopen N, Williams DR. Discrimination, other psychosocial stressors, and self-reported sleep duration and difficulties. Sleep 2014;37(1):147–56.

180. Bureau of Labor Statistics. American time use survey fact sheet. Washington, DC: Bureau of Labor-Statistics; 2013.

181. Rosekind MR, Gregory KB, Mallis MM, et al. The cost of poor sleep: workplace productivity loss and associated costs. J Occup Environ Med 2010;52(1):91–8.

182. Hui SK, Grandner MA. Trouble sleeping associated with lower work performance and greater healthcare costs: longitudinal data from Kansas state employee wellness program. J Occup Environ Med 2015;57(10):1031–8.

183. Hui SK, Grandner MA. Associations between poor sleep quality and stages of change of multiple health behaviors among participants of Employee Wellness Program. Prev Med Rep 2015;2:292–9.

184. Gurubhagavatula I, Nkwuo JE, Maislin G, et al. Estimated cost of crashes in commercial drivers supports screening and treatment of obstructive sleep apnea. Accid Anal Prev 2008;40(1):104–15.

185. Pack AI, Maislin G, Staley B, et al. Impaired performance in commercial drivers: role of sleep apnea and short sleep duration. Am J Respir Crit Care Med 2006;174(4):446–54.

186. Xie W, Chakrabarty S, Levine R, et al. Factors associated with obstructive sleep apnea among commercial motor vehicle drivers. J Occup Environ Med 2011;53(2):169–73.

187. Moore-Ede M, Heitmann A, Guttkuhn R, et al. Circadian alertness simulator for fatigue risk assessment in transportation: application to reduce frequency and severity of truck accidents. Aviat Space Environ Med 2004;75(3 Suppl):A107–18.

188. Paterson JL, Dorrian J, Clarkson L, et al. Beyond working time: factors affecting sleep behaviour in rail safety workers. Accid Anal Prev 2012;45(Suppl):32–5.

189. Darwent D, Dawson D, Roach GD. Prediction of probabilistic sleep distributions following travel across multiple time zones. Sleep 2010;33(2):185–95.

190. Dorrian J, Darwent D, Dawson D, et al. Predicting pilot's sleep during layovers using their own behaviour or data from colleagues: implications for biomathematical models. Accid Anal Prev 2012;45(Suppl):17–21.

191. Drury DA, Ferguson SA, Thomas MJ. Restricted sleep and negative affective states in commercial pilots during short haul operations. Accid Anal Prev 2012;45(Suppl):80–4.

192. Gander PH, Signal TL, van den Berg MJ, et al. In-flight sleep, pilot fatigue and Psychomotor Vigilance Task performance on ultra-long range versus long range flights. J Sleep Res 2013;22(6):697–706.

193. Holmes A, Al-Bayat S, Hilditch C, et al. Sleep and sleepiness during an ultra long-range flight operation between the Middle East and United States. Accid Anal Prev 2012;45(Suppl):27–31.

194. Powell DM, Spencer MB, Petrie KJ. Fatigue in airline pilots after an additional day's layover period. Aviat Space Environ Med 2010;81(11):1013–7.

195. Roach GD, Darwent D, Dawson D. How well do pilots sleep during long-haul flights? Ergonomics 2010;53(9):1072–5.

196. Roach GD, Petrilli RM, Dawson D, et al. Impact of lay over length on sleep, subjective fatigue levels,and sustained attention of long-haul airline pilots. Chronobiol Int 2012;29(5):580–6.

197. Roach GD, Sargent C, Darwent D, et al. Duty periods with early start times restrict the amount of sleep obtained by short-haul airline pilots. Accid Anal Prev 2012;45(Suppl):22–6.

198. Rajaratnam SM, Barger LK, Lockley SW, et al. Sleep disorders, health, and safety in police officers. JAMA 2011;306(23):2567–78.

199. Charles LE, Gu JK, Andrew ME, et al. Sleep duration and biomarkers of metabolic function among police officers. J Occup Environ Med 2011;53(8):831–7.

200. Fekedulegn D, Burchfiel CM, Hartley TA, et al. Shift work and sickness absence among police officers: the BCOPS study. Chronobiol Int 2013;30(7):930–41.

201. Gu JK, Charles LE, Burchfiel CM, et al. Long work hours and adiposity among police officers in a US northeast city. J Occup Environ Med 2012;54(11):1374–81.

202. McCanlies EC, Slaven JE, Smith LM, et al. Metabolic syndrome and sleep duration in police officers. Work 2012;43(2):133–9.

203. Neylan TC, Metzler TJ, Henn-Haase C, et al. Prior night sleep duration is associated with psychomotor vigilance in a healthy sample of police academy recruits. Chronobiol Int 2010;27(7):1493–508.

204. Aisbett B, Wolkow A, Sprajcer M, et al. Awake, smoky, and hot": providing an evidence-base for managing the risks associated with occupational stressors encountered by wildland firefighters. Appl Ergon 2012;43(5):916–25.

205. Vargas de Barros V, Martins LF, Saitz R, et al. Mental health conditions, individual and job characteristics and sleep disturbances among firefighters. J Health Psychol 2013;18(3):350–8.

206. Grandner MA, Pack AI. Sleep disorders, public health, and public safety. JAMA 2011;306(23):2616–7.

207. Sharwood LN, Elkington J, Meuleners L, et al. Use of caffeinated substances and risk of crashes in long distance drivers of commercial vehicles: case-control study. BMJ 2013;346:f1140.

208. Grundy A, Sanchez M, Richardson H, et al. Light intensity exposure, sleep duration, physical activity, and biomarkers of melatonin among rotating shift nurses. Chronobiol Int 2009;26(7):1443–61.

209. Ruggiero JS, Redeker NS, Fiedler N, et al. Sleep and psychomotor vigilance in female shift workers. Biol Res Nurs 2012;14(3):225–35.

210. Chang YS, Wu YH, Hsu CY, et al. Impairment of perceptual and motor abilities at the end of a night shift is greater in nurses working fast rotating shifts. Sleep Med 2011;12(9):866–9.

211. Chung MH, Kuo TB, Hsu N, et al. Recovery after three-shift work: relation to sleep-related cardiac neuronal regulation in nurses. Ind Health 2012; 50(1):24–30.

212. Demir Zencirci A, Arslan S. Morning-evening type and burnout level as factors influencing sleep quality of shift nurses: a questionnaire study. Croat Medj 2011;52(4):527–37.

213. Dorrian J, Paterson J, Dawson D, et al. Sleep,stress and compensatory behaviors in Australian nurses and midwives. Rev Saude Publica 2011;45(5): 922–30.

214. Eldevik MF, Flo E, Moen BE, et al. Insomnia, excessive sleepiness, excessive fatigue, anxiety, depression and shift work disorder in nurses having less than 11 hours in-between shifts. PLoS One 2013; 8(8):e70882.

215. Geiger-Brown J, Rogers VE, Han K, et al. Occupational screening for sleep disorders in 12-h shift nurses using the Berlin Questionnaire. Sleep Breath 2013;17(1):381–8.

216. Geiger-Brown J, Rogers VE, Trinkoff AM, et al. Sleep, sleepiness, fatigue, and performance of12-hour-shift nurses. Chronobiol Int 2012;29(2):211–9.

217. Geiger-Brown J, Trinkoff A, Rogers VE. The impact of work schedules, home, and work demands on self-reported sleep in registered nurses. J Occup Environ Med 2011;53(3):303–7.

218. Ulmer C, Wolman DM, Johns MME, Institute of Medicine committee on optimizing graduate medical trainee (resident) hours and work schedules to improve patient safety. Resident duty hours: enhancing sleep, supervision, and safety. Washington, DC: National Academies Press; 2009.

219. Amin MM, Graber M, Ahmad K, et al. The effects of a mid-day nap on the neurocognitive performance of first-year medical residents: a controlled interventional pilot study. Acad Med 2012;87(10): 1428–33.

220. Arora VM, Georgitis E, Woodruff JN, et al. Improving sleep hygiene of medical interns: can the sleep, alertness, and fatigue education in residency program help? Arch Intern Med 2007; 167(16):1738–44.

221. Kim HJ, Kim JH, Park K-D, et al. A survey of sleep deprivation patterns and their effects on cognitive functions of residents and interns in Korea. Sleep Med 2011;12(4):390–6.

222. Reed DA, Fletcher KE, Arora VM. Systematic review: association of shift length, protected sleeptime, and night float with patient care, residents' health, and education. Ann Intern Med 2010; 153(12):829–42.

223. Bilimoria KY, Chung JW, Hedges LV, et al. National cluster-randomized trial of duty-hour flexibility in surgical training. N Engl J Med 2016;374(8): 713–27.

224. Hale L, Do DP. Racial differences in self-reports of sleep duration in a population-based study. Sleep 2007;30(9):1096–103.

225. Hale L, Hill TD, Burdette AM. Does sleep quality mediate the association between neighborhood disorder and self-rated physical health? Prev Med 2010;51(3–4):275–8.

226. Hale L, Hill TD, Friedman E, et al. Perceived neighborhood quality, sleep quality, and health status: evidence from the Survey of the Health of Wisconsin. Soc Sci Med 2013;79:16–22.

227. Hill TD, Burdette AM, Hale L. Neighborhood disorder, sleep quality, and psychological distress: testing a model of structural amplification. Health Place 2009;15(4):1006–13.

228. Pirrera S, De Valck E, Cluydts R. Nocturnal road traffic noise: a review on its assessment and consequences on sleep and health. Environ Int 2010; 36(5):492–8.

229. Kawada T. Noise and health: sleep disturbance in adults. J Occup Health 2011;53(6):413–6.

230. Fonken LK, Kitsmiller E, Smale L, et al. Dim nighttime light impairs cognition and provokes depressive-like responses in a diurnal rodent. J Biol Rhythms 2012;27(4):319–27.

231. Hu RF, Jiang XY, Zeng YM, et al. Effects of ear plugs and eye masks on nocturnal sleep, melatonin and cortisol in a simulated intensive care unit environment. Crit Care 2010;14(2):R66.

232. Wood B, Rea MS, Plitnick B, et al. Light level and duration of exposure determine the impact of self-luminous tablets on melatonin suppression. Appl Ergon 2013;44(2):237–40.

233. Herljevic M, Middleton B, Thapan K, et al. Light-induced melatonin suppression: age-related reduction in response to short wavelength light. Exp Gerontol 2005;40(3):237–42.

234. Pigeon WR, Grandner MA. Creating an optimal sleep environment. In: Kushida CA, editor. Encyclopedia of sleep. Oxford (United Kingdom): Elsevier; 2013. p. 72–6.

235. Buxton OM, Ellenbogen JM, Wang W, et al. Sleep disruption due to hospital noises: a prospective evaluation. Ann Intern Med 2012;157(3):170–9.

236. Parmeggiani PL. Sleep behaviour and temperature. In: Parmeggiani PL, Velluti RA, editors. The physiologic nature of sleep. London: Imperial College Press; 2005. p. 387–405.

237. McCall WV, Boggs N, Letton A. Changes in sleep and wake in response to different sleeping surfaces: a pilot study. Appl Ergon 2012;43(2): 386–91.

238. Shanmugan B, Roux F, Stonestreet C, et al. Lower back pain and sleep: mattresses, sleep quality and daytime symptoms. Sleep Diagn Ther 2007; 2(5):36–40.

239. Verhaert V, Haex B, De Wilde T, et al. Ergonomics in bed design: the effect of spinal alignment on sleep parameters. Ergonomics 2011;54(2):169–78.

240. Troxel WM. It's more than sex: exploring the dyadic nature of sleep and implications for health. Psychosom Med 2010;72(6):578–86.

241. Troxel WM, Robles TF, Hall M, et al. Marital quality and the marital bed: examining the covariation between relationship quality and sleep. Sleep Med Rev 2007;11(5):389–404.

242. Troxel WM, Buysse DJ, Hall M, et al. Marital happiness and sleep disturbances in a multi-ethnic sample of middle-aged women. Behav Sleep Med 2009;7(1):2–19.

243. Troxel WM, Buysse DJ, Monk TH, et al. Does social support differentially affect sleep in older adults with versus without insomnia? J Psychosom Res 2010;69(5):459–66.

244. Troxel WM, Cyranowski JM, Hall M, et al. Attachment anxiety, relationship context, and sleep in women with recurrent major depression. Psychosom Med 2007;69(7):692–9.

245. Gradisar M, Wolfson AR, Harvey AG, et al. The sleep and technology use of Americans: findings from the National Sleep Foundation's 2011 Sleep in America poll. J Clin Sleep Med 2013;9(12): 1291–9.

246. Orzech K, Grandner MA, Roane BM, et al. Electronic media use within 2 hours of bedtime predicts sleep variables in college students. Sleep 2012; 35(Abstract Suppl):A73.

247. Chang AM, Aeschbach D, Duffy JF, et al. Evening use of light-emitting eReaders negatively affects sleep, circadian timing, and next-morning alertness. Proc Natl Acad Sci U S A 2015;112(4): 1232–7.

248. Weaver E, Gradisar M, Dohnt H, et al. The effect of presleep video-game playing on adolescent sleep. J Clin Sleep Med 2010;6(2):184–9.

249. NHTSA. Drowsy driving. Washington, DC: US Department of Transportation; 2011.

250. Strohl KP, Blatt J, Council F, et al. Drowsy driving and automobile crashes: NCSDR/NHTSA expert panel on driver fatigue and sleepiness. Washington, DC: National Highway Traffic Safety Administration; 1998.

251. Borman KR, Biester TW, Jones AT, et al. Sleep, supervision, education, and service: views of junior and senior residents. J Surg Educ 2011;68(6): 495–501.

252. Borman KR, Fuhrman GM. Resident duty hours: enhancing sleep, supervision, and safety": response of the Association of Program Directors in Surgery to the December 2008 report of the Institute of Medicine. Surgery 2009;146(3):420–7.

253. Sataloff RT. Resident duty hours: concerns and consequences. Ear Nose Throat J 2009;88(3): 812–6.

254. Federal Aviation Administration. Fact sheet-sleep apnea in aviation. Washington, DC: FAA; 2015.

255. McKnight-Eily LR, Liu Y, Wheaton AG, et al. Unhealthy sleep-related behaviors—12 States, 2009. MMWR Morb Mortal Wkly Rep 2011;60(8):233–8.

256. Lufi D, Tzischinsky O, Hadar S. Delaying school starting time by one hour: some effects on attention levels in adolescents. J Clin Sleep Med 2011;7(2): 137–43.

257. Moore M, Meltzer LJ. The sleepy adolescent: causes and consequences of sleepiness in teens. Paediatr Respir Rev 2008;9(2):114–20 [quiz:120-1].

258. Wahlstrom K. School start time and sleepy teens. Arch Pediatr Adolesc Med 2010;164(7):676–7.

259. Wolfson AR, Spaulding NL, Dandrow C, et al. Middle school start times: the importance of a good-night's sleep for young adolescents. Behav Sleep Med 2007;5(3):194–209.

260. Roenneberg T, Kuehnle T, Pramstaller PP, et al. A marker for the end of adolescence. Curr Biol 2004;14(24):R1038–9.

261. Barnes M, Davis K, Mancini M, et al. Setting adolescents up for success: promoting a policy to delay high school start times. J Sch Health 2016; 86(7):552–7.

262. Meltzer LJ, Shaheed K, Ambler D. Start later, sleep later: school start times and adolescent sleep in homeschool versus public/private school students. Behav Sleep Med 2016;14(2):140–54.

263. Millman RP, Boergers J, Owens J. Healthy school start times: can we do a better job in reaching our goals? Sleep 2016;39(2):267–8.

264. Minges KE, Redeker NS. Delayed school start times and adolescent sleep: a systematic review of the experimental evidence. Sleep Med Rev 2016;28:86–95.

265. Thacher PV, Onyper SV. Longitudinal outcomes of start time delay on sleep, behavior, and achievement in high school. Sleep 2016;39(2):271–81.

266. Wheaton AG, Chapman DP, Croft JB. School start times, sleep, behavioral, health, and academic outcomes: a review of the Literature. J Sch Health 2016;86(5):363–81.

267. Siebern AT, Manber R. Insomnia and its effective non-pharmacologic treatment. Med Clin North Am 2010;94(3):581–91.

268. Watson NF, Horn E, Duncan GE, et al. Sleep duration and area-level deprivation in twins. Sleep 2016;39(1):67–77.

269. Knutson KL, Van Cauter E, Rathouz PJ, et al. Association between sleep and blood pressure in midlife: the CARDIA sleep study. Arch Intern Med 2009;169(11):1055–61.

Neurobiology of Circadian Rhythm Regulation

Alan M. Rosenwasser, PhD[a],*, Fred W. Turek, PhD[b]

KEYWORDS

- Circadian • Pacemaker • Suprachiasmatic nucleus • Entrainment • Clock genes

KEY POINTS

- The suprachiasmatic nucleus (SCN) of the anterior hypothalamus has been firmly established as the master circadian pacemaker in mammals.
- The SCN circadian pacemaker is synchronized (entrained) by environmental light–dark cycles via photoreceptors and neural pathways distinct from those mediating visual perception.
- The cellular–molecular basis of circadian rhythm generation involves several circadian clock genes expressed not only in the SCN but also throughout the brain and peripheral tissues and organs.
- The SCN serves as a central pacemaker atop a hierarchically organized, anatomically distributed circadian timing system and entrains downstream circadian clocks via neural and neuroendocrine pathways.
- System-wide circadian coordination is necessary for optimal physiologic function and maintenance of physical and mental health.

IDENTIFICATION OF THE SUPRACHIASMATIC NUCLEUS CIRCADIAN PACEMAKER

The initial demonstrations that lesions of the suprachiasmatic nucleus (SCN) severely disrupt or abolish circadian rhythms in behavioral and endocrine functions were published in the early 1970s.[1,2] Following these initial demonstrations, extensive subsequent research involving lesions, in vivo and in vitro electrophysiology, functional metabolic mapping, fetal tissue transplant, and molecular analyses revealed that the SCN is capable of autonomous, self-sustained circadian rhythmicity at both the single-cell and tissue levels. These now-classic studies are summarized in the published report of a meeting held to evaluate the state of SCN research on the 25th anniversary of its discovery.[3]

SUPRACHIASMATIC NUCLEUS: A NETWORK OF CLOCK CELLS

Studies using a variety of in vitro models, including electrophysiological recording and optical monitoring of SCN cell and tissue cultures, have provided compelling evidence that circadian oscillation is fundamentally a cell-autonomous process, expressed in many, but probably not all, individual SCN neurons.[4–7]

Nevertheless, individual SCN clock cells normally interact to produce coherent circadian signals at the tissue (and behavioral) level.[8–10] Despite the capacity of individual SCN neurons for autonomous rhythmicity, recent studies have revealed that neuronal network interactions increase the frequency of rhythmic cells detected in culture, as well as the amplitude of their

[a] Department of Psychology, School of Biology and Ecology, Graduate School of Biomedical Science and Engineering, University of Maine, 5742 Little Hall, Orono, ME 04467, USA; [b] Department of Neurobiology, Center for Sleep and Circadian Biology, Northwestern University, 2205 Tech Drive, Hogan Hall 2-160, Evanston, IL 60208, USA
* Corresponding author.
E-mail address: alanr@maine.edu

Sleep Med Clin 17 (2022) 141–150
https://doi.org/10.1016/j.jsmc.2022.02.006
1556-407X/22/© 2022 Elsevier Inc. All rights reserved.

oscillation, and contribute to the overall robustness of SCN pacemaker function.[11,12]

Early studies suggested that SCN clock cells could maintain intercellular synchrony in the absence of sodium-dependent action potentials,[13,14] suggesting that gap junctions, glial coupling, calcium-dependent signaling, or local diffusible signals might be responsible for synchronizing the network of clock cells.[15] In contrast, however, more recent studies have found that blocking action potentials in SCN tissue slices or cell cultures can disrupt intercellular phase synchrony,[10] thus reviving interest in the possible synchronizing role of synaptic transmission. Both g-aminobutyric acid (GABA) and vasoactive intestinal peptide (VIP) neurotransmission, among other signaling mechanisms, have now been implicated in the maintenance of coupling among SCN clock cells, as well as among subpopulations of SCN clock cells.[16,17]

MOLECULAR BASIS OF THE SUPRACHIASMATIC NUCLEUS CIRCADIAN PACEMAKER

A critical role for protein synthesis in the mammalian circadian pacemaker was established in the late 1980s,[18,19] and elucidation of the fundamental molecular genetic oscillatory mechanism began in earnest about 10 years later. The first mammalian circadian clock gene, Clock, was identified in a forward-genetics mutagenesis screen,[20] and this discovery was followed quickly by the identification of several other core molecular clock components, some of which were homologous to previously discovered circadian clock genes in the fruit fly.[21,22] In addition to Clock, other recognized mammalian clock genes include the 3 period (Per) genes (Per1, Per2, and Per3), 2 cryptochrome genes (Cry1 and Cry2), Bmal1 (also known as Arntl1 and Mop3), CK1e (Casein kinase 1 epsilon), Rev-erba, and Fxbl3, all of which are expressed in SCN neurons. The specific functions of these various genes within the interlocking molecular feedback loops that generate circadian signals at the cellular level have been reviewed extensively elsewhere, and are not discussed here.

Mutations or deletions of any of these genes produce alterations in circadian phenotype at the behavioral level. The most devastating effects on clock function are seen in Bmal1-knockout mice, which express immediate loss of rhythmicity in the absence of a light–dark cycle.[21,22] In contrast, the original Clock mutation, which codes for a dominant-negative CLOCK protein, dramatically lengthens free-running period and often leads to a gradual loss of rhythmicity under long-term free-running conditions.[21,22] Surprisingly, however, unlike the original Clock mutation, Clock-null (knockout) mice express robust and persisting circadian rhythms, with only a modest shortening of circadian period[23]; it was subsequently found that NPAS2 can substitute for CLOCK as a dimerization partner for BMAL1 within the SCN, thus maintaining circadian pacemaker function.[24] Regarding the Per genes, several distinct mutations have been studied by different laboratories, but in general, Per1 or Per2 disruption shortens circadian period and reduces the robustness of free-running rhythms.[25,26] Similarly, Cry-mutant mice also exhibit alterations in the free-running period, whereas Cry1/Cry2 double mutants are rendered arrhythmic.[27,28] In contrast to other clock genes, the circadian clock function of Ck1e was discovered by genetic analysis of a spontaneous single-gene mutation that dramatically shortens free-running period in the hamster, originally called the tau mutation.[29] Cloning of the tau gene revealed its identity as Ck1e, and subsequent transgenic insertion of this allele into mice recapitulated the hamster short-period phenotype, whereas deletion of Ck1e in mice lengthened the circadian period.[30] More recently, mutations of the Fxbl3 gene have been shown to lengthen the free-running period.[31,32] Similar to Ck1e, Fxbl3 influences circadian period by regulating the post-translational stability of other clock proteins such as PER and CRY.[33] Of course, for the molecular clock to drive circadian rhythmicity in physiology and behavior, clock gene expression must be linked to intracellular signaling pathways regulating neuronal membrane potential and, ultimately, firing rate. Remarkably, recent research demonstrates that ionic events at the cell membrane influence the molecular clock via some of the same intracellular signals that convey clock signals to the membrane, and in some cases, these ionic currents may be necessary for self-sustainment of the molecular clock.[34] Such results—at a minimum—serve to blur the distinction between the core clock mechanisms and the so-called hands of the clock.

In addition to their effects on circadian behavior, some circadian clock gene mutations also affect sleep–wake homeostasis, and several forms of affective behavior, suggesting possible molecular links between the circadian, sleep regulatory, and motivational systems of the brain.[35–37]

FUNCTIONAL ARCHITECTURE OF THE SUPRACHIASMATIC NUCLEUS

Although the SCN was initially characterized as being composed of distinct ventrolateral and dorsomedial subdivisions,[38] this scheme has been recast to include SCN core and shell subnuclei, a concept that may better accommodate species differences in the anatomic distribution of neuropeptides, afferent terminal fields, and gene expression patterns in the SCN.[39] The SCN core is associated with a high concentration of VIP-positive and gastrin-releasing peptide (GRP)–positive neurons, whereas the shell is associated with the presence of arginine vasopressin–positive neurons. Beyond this basic organization, however, clear species differences have been noted, and it has been argued that the popular distinction between SCN core and shell may be such an extreme oversimplification as to impede understanding of the functional organization of this critical structure.[40,41]

Although the specific functions of chemically defined SCN cell populations are not fully known, VIP and GRP neurons of the SCN core seem to collate afferent signals relevant to pacemaker entrainment, whereas vasopressinergic (or other) neurons of the SCN shell may have the primary responsibility of generation of self-sustaining circadian oscillations.[42] A preeminent role for the SCN core in pacemaker entrainment is supported by findings that major SCN afferent systems converge in the core subnucleus, administration of SCN core peptides such as VIP and GRP can mimic both light-induced phase shifting and *Per* gene expression in the SCN in vivo and in vitro, and light-evoked changes in SCN physiology and gene expression spreads over time from core to shell. Conversely, evidence for a preeminent role of the SCN shell in pacemaking includes findings that the core projects robustly to the shell, but not vice versa, spontaneous circadian rhythmicity in neuronal activity, neuropeptide release, and gene expression is seen more reliably in the shell than in the core, and spontaneous rhythmicity in SCN gene expression seems to flow from the most dorsomedial toward more central–lateral regions over the course of the circadian cycle. On the other hand, the view that SCN core and shell underlie discrete entrainment and pacemaking functions is probably too simplistic because (1) several arousal-related afferents of limbic and brainstem origin target the SCN shell,[39] (2) in vitro studies have revealed independent free-running rhythmicity in the secretion of core and shell peptides from the same tissue explant,[43] and (3) SCN core and shell can exhibit stable dissociation of rhythmic gene expression in vivo under certain conditions.[44] Furthermore, studies using microlesions indicate that the integrity of the SCN core is essential for the maintenance of high-amplitude behavioral and molecular-level rhythmicity, suggesting that rhythmic signals from the core serve a permissive gate-like role in sustaining oscillatory function in the shell.[42]

LIGHT INPUT TO THE SUPRACHIASMATIC NUCLEUS: THE RETINOHYPOTHALAMIC TRACT

Although stimuli such as temperature, sound, food, and social cues seem to contribute to phase control, the 24-h environmental light–dark cycle is the primary cue for circadian entrainment in most mammalians (and other vertebrate taxa). A specialized retinal projection system, referred to as the retinohypothalamic tract (RHT), is both necessary and sufficient for photic entrainment of the circadian pacemaker[45,46] (**Fig. 1**). The RHT originates from a distinct subset of retinal ganglion cells, separate from those giving rise to the primary visual pathways,[47] and terminates mainly in the SCN, as well as more sparsely in the anterolateral hypothalamus, subparaventricular zone, and supraoptic region.[48,49] In addition, RHT axon collaterals also project to the thalamic intergeniculate leaflet (IGL), which, as discussed later, is an important component of the circadian system.

Remarkably, retinally degenerate strains of mice, in which nearly all classic photoreceptors (ie, rods and cones) are lost by early adulthood, exhibit normal circadian responses to light.[50] More recently, similar findings have been reported in genetically engineered mice with a total developmental absence of both rods and cones, demonstrating conclusively that circadian light entrainment can be mediated by a novel, nonrod, noncone photoreceptor system.[51] Circadian entrainment in the absence of rods and cones is maintained by a population of intrinsically photosensitive retinal ganglion cells that use the peptide melanopsin as a photopigment.[52,53] Nevertheless, circadian entrainment is maintained in melanopsin-knockout mice[54,55] and is only fully abolished when both classical and melanopsin-based photoreception is eliminated demonstrating redundancy in the circadian photoreception system in the retina.[56–58]

RHT terminals release the excitatory amino acid neurotransmitter, glutamate, which acts through both W-methyl-D-aspartate (NMDA) and non-NMDA receptors and a variety of intracellular signaling pathways to increase *Per* gene expression. These changes in gene expression, when superimposed on the ongoing circadian transcription–translation cycle, correspond functionally to phase shifts of the circadian oscillator.[59–62] In addition to glutamate, RHT terminals also release 2 identified peptide cotransmitters,

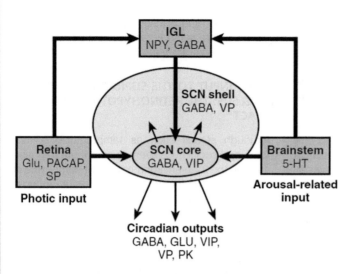

Fig. 1. Overview of functional neuroanatomic pathways in the mammalian circadian system. Major SCN afferent systems originating in the retina and raphe nuclei also target the intergeniculate leaflet (IGL) of the thalamus, which itself projects to the SCN. Retinal projections to the SCN and IGL mediate photic input to the circadian system, whereas raphe projections to the SCN and IGL mediate the effects of certain nonphotic, behavioral state–related signals. Furthermore, raphe-IGL-SCN circuits also modulate and integrate photic and nonphotic signaling to the SCN pacemaker. SCN outputs mainly target the hypothalamus and diencephalon and seem to include both neural efferents and secreted paracrine signals. 5-HT, 5-hydroxy-tryptamine; GLU, glutamate; NPY, neuropeptide Y; PACAP, pituitary adenyl cyclase-activating peptide; PK, prokineticin; SP, substance P; VP, arginine vasopressin; VIP, vasoactive intestinal polypeptide.

substance P (SP) and pituitary adenyl cyclase–activating peptide (PACAP). SP seems to play an important role in RHT transmission because selective SP antagonists block light-induced phase shifting and immediate-early gene expression in vivo, as well as glutamate receptor–mediated phase shifting in vitro, whereas SP administration can itself induce circadian phase shifts.[63–65] In contrast, PACAP administration has been reported either to antagonize or to mimic the effects of glutamate on circadian phase shifting and *Per* gene expression in vitro, depending on the dose and the circadian phase of administration.[66–68]

OTHER FUNCTIONAL INPUTS TO THE SUPRACHIASMATIC NUCLEUS

An additional major SCN afferent system arises from the IGL, a distinct retinorecipient region of the lateral geniculate complex, intercalated between the dorsal and ventral lateral geniculate nuclei[69–71] (see **Fig. 1**). The projection from the IGL to the SCN is referred to as the geniculohypothalamic tract (GHT), and GHT neurons release both neuropeptide Y and GABA. Retinal signals are conveyed to the IGL in part by axon collaterals of RHT neurons,[72] and GHT and RHT terminal fields are largely coextensive within the SCN core. Thus, the IGL/GHT system provides a secondary, indirect pathway by which light signals can reach the circadian pacemaker. Although the IGL is clearly not necessary for photic entrainment, lesions of the IGL/GHT system result in subtle modifications in the photic control of circadian phase and period.[70,71] Furthermore, the IGL may have a significant role in entrainment under more naturalistic lighting conditions (eg, regimens including twilight transitions, seasonally changing photoperiod, or simulated moonlight), relative to the square-wave light–dark cycles commonly used in the laboratory.[72]

In addition to providing a secondary, indirect source of photic signaling to the circadian clock, the IGL also plays a preeminent role in the regulation of the circadian system by nonphotic, arousal-related stimuli. Thus, IGL lesions abolish the phase-shifting effects of novelty-induced wheel running and benzodiazepine administration in hamsters, as well as the period-shortening effect of running-wheel access in rats and the entrainment effect of scheduled daily treadmill activity in mice.[73–78] More recently, evidence has been presented that IGL neurons may mediate the effects of metabolic signals on the SCN pacemaker.[79,80] A third major afferent system converging mainly on the SCN core originates from the serotonergic midbrain raphe, especially the median raphe nucleus[81–84] (see **Fig. 1**). In addition, ascending serotonergic projections originating in the dorsal raphe nucleus innervate the IGL, providing a second route for serotonergic regulation of the SCN circadian pacemaker.[81,82] As for the IGL itself, extensive evidence has implicated serotonergic projections to the SCN and IGL in modulation of photic effects on the circadian pacemaker, as well as in the mediation of nonphotic effects on the pacemaker. These effects seem to be mediated via 5-hydroxytryptamine (5-HT)$_{1A}$ and 5-HT$_7$ receptors within the SCN, the IGL, and the raphe nuclei and by 5-HT$_{1B}$ receptors located presynaptically on RHT terminals.[85–89]

In addition to the RHT, GHT, and 5-HT projections, several other identified pathways provide afferent input to the circadian system, including noradrenergic projections from the locus coeruleus, cholinergic projections from the basal forebrain and pontine tegmentum, and histaminergic projections from the posterior hypothalamus.[90,91] Similar to serotonergic projections, noradrenergic and cholinergic projections also innervate the IGL, providing an alternate pathway by which these transmitter systems could alter SCN function. However, unlike the RHT, GHT, and 5-HT projections to the SCN, which form generally overlapping terminal fields in the SCN core, noradrenergic, cholinergic, and histaminergic SCN inputs preferentially target the SCN shell. Beyond these systems, a recent review concluded that the SCN receives direct monosynaptic projections from at least 35 distinct brain areas,[41] revealing enormous potential for circadian pacemaker modulation by a wide range of extrinsic and intrinsic stimuli.

SUPRACHIASMATIC NUCLEUS OUTPUT PATHWAYS

Perhaps surprisingly, first-order SCN efferents innervate a relatively small number of target areas concentrated mainly in the diencephalon and basal forebrain.[92,93] These SCN targets then relay circadian timing signals to autonomic and neuroendocrine systems, as well as to central structures regulating affective, sensory, and motor processes, as well as to sleep-regulatory brain regions.[94] SCN efferents emerge from both the core and shell subnuclei and release several neurotransmitters and peptides including GABA, glutamate, and vasopressin (see **Fig. 1**). Remarkably, anatomically distinct populations of SCN neurons seem to innervate specific efferent targets, providing multiple waves of neuronal signals that regulate circadian phase in a target-specific manner. Despite earlier evidence that neuronal efferents were exclusively responsible for conveying SCN output signals,[95] it now appears that the SCN regulates certain rhythmic processes via diffusible paracrine signals. Evidence for a diffusible SCN output signal was first suggested by the finding that surgical isolation of the hamster SCN within a hypothalamic island abolished SCN-dependent neuroendocrine responses but allowed for persisting locomotor activity rhythms in the same animals.[96] The hypothesis for paracrine signaling from the SCN in the regulation of rhythmic processes was strengthened considerably by the finding that transplant of SCN tissue encased within a semipermeable capsule could restore locomotor but not neuroendocrine rhythms to SCN-lesioned arrhythmic hosts.[97] Several diffusible candidate molecules have now been implicated as circadian output signals, including prokineticin-2, tumor necrosis factor-a, and vasopressin.[97]

MULTIOSCILLATOR NATURE OF THE CIRCADIAN SYSTEM

The evidence reviewed earlier in this study amply justifies the use of the term pacemaker to describe the SCN's role in circadian rhythmicity. Nevertheless, the larger circadian system is now known to be composed of a multiplicity of circadian oscillators distributed widely in the brain and body. Although extensive physiologic studies conducted in the premolecular era revealed several varieties of rhythmic dissociation and disruption that strongly implied the existence of a multioscillatory circadian system,[98] these studies provided little evidence regarding the anatomic localization and distribution of the circadian system.

After the elucidation of the core clock genes, it soon became apparent that the expression of these genes was not restricted to the SCN but was in fact widely distributed in the brain and periphery. Nevertheless, it was generally believed that non-SCN cellular oscillators were highly damped and possessed little or no capacity for self-sustainment in the absence of periodic SCN input. More recently, however, the finding that circadian clock genes express persistent rhythmically in several surgically isolated brain regions[99,100] and in numerous cultured peripheral tissues and cell types[101,102] has provided compelling evidence for a whole-body, anatomically distributed network of cellular- and tissue-level circadian clocks. Thus, the current conception of the circadian system is that the SCN pacemaker entrains rhythmicity in downstream central and peripheral clocks via neural and neuroendocrine signals, as well as less directly via its control of rhythmic feeding, activity, and body temperature,[103] which in turn entrain other behavioral, physiologic, and cellular rhythms (**Fig. 2**). In this way, a broad network of direct and indirect controls ensures that the SCN and other central and peripheral clocks maintain specific, and presumably optimal, phase relationships with the external and internal environment, resulting in the overall temporal coordination of the system.

What is the advantage of a distributed system of independent circadian clocks, as opposed to a passive system that strongly depends on SCN signals for the sustainment of periodicity? Perhaps the advantage lies in the ability of such a system

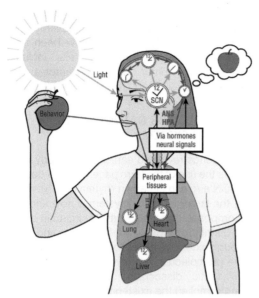

Fig. 2. The multioscillatory circadian timing system includes a large number of autonomously rhythmic circadian clock cells distributed within both central and peripheral tissues. The circadian pacemaker resides in the SCN, is entrained by light–dark cycles and other environmental stimuli, and in turn, serves to entrain and synchronize peripheral clocks. Some peripheral tissues can exhibit persistent autonomous rhythmicity, whereas others may be damped in the absence of periodic SCN signals. Together, SCN and non-SCN central neural oscillators result in rhythmic behavior (such as food intake and motor activity), autonomic nervous system (ANS) function, and hypothalamic–pituitary–adrenal (HPA) axis hormone secretion. These behavioral and physiologic rhythms in turn can give rise to other rhythmic signals (eg, glucose availability, corticosterone levels, and body temperature) that serve to maintain phase synchrony among peripheral oscillators, probably in a tissue-specific manner. In turn, the activity of peripheral oscillators may give rise to rhythmic signals (eg, peripheral hormones, autonomic afferents, and metabolic signals) that contribute to the synchronization of the SCN pacemaker and other central oscillators.

to display a degree of plasticity in internal phase relationships under certain environmental conditions, such as when sleep and wakefulness occur at abnormal clock times or when feeding is restricted to atypical temporal windows. Under such conditions, a system of largely self-sustaining clocks can maintain largely undamped rhythmicity at the cellular and tissue levels. Thus, although temporal coordination throughout the circadian system is generally assumed to be physiologically optimal, the overall circadian system may be designed to allow downstream oscillators to display adaptive phase adjustments under

certain natural circumstances. Of course, such plasticity may become maladaptive when humans choose to chronically disconnect their feeding and/or sleep–wake cycles from the SCN, as so often occurs in the current 24/7 society.

THE CIRCADIAN TIMING SYSTEM IN HEALTH AND DISEASE

This new picture of the circadian timing system has raised important questions about the potential adverse health effects that may be associated with a loss of normal synchronization between and among central and peripheral oscillations. Thus, circadian disruption at the molecular and systemic levels has been linked to sleep disorders, obesity and diabetes, heart disease, cancer, and psychiatric disorders.[103–106] Given estimates that approximately 10% to 20% of the entire genome is expressed rhythmically in any given tissue or organ,[107,108] many other mechanisms linking circadian synchrony and desynchrony to health and disease will undoubtedly emerge in the next few years and beyond.

Circadian dysregulation certainly occurs quite often in humans, who can over-ride their circadian clock and exert substantial volitional control over their sleep–wake and feeding cycles. Under such circumstances, abnormal phase relationships are expressed between sleep–wake behaviors (and other rhythmic processes tightly linked to sleep or wake states, as well as feeding or fasting states) and the circadian clock (and rhythmic processes tightly linked to those behavioral processes). Although the internal desynchronies that occur with jet lag and shift work may be the most dramatic, they are not the only examples of real-world circadian disruption. Indeed, social constraints, work schedules, and the use of artificial lighting may result in the widespread occurrence of social jet lag even in people living under relatively stable entrained conditions but who phase shift their sleep and feeding times on weekends and holidays relative to the weekdays.[109] Regardless of work or travel schedules, humans in the modern, round-the-clock society are certainly becoming less strictly diurnal, opposing millions of years of evolutionary selection.

SUMMARY

The SCN contains a master circadian pacemaker that entrains, coordinates, and contributes to the sustainment of a large population of cellular- and tissue-level circadian clocks located throughout the brain and body. Furthermore, the SCN itself contains a large number of normally coupled, but potentially autonomous, cellular oscillators that interact to underlie its pacemaker function. These cellular oscillations are generated by a set of circadian clock genes that interact via negative and positive feedback and ultimately drive circadian expression of a large number of clock-controlled genes, which in turn regulate downstream cellular and physiologic processes. Anatomically, the SCN is characterized by a complex regional organization that is not fully understood. The SCN pacemaker is entrained by several convergent afferent pathways that signal photic and nonphotic stimuli that mediate pacemaker entrainment to periodic environmental events. SCN outputs serve to synchronize non-SCN clocks and to impose rhythmicity on otherwise nonrhythmic processes. While it is becoming increasingly clear that proper coordination of the overall circadian system is critical for maintenance of health and well-being, it may also be the case that adaptive uncoupling among circadian clocks may allow for temporal adaptation to challenging environments.

CLINICS CARE POINTS

- Evaluation of sleep patterns and circadian integrity should be included in virtually all clinical assessments, across disease categories.

DISCLOSURE

The author has nothing to disclose.

REFERENCES

1. Moore RY, Eichler VB. Loss of a circadian adrenal corticosterone rhythm following suprachiasmatic lesions in the rat. Brain Res 1972;42(1):201–6.
2. Stephan FK, Zucker I. Circadian rhythms in drinking behavior and locomotor activity of rats are eliminated by hypothalamic lesions. Proc Natl Acad Sci U S A 1972;69(6):1583–6.
3. Weaver DR. The suprachiasmatic nucleus: a 25- year retrospective. J Biol Rhythms 1998;13(2):100–12.
4. Welsh DK, Logothetis DE, Meister M, et al. Individual neurons dissociated from rat suprachiasmatic nucleus express independently phased circadian firing rhythms. Neuron 1995;14:697–706.
5. Herzog ED, Geusz ME, Khalsa SB, et al. Circadian rhythms in mouse suprachiasmatic nucleus explants on multimicroelectrode plates. Brain Res 1997;757:285–90.
6. Colwell CS. Circadian modulation of calcium levels in cells in the suprachiasmatic nucleus. Eur J Neurosci 2000;12:571–6.
7. Kuhlman SJ, Quintero JE, McMahon DG. GFP fluorescence reports Period 1 gene regulation in the mammalian biological clock. Neuroreport 2000; 11:1479–82.
8. Low-Zeddies SS, Takahashi JS. Chimera analysis of the Clock mutation in mice shows that complex cellular integration determines circadian behavior. Cell 2001;105:25–42.
9. Shirakawa T, Honma S, Honma K. Multiple oscillators in the suprachiasmatic nucleus. Chronobiol Int 2001;18:371–87.
10. Yamaguchi S, Isejima H, Matsuo T, et al. Synchronization of cellular clocks in the suprachiasmatic nucleus. Science 2003;302:1408–12.
11. Welsh DK, Takahashi JS, Kay SA. Suprachiasmatic nucleus: cell autonomy and network properties. Annu Rev Physiol 2010;72:551–77.
12. Mohawk JA, Takahashi JS. Cell autonomy and synchrony of suprachiasmatic nucleus circadian oscillators. Trends Neurosci 2011;34:349–58.
13. Schwartz W, Gross RA, Morton MT. The suprachiasmatic nuclei contain a tetrodotoxin-resistant circadian pacemaker. Proc Natl Acad Sci U S A 1987;84:1694–8.
14. Shibata S, Moore RY. Tetrodotoxin does not affect circadian rhythms in neuronal activity and metabolism in rodent suprachiasmatic nucleus in vitro. Brain Res 1993;606:259–66.
15. Miche S, Colwell CS. Cellular communication and coupling within the suprachiasmatic nucleus. Chronobiol Int 2001;18:579–600.
16. Aton SJ, Herzog ED. Come together, right … now: synchronization of rhythms in a mammalian circadian clock. Neuron 2005;48:531–4.
17. Herzog ED. Neurons and networks in daily rhythms. Nat Rev Neurosci 2007;8:790–802.
18. Takahashi JS, Turek FW. Anisomycin, an inhibitor of protein synthesis, perturbs the phase of a mammalian circadian pacemaker. Brain Res 1987;405: 199–203.
19. Inouye ST, Takahashi JS, Wollnik F, et al. Inhibitor of protein synthesis phase shifts a circadian pacemaker in the mammalian SCN. Am J Physiol 1988;255:R1055–8.
20. Vitaterna MH, King DP, Chang A-M, et al. Mutagenesis and mapping of a mouse gene, Clock, essential for circadian behavior. Science 1994;264: 719–25.
21. Allada R, Emery P, Takahashi JS, et al. Stopping time: the genetics of fly and mouse circadian clocks. Annu Rev Neurosci 2001;24:1091–119.
22. Ko CH, Takahashi JS. Molecular components of the mammalian circadian clock. Hum Mol Genet 2006; 15:R271–7.

23. Debruyne JP, Noton E, Lambert CM, et al. A clock shock: mouse CLOCK is not required for circadian oscillator function. Neuron 2006;50:465–77.

24. DeBruyne JP, Weaver DR, Reppert SM. CLOCK and NPAS2 have overlapping roles in the suprachiasmatic circadian clock. Nat Neurosci 2007;10: 543–5.

25. Shearman LP, Zylka MJ, Weaver DR, et al. Two period homologs: circadian expression and photic regulation in the suprachiasmatic nuclei. Neuron 1997;19:1261–9.

26. Zheng B, Albrecht U, Kaasik K, et al. Nonredundant roles of the mPer1 and mPer2 genes in the mammalian circadian clock. Cell 2001;105: 683–94.

27. Miyamoto Y, Sancar A. Circadian regulation of cryptochrome genes in the mouse. Brain Res Mol Brain Res 1999;71:238–43.

28. Van der Horst GT, Muijtjens M, Kobayashi K, et al. Mammalian Cry1 and Cry2 are essential for maintenance of circadian rhythms. Nature 1999;398:627–30.

29. Lowrey PL, Shimomura K, Antoch MP, et al. Positional syntenic cloning and functional characterization of the mammalian circadian mutation tau. Science 2000;288:483–92.

30. Meng QJ, Logunova L, Maywood ES, et al. Setting clock speed in mammals: the CK1 epsilon tau mutation in mice accelerates circadian pacemakers by selectively destabilizing PERIOD proteins. Neuron 2008;58:78–88.

31. Godinho SI, Maywood ES, Shaw L, et al. The afterhours mutant reveals a role for Fbxl3 in determining mammalian circadian period. Science 2007;316: 897–900.

32. Siepka SM, Yoo SH, Park J, et al. Circadian mutant Overtime reveals F-box protein FBXL3 regulation of cryptochrome and period gene expression. Cell 2007;129:1011–23.

33. Maywood ES, Chesham JE, Meng QJ, et al. Tuning the period of the mammalian circadian clock: additive and independent effects of CK1epsilonTau and Fbxl3Afh mutations on mouse circadian behavior and molecular pacemaking. J Neurosci 2010;31: 1539–44.

34. Colwell CS. Linking neural activity and molecular oscillations in the SCN. Nat Rev Neurosci 2010; 12:553–69.

35. Naylor E, Bergmann BM, Krauski K, et al. The circadian clock mutation alters sleep homeostasis in the mouse. J Neurosci 2000;20:8138–43.

36. Tafti M, Franken P. Functional genomics of sleep and circadian rhythm. Invited review: genetic dissection of sleep. J Appl Physiol 2002;92:1339–47.

37. Rosenwasser AM. Circadian clock genes: noncircadian roles in sleep, addiction, and psychiatric disorders? Neurosci Biobehav Rev 2010;34: 1249–55.

38. Moore RY. Entrainment pathways and the functional organization of the circadian system. Prog Brain Res 1996;111:103–19.

39. Moore RY, Silver R. Suprachiasmatic nucleus organization. Chronobiol Int 1998;15:475–87.

40. Morin LP. SCN organization reconsidered. J Biol Rhythms 2007;22:3–13.

41. Morin LP. Neuroanatomy of the extended circadian rhythm system. Exp Neurol 2013;243:4–20.

42. Antle MC, Silver R. Orchestrating time: arrangements of the brain circadian clock. Trends Neurosci 2005;28:145–51.

43. Shinohara K, Honma S, Katsuno Y, et al. Two distinct oscillators in the rat suprachiasmatic nucleus in vitro. Proc Natl Acad Sci U S A 1995;92: 7396–400.

44. de la Iglesia HO, Cambras T, Schwartz WJ, et al. Forced desynchronization of dual circadian oscillators within the rat suprachiasmatic nucleus. Curr Biol 2004;14:796–800.

45. Johnson RF, Moore RY, Morin LP. Loss of entrainment and anatomical plasticity after lesions of the hamster retinohypothalamic tract. Brain Res 1998; 460:297–313.

46. Golombek DA, Rosenstein RE. Physiology of circadian entrainment. Physiol Rev 2010;90:1063–102.

47. Moore RY, Speh JC, Card JP. The retinohypothalamic tract originates from a distinct subset of retinal ganglion cells. J Comp Neurol 1995;352:351–66.

48. Johnson RF, Morin LP, Moore RY. Retinohypothalamic projects in the hamster and rat demonstrated using cholera toxin. Brain Res 1998;462:301–12.

49. Levine JD, Weiss ML, Rosenwasser AM, et al. Retinohypothalamic tract in the female albino rat: a study using horseradish peroxidase conjugated to cholera toxin. J Comp Neurol 1991;306:344–60.

50. Foster RG, Argamaso S, Coleman S, et al. Photoreceptors regulating circadian behavior: a mouse model. J Biol Rhythms 1993;8(Suppl):S17–23.

51. Freedman MS, Lucas RJ, Soni B, et al. Regulation of mammalian circadian behavior by non-rod, non-cone, ocular photoreceptors. Science 1999;284: 502–4.

52. Hattar S, Liao HW, Takao M, et al. Melanopsin-containing retinal ganglion cells: architecture, projections, and intrinsic photosensitivity. Science 2002; 295:1065–70.

53. Berson DM, Dunn FA, Takao M. Phototransduction by retinal ganglion cells that set the circadian clock. Science 2002;295:1070–3.

54. Ruby NF, Brennan TJ, Xie X, et al. Role of melanopsin in circadian responses to light. Science 2002; 298:2211–3.

55. Panda S, Sato TK, Castrucci AM, et al. Melanopsin (Opn4) requirement for normal light-induced circadian phase shifting. Science 2002;298: 2213–6.

56. Hattar S, Lucas RJ, Mrosovsky N, et al. Melanopsin and rod-cone photoreceptive systems account for all major accessory visual functions in mice. Nature 2003;424:76–81.

57. Drouyer E, Rieux C, Hut RA, et al. Responses of suprachiasmatic nucleus neurons to light and dark adaptation: relative contributions of melanopsin and rod-cone inputs. J Neurosci 2007;27:9623–31.

58. Guler AD, Altimus CM, Ecker JL, et al. Multiple photoreceptors contribute to nonimage-forming visual functions predominantly through melanopsin-containing retinal ganglion cells. Cold Spring Harb Symp Quant Biol 2007;72:509–15.

59. Gillette MU. Regulation of entrainment pathways by the suprachiasmatic circadian clock: sensitivities to second messengers. Prog Brain Res 1996;111: 121–32.

60. Kornhauser JM, Ginty DD, Greenberg ME, et al. Light entrainment and activation of signal transduction pathways in the SCN. Prog Brain Res 1996; 111:133–46.

61. Shigeyoshi Y, Taguchi K, Yamamoto S, et al. Light-induced resetting of a mammalian circadian clock is associated with rapid induction of the mPer1 transcript. Cell 1997;91:1043–53.

62. Moriya T, Horikawa K, Akiyama M, et al. Correlative association between N-methyl-D-aspartate receptor-mediated expression of period genes in the suprachiasmatic nucleus and phase shifts in behavior with photic entrainment of clock in hamsters. Mol Pharmacol 2000;58:1554–62.

63. Challet E, Dugovic C, Turek FW, et al. The selective neurokinin 1 receptor antagonist R116301 modulates photic responses of the hamster circadian system. Neuropharmacology 2001;40:408–15.

64. Kim DY, Kang HC, Shin HC, et al. Substance P plays a critical role in photic resetting of the circadian pacemaker in the rat hypothalamus. J Neurosci 2001;21:4026–31.

65. Piggins HD, Rusak B. Effects of microinjections of substance P into the suprachiasmatic nucleus region on hamster wheel-running rhythms. Brain Res Bull 1997;42:451–5.

66. Chen D, Buchanan GF, Ding JM, et al. Pituitary adenylate cyclase-activating peptide: a pivotal modulator of glutamatergic regulation of the suprachiasmatic circadian clock. Proc Natl Acad Sci U S A 1999;96:13468–73.

67. Harrington ME, Hoque S, Hall A, et al. Pituitary adenylate cyclase activating peptide phase shifts circadian rhythms in a manner similar to light. J Neurosci 1999;19:6637–42.

68. Hannibal J, Jamen F, Nielsen HS, et al. Dissociation between light-induced phase shift of the circadian rhythm and clock gene expression in mice lacking the pituitary adenylate cyclase activating polypeptide type 1 receptor. J Neurosci 2001;21:4883–90.

69. Moore RY, Card JP. Intergeniculate leaflet: an anatomically and functionally distinct subdivision of the lateral geniculate complex. J Comp Neurol 1994;344:403–30.

70. Morin LP. The circadian visual system. Brain Res Rev 1994;67:102–27.

71. Harrington ME. The ventral lateral geniculate nucleus and the intergeniculate leaflet: interrelated structures in the visual and circadian systems. Neurosci Biobehav Rev 1997;21:705–27.

72. Pickard GE. Bifurcating axons of retinal ganglion cells terminate in the hypothalamic suprachiasmatic nucleus and in the intergeniculate leaflet of the thalamus. Neurosci Lett 1982;55: 211–7.

73. Wickland CR, Turek FW. Lesions of the thalamic intergeniculate leaflet block activity-induced phase shifts in the circadian activity rhythm of the golden hamster. Brain Res 1994;660:293–300.

74. Janik D, Mrosovsky N. Intergeniculate leaflet lesions and behaviorally-induced shifts of circadian rhythms. Brain Res 1994;651:174–82.

75. Johnson R, Smale L, Moore RY, et al. Lateral geniculate lesions block circadian phase-shift responses to a benzodiazepine. Proc Natl Acad Sci U S A 1988;85:5301–4.

76. Meyer EL, Harrington ME, Rahmani T. A phase-response curve to the benzodiazepine chlordiazepoxide and the effect of geniculo-hypothalamic tract ablation. Physiol Behav 1993;53:237–43.

77. Kuroda H, Fukushima M, Nakai M, et al. Daily wheel running activity modifies the period of free-running rhythm in rats via intergeniculate leaflet. Physiol Behav 1997;61:633–7.

78. Marchant EG, Watson NV, Mistlberger RE. Both neuropeptide Y and serotonin are necessary for entrainment of circadian rhythms in mice by daily treadmill running schedules. J Neurosci 1997;17:7974–87.

79. Pekala D, Blasiak T, Raastad M, et al. The influence of orexins on the firing rate and pattern of rat intergeniculate leaflet neurons-electrophysiological and immunohistological studies. Eur J Neurosci 2011; 34:1406–18.

80. Saderi N, Cazarez-Marquez F, Buijs FN, et al. The NPY intergeniculate leaflet projections to the suprachiasmatic nucleus transmit metabolic conditions. Neuroscience 2013;246:291–300.

81. Meyer-Bernstein EL, Morin LP. Differential serotonergic innervation of the suprachiasmatic nucleus and the intergeniculate leaflet and its role in circadian rhythm modulation. J Neurosci 1996;16: 2097–111.

82. Morin LP. Serotonin and the regulation of mammalian circadian rhythmicity. Ann Med 1999;31:12–33.

83. Rea MA, Pickard GE. Serotonergic modulation of photic entrainment in the Syrian hamster. Biol Rhythm Res 2000;31:284–314.

84. Mistlberger RE, Antle MC, Glass JD, et al. Behavioral and serotonergic regulation of circadian rhythms. Biol Rhythm Res 2000;31:240–83.

85. Ehlen JC, Grossman GH, Glass JD. In vivo resetting of the hamster circadian clock by 5-HT7 receptors in the suprachiasmatic nucleus. J Neurosci 2001;21:5351–7.

86. Mintz EM, Gillespie CF, Marvel CL, et al. Serotonergic regulation of circadian rhythms in Syrian hamsters. Neuroscience 1997;79:563–9.

87. Prosser RA. Serotonergic actions and interactions on the SCN circadian pacemaker: in vitro investigations. Biol Rhythm Res 2000;31:315–39.

88. Pickard GE, Rea MA. TFMPP, a 5HT1B receptor agonist, inhibits light-induced phase shifts of the circadian activity rhythm and c-Fos expression in the mouse suprachiasmatic nucleus. Neurosci Lett 1997;231:95–8.

89. Smith BN, Sollars PJ, Dudek FE, et al. Serotonergic modulation of retinal input to the mouse suprachiasmatic nucleus mediated by 5-HT1B and 5-HT7 receptors. J Biol Rhythms 2001;16:25–38.

90. Rosenwasser AM. Neurobiology of the mammalian circadian system: oscillators, pacemakers, and pathways. Prog Psychobiol Physiol Psychol 2003; 18:1–38.

91. Rosenwasser AM, Turek FW. Physiology of the mammalian circadian system. In: Kryger MH, Roth T, Dement WC, editors. Principles and practice of sleep medicine. 5th edition. St Louis (MO): Elsevier-Saunders; 2011. p. 390–401.

92. Kalsbeek A, Perreau-Lenz S, Buijs RM. A network of (autonomic) clock outputs. Chronobiol Int 2006; 23:521–35.

93. Kalsbeek A, Palm IF, La Fleur SE, et al. SCN outputs and the hypothalamic balance of life. J Biol Rhythms 2006;21:458–69.

94. Rosenwasser AM. Functional neuroanatomy of sleep and circadian rhythms. Brain Res Rev 2009;61:281–306.

95. LeSauter J, Silver R. Output signals of the SCN. Chronobiol Int 1998;15:535–50.

96. Hakim H, DeBernardo AP, Silver R. Circadian locomotor rhythms, but not photoperiodic responses, survive surgical isolation of the SCN in hamsters. J Biol Rhythms 1991;6:97–113.

97. Silver R, LeSauter J, Tresco PA, et al. A diffusible coupling signal from the transplanted suprachiasmatic nucleus controlling circadian locomotor rhythms. Nature 1996;382:810–3.

98. Rosenwasser AM, Adler NT. Structure and function in circadian timing systems: evidence for multiple coupled circadian oscillators. Neurosci Biobehav Rev 1986;10:431–48.

99. Abe M, Herzog ED, Yamazaki S, et al. Circadian rhythms in isolated brain regions. J Neurosci 2002;22:350–6.

100. Granados-Fuentes D, Tseng A, Herzog ED. A circadian clock in the olfactory bulb controls olfactory responsivity. J Neurosci 2006;26:12219–25.

101. Yoo SH, Yamazaki S, Lowrey PL, et al. PERIOD2::LUCIFERASE real-time reporting of circadian dynamics reveals persistent circadian oscillations in mouse peripheral tissues. Proc Natl Acad Sci U S A 2004;101:5339–46.

102. Welsh DK, Yoo SH, Liu AC, et al. Bioluminescence imaging of individual fibroblasts reveals persistent, independently phased circadian rhythms of clock gene expression. Curr Biol 2004;14:2289–95.

103. Hastings MH, Reddy AB, Maywood ES. A clockwork web: circadian timing in brain and periphery, in health and disease. Nat Rev Neurosci 2003;4:649–61.

104. Takahashi JS, Hong HK, Ko CH, et al. The genetics of mammalian circadian order and disorder: implications for physiology and disease. Nat Rev Genet 2008;9:764–75.

105. Karatsoreos IN. Effects of circadian disruption on mental and physical health. Curr Neurol Neurosci Rep 2012;12:218–25.

106. Zelinski EL, Deibel SH, McDonald RJ. The trouble with circadian clock dysfunction: multiple deleterious effects on the brain and body. Neurosci Biobehav Rev 2014;40:80–101.

107. Akhtar RA, Reddy AB, Maywood ES, et al. Circadian cycling of the mouse liver transcriptome, as revealed by cDNA microarray, is driven by the suprachiasmatic nucleus. Curr Biol 2002;12:540–50.

108. Panda S, Antoch MP, Miller BH, et al. Coordinated transcription of key pathways in the mouse by the circadian clock. Cell 2002;109:307–20.

109. Wittmann M, Dinich J, Merrow M, et al. Social jetlag: misalignment of social and biological time. Chronobiol Int 2006;23:497–509.

Sleep-Wake Neurochemistry

Sebastian C. Holst, PhD[a],*, Hans-Peter Landolt, PhD[b,c]

KEYWORDS

- Neurotransmitters • Neuromodulators • Glutamate • Acetylcholine • Norepinephrine • Dopamine
- GABA • Adenosine

KEY POINTS

- Behavioral states alternate between wakefulness, rapid eye movement, and non-rapid eye movement sleep.
- Waking and sleep states are highly complex processes, elegantly fine-tuned by cerebral neurochemical changes in the neurotransmitters and neuromodulators glutamate, acetylcholine, γ-aminobutyric acid, norepinephrine, dopamine, serotonin, histamine, hypocretin, melanin-concentrating hormone, adenosine, and melatonin.
- No single neurotransmitter or neuromodulator, but rather their complex interactions within organized neuronal ensembles, regulate waking and sleep states and drive their transitions.
- Dysregulation or medications interfering with these neurochemical systems can lead to sleep-wake disorders and functional changes of wakefulness and sleep.
- The neurochemical pathways presented here provide a conceptual framework for the understanding of the effects of currently used medications on wakefulness and sleep.

INTRODUCTION

Based on behavioral and (neuro) physiologic characteristics derived from polysomnographic recordings, the 3 distinct vigilance states of wakefulness, rapid eye movement (REM) sleep, and non-REM (NREM) sleep can be unambiguously defined in mammals. Wakefulness with eyes closed is typically associated with electroencephalographic (EEG) activity in the alpha range (8–12 Hz) and with high-frequency, desynchronized activity greater than 40 Hz. In a normal sleep episode, voluntary muscle control is gradually lost and NREM and REM sleep episodes alternate in a cyclic pattern. In NREM sleep, the EEG shows slow, high-amplitude activity reflecting widespread, synchronous oscillations of neurons exhibiting alternating periods of firing and silence (burst-pause firing pattern).[1] The so-called EEG delta activity (<4.5 Hz) is under tight homeostatic control and exhibits a declining trend in the course of the night, which reflects the dissipation of sleep need and the decline in sleep intensity.[2] The EEG in REM sleep (sometimes called paradoxic sleep) is partly reminiscent of EEG activity in drowsy wakefulness, yet it is characterized by muscle atonia with occasional muscle twitches and REMs.

Distinct neurotransmitter nuclei and neuronal pathways modulate and maintain these 3 behavioral states. First insights were reported by Constantin von Economo[3] (1876–1931) who studied patients with a particular type of viral encephalitis, encephalitis lethargica. von Economo discovered that the encephalitis was associated with lesions

This article previously appeared in *Sleep Med Clin* 13 (2018) 137–146.
[a] Neuroscience and Rare Diseases Discovery and Translational Area, Roche Pharmaceutical Research and Early Development, Roche Innovation Center Basel, Grenzacherstrasse 124, Basel 4070, Switzerland; [b] Institute of Pharmacology and Toxicology, University of Zürich, Winterthurerstrasse 190, Zürich 8057, Switzerland; [c] Zürich Center for Interdisciplinary Sleep Research (ZiS), University of Zürich, Zürich, Switzerland
* Corresponding author.
E-mail address: sebastian.holst@roche.com

Sleep Med Clin 17 (2022) 151–160
https://doi.org/10.1016/j.jsmc.2022.03.002
1556-407X/22/© 2022 Elsevier Inc. All rights reserved.

to distinct brain areas in the midbrain and brainstem reticular formation. Lesions of the ventral periaqueductal gray and posterior hypothalamus were associated with severe hypersomnia, whereas lesions of the hypothalamic anterior preoptic area extending into the basal ganglia were associated with insomnia. These findings were the first in a series of fundamental studies, eventually leading to the postulation of an ascending reticular activating system (ARAS).[4] The ARAS arises from a network of neuronal clusters in the brainstem, which activates forebrain, thalamus, and cortex, mainly in wakefulness but to some extent also in REM sleep. Today, the ARAS is no longer seen as a loose reticular system but, instead, as consisting of a network of individual nuclei expressing distinct neurotransmitters that promote arousal (**Fig. 1**). The key modulatory neurotransmitters of the ascending activating system include acetylcholine (ACh), several monoamines (norepinephrine [NE], serotonin [5-hydroxytryptamine, 5-HT], histamine [His], dopamine [DA]), and the slow-acting neuropeptide hypocretin (Hcrt; aka orexin). Together with glutamate,[5] adenosine, and gamma-aminobutyric acid (GABA), these neurochemicals play important roles in promoting waking and sleep states, which provide a useful conceptual framework to understand the effects of medications on wakefulness and sleep. With the recent advent of powerful optogenetic and chemogenetic tools, experimental in vivo control of neuronal activity by stimulating or inhibiting distinct neuronal ensembles permitted exciting new insights into the causal underpinnings of brain state transitions. A comprehensive summary of these insights is beyond the scope of this article; this has been the topic of excellent recent overviews.[6,7] Nevertheless, some recent progress in current understanding of sleep-wake neurochemistry made by investigating sleep-wake circuits with optogenetic techniques are covered.

The Neurochemical Underpinnings of Wakefulness

Acetylcholine

ACh-releasing nuclei in the pedunculopontine (PPT) and laterodorsal tegmental nuclei (LDT) of the pons project primarily to the basal forebrain (BF), as well as to the thalamic relay and reticular cells. This pathway is crucial for gating thalamic signaling to the cortex and is importantly involved in the promotion of both wakefulness and REM sleep. A second cluster of ACh-releasing neurons is located in the BF, which projects widely to the cortex. ACh activates ionotropic nicotinic receptors and metabotropic muscarinic receptors. Nicotinic receptors are expressed in presynaptic and postsynaptic membranes. When they are activated, sodium and calcium ions rapidly enter the cells, leading to membrane depolarization. Muscarinic receptors are part of the superfamily of G protein–coupled receptors (GPCRs). Five types of muscarinic receptors are currently known. The M_1, M_3, and M_5 receptors are coupled with G_q proteins that activate phospholipase C and adenylyl cyclase. They are expressed in the cortex and striatum, as well as other brain regions. M_2 and M_4 are coupled to $G_{i/o}$ proteins, and their activation inhibits adenylyl cyclase. These receptors are found, among other regions, in the BF, where they act as autoreceptors and are thought to control ACh synthesis and release. The cholinergic neurons in the central nervous system (CNS) are active mainly in wakefulness and REM sleep and have a firing rate in the theta range.[8] They promote cortical arousal and REM sleep, while reducing NREM sleep.[9–11]

Recent optogenetic studies in mice have improved our understanding of the role of ACh and other wake-promoting neurotransmitters in controlling vigilance states. With this method, selected neurons are genetically modified to express channelrhodopsin-2 (ChR2), a light-activated nonspecific cation channel. When ChR2 is activated by a light pulse, influx of cations such as Ca^{21} is triggered and the ChR2-expressing cells are activated.[12] Optogenetic activation of the cholinergic PPT or LDT neurons in mice during NREM sleep leads to a rapid transition into REM sleep, yet not into wakefulness.[13] On the other hand, optogenetic stimulation of PPT or LDT neurons during wakefulness is associated with moderate arousal.[13] Interestingly, activation of ChR2-expressing cholinergic neurons of the BF during wakefulness also promotes arousal, whereas activation during NREM sleep leads to transition, at roughly equal amount, into wakefulness and REM sleep.[14] These observations suggest that the cholinergic neurons in the brainstem are more involved in regulating transitions into REM sleep, whereas the cells of the BF are more linked to general arousal.

Another recent study using optogenetics could corroborate that the ACh neurons of the BF contribute to arousal and the promotion of wakefulness.[15] Nevertheless, by also stimulating the glutamatergic and GABAergic neurons of the BF, it was found that the 3 neuronal cell groups exert similar effects on arousal.[15] Interestingly, activation of BF GABAergic neurons substantially enhanced wakefulness. However, when BF glutamatergic and cholinergic neurons were activated, the effects on

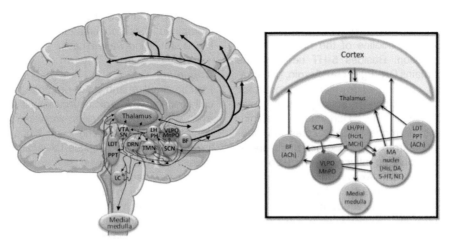

Fig. 1. Anatomic locations of major neurotransmitter nuclei (*left*) and simplified overview of their major connections relevant for sleep-wake regulation (*right*). Wakefulness (*orange*): cholinergic (ACh) tegmental (LDT or PPT) neurons and monoaminergic (MA) neurons of upper brainstem and hypothalamus innervate thalamus and basal forebrain (BF). The MA neurons have a pronounced role and directly innervate the cerebral cortex. Hypocretin (Hcrt) neurons of lateral or posterior hypothalamus (LH or PH) reinforce the activity of this ascending arousal pathways and directly excite the (BF). NREM sleep (*purple*): GABAergic VLPO and MnPO nuclei, which inhibit the ascending arousal pathways, are active in NREM sleep. REM sleep (*cyan*): ACh-ergic neurons of LDT or PPT promote REM sleep, during which NE and 5-HT neurons are silent. Entry into REM is inhibited by Hcrt neurons and facilitated by the VLPO. Connections from the SCN are important in regulating the timing of wakefulness and sleep. Black arrows indicate an excitatory connection. Red squares and lines indicate an inhibitory connection. Please refer to main text for full list of abbreviations.

arousal were minor.[15–18] In conclusion, although ACh neurons of the BF likely modulate wakefulness, it now seems that subgroups of BF GABAergic neurons may be more important than cholinergic neurons for the regulation of arousal.

Monoamines

The monoamines promoting arousal and maintaining wakefulness include NE, 5-HT, DA, and His. The primary site of production and release of NE is the locus coeruleus (LC), of 5-HT the raphe nucleus (DRN), of DA the ventral tegmental area (VTA) and substantia nigra (SN), and of His the hypothalamic tuberomammillary nucleus (TMN). With the exception of the dopaminergic cell groups, all these nuclei fire at high rates in wakefulness, lower rates in NREM sleep, and are virtually silent in REM sleep.[19–21] They have widespread CNS projections and innervate cortex, brainstem, ventrolateral preoptic (VLPO) nucleus, thalamus, and the BF, making them ideally located to promote and sustain wakefulness.

Norepinephrine

The LC is an important small cell cluster involved in the regulation of arousal.[20] It is located in the brainstem and consists of roughly 25,000 NE neurons. NE can activate both the α and β families of adrenergic receptors, which are part of the GPCR superfamily. Adrenergic receptors are divided into 3 main types: α_1 (mainly G_q coupled), α_2 (inhibitory autosynaptic and postsynaptic receptors, $G_{i/o}$ coupled), and b receptors (G_s coupled), which are all widely expressed in the CNS.[22] Optogenetic stimulation of the noradrenergic neurons in the LC is associated with immediate transitions from sleep to wakefulness and increased locomotor activity,[23] highlighting the role of the LC in maintaining behavioral arousal. Recent evidence also suggests a role for NE in the sleep-driven macroscopic pathway referred to as the glymphatic system. This system is governed by a flow of cerebrospinal fluid into the brain through perivascular (also known as Virchow-Robin) spaces, which enables the removal of macroscopic waste products from the brain parenchyma in NREM sleep.[24,25] Increased glymphatic function in NREM sleep results from an increased interstitial space volume fraction, which seems to be driven by reduced LC-derived NE-ergic tone.[25] However, the increase in interstitial space that enables glymphatic flow during sleep may not solely be driven by NE. The size of the interstitial space can also be reduced by a wake-promoting cocktail of monoamines, ACh, and Hcrt and even by altering the concentrations of potassium, calcium, and magnesium ions in the cerebrospinal fluid.[26,27]

Serotonin

The major nuclei releasing 5-HT, the DRN, are located along the midline of the brainstem and reticular formation. Besides 5-HT neurons, the DRN also contains DA-ergic, GABAergic, glutamatergic, and neuropeptide-releasing neurons. Moreover, the DRN is innervated by GABA, glutamate, ACh, NE, His, Hcrt, and melanin-concentrating hormone (MCH)-expressing neurons originating from several other brain areas, rendering serotonergic influences on sleep-wake regulation highly complex in nature. Furthermore, the 5-HT receptors are subdivided into 7 distinct families: 5-HT to $5-HT_7$ receptors. Similar to the other monoamines, all 5-HT receptors, except the ligand-gated $5-HT_3$ ion channel, belong to the GPCR superfamily. The 5-HT! and $5-HT_5$ receptors are coupled to $G_{i/o}$ protein, the $5-HT_2$ receptor is coupled to G_q protein, and the $5-HT_4$, $5-HT_6$, and $5-HT_7$ receptors are coupled to G_s protein. The many 5-HT receptor subtypes and the widespread effects of 5-HT in the CNS have made it challenging to elucidate the distinct roles for 5-HT in sleep-wake regulation.[28] Intriguingly, $5-HT_{1A}$ and $5-HT_{1B}$ receptor knockout mice have enhanced amounts of REM sleep,[29,30] whereas mutant mice without $5-HT_{2A}$ or $5-HT_{2C}$ receptors show enhanced durations of wakefulness and reduced NREM sleep.[31,32] Overall, the current evidence suggests that 5-HT transmission generally promotes wakefulness, inhibits REM sleep, and can interfere with slow wave sleep.[33] Optogenetic stimulation of DRN 5-HT neurons has been attempted and found to enhance patience in an anticipated-reward paradigm.[34] With respect to sleep-wake regulation, optogenetic activation of DRN 5-HT neurons has not been examined. However, it was recently shown that optogenetic activation of DRN DA neurons promote wakefulness and contribute to the regulation of sleep-wake states.[35]

Histamine

The TMN is a small His-releasing cell cluster found inferior to the hypothalamus. The TMN shows a projection pattern that is similar to the LC and the DRN, including strong reciprocal innervation with the VLPO.[36] Three types of His-ergic GPCRs have so far been classified in the brain: H_1, H_2, and H_3 receptors that are coupled to G_q, G_s, and G_i proteins. It is well known that antihistamines are sedative, which is a common side effect of early H1 receptor antagonists (eg, diphenhydramine) in the treatment of allergies. The release of His within the TMN by optogenetic photostimulation activates H3 autoreceptors and suppresses inhibitory GABAergic inputs to TMN.[37] Moreover, His from the TMN enhanced the inhibition of the VLPO. Combined, these observations support a role for His in stabilizing wakefulness.

Dopamine

Psychostimulant and wake-promoting agents typically enhance DA-ergic neurotransmission.[38] However, with respect to sleep-wake regulation, this neurotransmitter has long been thought to be of limited importance because DA-ergic neurotransmission in cats showed only minor alterations across the sleep-wake cycle. By contrast, more recent evidence in rats revealed that extracellular DA levels in the medial prefrontal cortex and parts of the nucleus accumbens (NAc) of the ventral striatum are high in wakefulness and REM sleep and significantly lower in NREM sleep.[39,40] Thus, similar to the other monoamines, DA may indeed play an important role in regulating wakefulness and sleep. Five types of DA-ergic GPCRs are known. The D_1-like (D_1 and D_5) DA receptors are coupled to G_s protein and are mainly stimulatory. On the contrary, the D_2-like (D_2, D_3, and D_4) DA receptors are coupled to inhibitory G_i protein. Importantly, D_1 and D_2 receptors form functional heteromers with adenosine A1 and A2A receptors (see later discussion), such that the binding of adenosine results in reduced dopaminergic signaling.

Both distinct subtypes of DA and adenosine receptors are primarily expressed in the NAc, a brain region recently suggested to play a crucial role in sleep-wake regulation.[6] The NAc is innervated by DA projections of the mesolimbic pathway originating in the VTA. By integrating signals from cortex, thalamus, amygdala, and midbrain, the NAc is able to inhibit several other arousal pathways via GABAergic interneurons. Experimental inhibition and activation of the NAc, thus, promote wakefulness and sleep.[41–43] Several studies interrogated DA-ergic neurotransmission by optogenetics, in particular with respect to reward and addiction. However, a recent study in rats elegantly showed that destruction of DA afferents in the SN pars compacta (SNc), projecting via the nigrostriatal pathway to the dorsal striatum, enhanced wakefulness and induced sleep-wake fragmentation.[44] The investigators then optogenetically stimulated the SNc DA neurons, which resulted in increased firing and enhanced sleep,[44] suggesting that the nigrostriatal DA-ergic pathway promotes sleep. Taken together, it is likely that distinct roles for DA in sleep-wake regulation are region specific and pathway specific and probably also dose dependent.

Neuropeptides

Approximately 100 neuropeptides have been described in the human brain.[45] They typically act via GPCRs, exert long-lasting dynamic modulatory effects at the synapse, and do not cross the blood-brain barrier. These characteristics make them difficult targets for pharmacologic interventions.

Hypocretin

Several neuropeptides, including Hcrt, MCH, galanin, oxytocin, neuropeptide Y, somatostatin, ghrelin, and substance P, play important roles in regulating mood, reward, arousal, and sleep.[46] With respect to sleep-wake regulation, Hcrt and MCH especially deserve mention. These peptides are released from a small cluster of neurons found solely in the lateral hypothalamus (LH). The MCH contributes mainly to the promotion and maintenance of sleep[47] (see later discussion).

The Hcrt-producing neurons project to all previously described nuclei of the arousal pathways, especially to LC, DRN, and TMN. They also release glutamate and play important roles in maintaining arousal and stabilizing the wake state. Similar to the other wake-promoting systems, the Hcrt neurons are mainly active in wakefulness, especially when animals are exploring, and become silent in REM sleep and NREM sleep.[48] The Hcrt binds to 2 subtypes of GPCRs, referred to as Hcrt-1 and Hcrt-2 receptors. Activation of these receptors increases intracellular calcium levels. The loss of Hcrt neurons causes narcolepsy with cataplexy, which is characterized by behavioral state instability, most likely caused by an insufficient inhibition of the circuits regulating REM sleep and NREM sleep.[49,50] Supporting the wake-promoting role of Hcrt, optogenetic activation of Hcrt neurons triggers brief awakenings from both REM sleep and NREM sleep, an effect that is diminished with increasing sleep pressure.[51,52] Combined, these findings suggest that sleep-dependent processes feedback to Hcrt neurons and inhibit their wake-promoting actions.

The Neurochemical Underpinnings of Sleep

Neuropeptides: melanin-concentrating hormone

The MCH-expressing neurons in the LH are intermingled with Hcrt neurons and also produce GABA. These neurons innervate many of the Hcrt-target regions, including the LC and the DRN.[53] However, in contrast to Hcrt, the MCH projections are inhibitory and fire at high rates in REM sleep, are less active in NREM sleep, and remain almost silent in wakefulness.[54] Thus, MCH neurons likely promote REM sleep and inhibit wakefulness. Indeed, MCH-deficient mice spend less time in both REM and NREM sleep.[55] On the contrary, when the MCH neurons are optogenetically

activated, either REM sleep alone[56,57] or both REM sleep and NREM sleep[58] were found to be enhanced. Although more research is warranted, it seems evident that MCH neurons inhibit wakefulness and functionally oppose Hcrt neurons in regulating the transition between wakefulness and sleep states.[57]

Adenosine

Adenosine, via the well-known adenosine antagonist caffeine, is likely the world's most readily consumed psychostimulant. Adenosine and adenosine receptors have long been suggested to play a key role for sleep-wake regulation.[59-62] Compelling evidence now suggests that the neuromodulator adenosine contributes to the regulation of the increase in sleep pressure during wakefulness and the decrease in sleep propensity during sleep. Four subtypes of G protein–coupled adenosine receptors have been identified to mediate adenosine's cellular effects: A1, A2A, A_{2B}, and A_3 receptors. Activation of A_1 and A_3 receptors inhibits adenylyl cyclase by coupling to $G_{i/o}$ protein, whereas A_{2A} and A_{2B} receptors mediate their effects by increased adenylyl cyclase activity through coupling to G_s protein.[63] The A1 and A2A receptors are strongly expressed in the brain, yet their local expression patterns vary. By contrast, A_{2B} and A_3 receptors are expressed with only low abundance in cerebral structures, and their roles in sleep-wake regulation are not well established. Recently, adenosine was demonstrated to also play a key role for in circadian regulation, where adenosine seems to integrate signaling from both light and prior sleep to regulate circadian timing.[64] Moreover, adenosine has many properties of a presumed endogenous sleep-regulating substance; however, its short half-life of less than a minute has made it a challenging target of research. It has long been known that adenosine, when infused into the intracerebroventricular space, promotes sleep.[65] Moreover, extracellular adenosine levels in the brain of animal models are typically higher in the active phase (dominated by wakefulness) when compared with a phase of rest (dominated by sleep). Similarly, adenosine in the BF is increased by sleep deprivation and normalized by recovery sleep.[66,67] Intriguingly, lesion and pharmacologic studies revealed that accumulation of adenosine in the BF is not necessary for sleep induction, nor are BF cholinergic neurons essential for sleep drive, highlighting the resilience of sleep regulation in the CNS.[68] Nevertheless, adenosine is today believed to play a central role in sleep-wake regulation. Not only by integrating circadian and homeostatic processes[64] but also via distinct effects of its receptors with A2A centrally involved in the promotion of sleep by suppressing arousal and A1 mediates physiologic sleep need and coordinates the response to sleep deprivation.[61]

Gamma-aminobutyric acid

Constantin von Economo[3] was the first to describe that lesions to the hypothalamic anterior preoptic area were associated with symptoms of insomnia. Today, it is widely accepted that the VLPO, as well as its neighboring region, the median preoptic area (MnPO), contain high densities of neurons that are active in and even a few minutes before initiation of NREM sleep. The VLPO or MnPO neurons fire less in REM sleep and are almost silent in wakefulness.[69,70] Lesions to the VLPO in cats dramatically reduce sleep.[71] The VLPO neurons are well positioned to innervate arousal systems of brainstem and hypothalamus, including the DRN, LC, LDT, PPT, SNc, VTA, TMN, and Hcrt-producing neurons in the LH.[5] The VLPO contains GABAergic, as well as galaninergic projections, both associated with inhibitory transmission on effector targets.[6] Specific activation of GABAergic neurons in the VLPO enhance NREM sleep, while reducing wakefulness.[72]

Apart from VLPO or MnPO, novel GABAergic structures and pathways that are active in NREM sleep have been discovered in recent years, yet their specific roles in sleep-wake regulation are not yet well established.[6] The actions of GABA are mediated via ligand-gated ion channels referred to as GABAA and GABAC receptors, as well as via Gi protein–coupled GABAB receptors that promote potassium ion conductance on their activation. The pharmacologic properties of GABA receptors are well investigated, although extremely complex. The $GABA_A$ receptor is the target for the clinically widely used sleep-inducing medications, benzodiazepines and Z-drugs (nonbenzodiazepine structure). This receptor subtype consists of a chloride ion channel composed of 5 subunits assembled from a symphony of α, β, γ, and other less frequent subunit variants.[73] In conclusion, GABAergic neurons of the VLPO, together with the MnPO, seem to regulate inhibitory inputs to the ARAS and to promote the transition from wakefulness to sleep and the maintenance of NREM sleep.

Melatonin

The endogenous biological master clock regulating the daily sleep-wake cycle is localized in the suprachiasmatic nucleus (SCN) of the hypothalamus. The SCN is a small neuronal cluster consisting of roughly 20,000 neurons.[74] The SCN functions as an endogenous zeitgeber with a roughly 24-hour periodicity, operating virtually independently of prior sleep and wakefulness. The SCN is primarily entrained by light, which is detected by retinal ganglion cells and transmitted via melanopsin-releasing neurons of the retinohypothalamic tract.[75,76] Nevertheless, other zeitgebers, such as temperature[77] and feeding,[78] also modulate the endogenous clock. The actual timekeeping is maintained by interconnected SCN neurons and transcriptional or translational feedback loops of core and associated clock genes.[74,79]

The SCN has projections to the pineal gland and other hypothalamic nuclei, including the dorsomedial hypothalamic (DMH) nucleus. The DMH seems especially important for the SCN in modulating sleep-wake timing, because abolition of DMH neurons also abolishes sleep-wake timing in experimental animals.[80] The DMH extends strong glutamatergic and GABAergic projections to the LH and VLPO, respectively, which allow the SCN to regulate sleep and wakefulness.[81] An important regulator of SCN function is melatonin. Melatonin is often referred to as the hormone of darkness. When compared with the biological day, its concentration is elevated about 10-fold during the biological night in both diurnal and nocturnal species. Melatonin binds to MT_1 (aka MT_{1A}) and MT_2 (MT_{1B}) melatonin receptors, which are GPCRs linked to $G_{i/o}$ protein, inhibiting the production of cyclic adenosine monophosphate. Melatonin receptors are highly expressed in the SCN. Their signaling cascade activated by melatonin is complex and not yet fully understood.[82] Nevertheless, the US Food and Drug Administration recently approved the MT_1-MT_2 receptor agonist ramelteon for treatment of insomnia. In addition, agomelatine, an MT_1-MT_2 receptor agonist and selective 5-HT2B/C receptor antagonist, shifts the phase of the circadian system and may improve sleep. Nevertheless, its usefulness for primary sleep disorders remains debated.[83]

The roles for melatonin in sleep-wake regulation were recently highlighted in a diurnal zebra-fish model, in which the synthesis of melatonin was genetically abolished.[84] The mutant fish showed a general loss of circadian rhythmicity and strongly reduced sleep compared with normal fish when kept in constant dark conditions. These findings suggest that melatonin modulates not only circadian but also homeostatic aspects of sleep-wake regulation. Interestingly, melatonin may induce sleep by the production of adenosine. Thus, when adenosine receptors were activated in the fish mutants, their wake-phenotype could be rescued, further strengthening the association of melatonin with sleep-wake homeostasis. Despite the basic importance of these data, the simple nervous system of zebrafish may not be directly comparable to humans, and melatonin may play even more complex roles in mammalian sleep-wake regulation.

Synopsis and Perspectives

Clinical observations and research spanning from patients with sleep-wake disorder to genetically engineered animal models have consistently identified the ascending arousal pathways, the VLPO, and the SCN as important players in the regulation of wakefulness and sleep (see **Fig. 1**). In waking, distinct cell clusters of the brainstem, BF, and hypothalamus activate the thalamus, hypothalamus, cortex, and spinal cord motor neurons. Concurrently, the sleep-promoting center of the VLPO is inhibited by the SCN, thereby promoting cortical arousal. In REM sleep, REM-on brainstem nuclei containing ACh, glutamate, and GABA promote activity in BF and cortex and induce muscle atonia and REMs. On the contrary, MCH-containing hypothalamic neurons suppress REM-off brain centers, including the ventrolateral part of the periaqueductal gray matter (vlPAG), LPT, DRN, and LC. In NREM sleep, GABA and galanin-containing VLPO neurons inhibit arousal nuclei in the brainstem, hypothalamus, and BF. The endogenous sleep regulatory substance adenosine can actively excite sleep active cells and integrate homeostatic and circadian sleep processes.

In NREM sleep, DRN 5-HT-ergic and LC NE-ergic neurons inhibit cholinergic LDT and PPT cells. These DRN and LC neurons become silent in REM sleep, which enables the cholinergic LDT and PPT neurons, in synchrony with GABAergic innervation, to generate the REM sleep state.

The pathways previously presented provide a conceptual framework of the neurochemical bases of sleep-wake regulation and the currently available pharmacologic interventions to treat sleep-wake disorders. Powerful new methods to interrogate sleep-wake regulating circuits have recently revealed additional molecular, cellular, and network mechanisms and pathways in sleep-wake regulation, which may lead to an extension of the traditional views of sleep-wake neurochemistry.[6,7] For example, the glutamatergic medial parabrachial nucleus in the dorsal pontine tegmentum regulates arousal,[85] and the GABAergic parafacial zone in the pontomedullary junction promotes sleep.[86] Furthermore, novel studies in humans and animals using different methodologies further suggest diverse additional brain regions, neuronal structures, and receptors as important regulators of wakefulness and sleep.[87–92] These insights highlight the complexity of the mammalian brain and the sophisticated and fine-tuned regulation of wakefulness and sleep. Future progress is needed to pave the way for the development of novel rational sleep-wake therapeutics.

DISCLOSURE

The authors' research has been supported by the Swiss National Science Foundation (320030_163439), Zürich Center for Interdisciplinary Sleep Research, Clinical Research Priority Program "Sleep & Health" of the University of Zürich, Zürich Center for Integrative Human Physiology, Neuroscience Center Zürich, and Novartis Foundation (08C42) for Medical-Biological Research (to H.P. Landolt).

REFERENCES

1. Steriade M, McCormick D, Sejnowski T. Thalamo cortical oscillations in the sleeping and aroused brain. Science 1993;262(5134):679–85.
2. Achermann P, Borbely AA. Sleep homeostasis and models of sleep regulation. In: Kryger MH, Roth T, Dement WC, editors. Principles and practice of sleep medicine. 5th edition. St Louis (MO): Saunders; 2011. p. 431–44.
3. von Economo C. Sleep as a problem of localization. J Nerv Ment Dis 1930;71(3):249.
4. Moruzzi G, Magoun HW. Brain stem reticular formation and activation of the EEG. Electroencephalogr Clin Neurophysiol 1949;1(1):455–73.
5. Saper CB, Fuller PM. Wake-sleep circuitry: an over view. Curr Opin Neurobiol 2017;44:186–92.
6. Luppi PH, Fort P. Neuroanatomical and neurochemical bases of vigilance states. Handb Exp Pharma Col 2018. https://doi.org/10.1007/164_2017_84. Available at.
7. Tyree SM, de Lecea L. Optogenetic investigation of arousal circuits. Int J Mol Sci 2017;18:e1773.
8. Lee MG. Cholinergic basal forebrain neurons burst with theta during waking and paradoxical sleep. J Neurosci 2005;25(17):4365–9.
9. Baghdoyan HA, Lydic R. M2 muscarinic receptor subtype in the feline medial pontine reticular formation modulates the amount of rapid eye movement sleep. Sleep 1999;22(7):835–47.
10. Nissen C, Power AE, Nofzinger EA, et al. M1 muscarinic acetylcholine receptor agonism alters sleep without affecting memory consolidation. J Cogn Neurosci 2006;18(11):1799–807.
11. Zhang L, Samet J, Caffo B, et al. Cigarette smoking and nocturnal sleep architecture. Am J Epidemiol 2006;164(6):529–37.

12. Boyden ES, Zhang F, Bamberg E, et al. Millisecond-timescale, genetically targeted optical control of neural activity. Nat Neurosci 2005;8(9): 1263–8.

13. Van Dort CJ, Zachs DP, Kenny JD, et al. Optogenetic activation of cholinergic neurons in the PPT or LDT induces REM sleep. Proc Natl Acad Sci U S A 2015;112(2):584–9.

14. Han Y, Shi YF, Xi W, et al. Selective activation of cholinergic basal forebrain neurons induces immediate sleep-wake transitions. Curr Biol 2014;24(6): 693–8.

15. Xu M, Chung S, Zhang S, et al. Basal forebrain cir cuit for sleep-wake control. Nat Neurosci 2015;18(11). https://doi.org/10.1038/nn.4143. Available at.

16. Anaclet C, Pedersen NP, Ferrari LL, et al. Basal forebrain control of wakefulness and cortical rhythms. Nat Commun 2015;6. https://doi.org/10.1038/ncomms9744.

17. Chen L, Yin D, Wang TX, et al. Basal Forebrain cholinergic neurons primarily contribute to inhibition of electroencephalogram delta activity, rather than inducing behavioral wakefulness in mice. Neuropsychopharmacology 2016;41(8):2133–46.

18. Kim T, Thankachan S, McKenna JT, et al. Cortically projecting basal forebrain parvalbumin neurons regulate cortical gamma band oscillations. Proc Natl Acad Sci U S A 2015;112(11):3535–40.

19. Jacobs BL, Fornal CA. Activity of serotonergic neurons in behaving animals. Neuropsychopharmacology 1999;21(2 Suppl):9S–15S.

20. Takahashi K, Kayama Y, Lin JS, et al. Locus coeruleus neuronal activity during the sleep-waking cycle in mice. Neuroscience 2010;169(3):1115–26.

21. Takahashi K, Lin J-S, Sakai K. Neuronal activity of histaminergic tuberomammillary neurons during wake-sleep states in the mouse. J Neurosci 2006; 26(40):10292–8.

22. Ramos BP, Arnsten AFT. Adrenergic pharmacology and cognition: focus on the prefrontal cortex. Pharmacol Ther 2007;113(3):523–36.

23. Carter ME, Yizhar O, Chikahisa S, et al. Tuning arousal with optogenetic modulation of locus coeruleus neurons. Nat Neurosci 2010;13(12):1526–35.

24. Hauglund NL, Pavan C, Nedergaard M. Cleaning the sleeping brain–the potential restorative function of the glymphatic system. Curr Opin Physiol 2020; 15:1–6.

25. Xie L, Kang H, Xu Q, et al. Sleep drives metabolite clearance from the adult brain. Science 2013; 342(6156):373–7.

26. Ding F, O'donnell J, Xu Q, et al. Changes in the composition of brain interstitial ions control the sleep-wake cycle. Science 2016;352(6285):550–5.

27. Landolt HP, Holst SC. Ionic control of sleep and wakefulness. Science 2016;352(6285):517–8.

28. Landolt H-P, Wehrle R. Antagonism of serotonergic 5-HT2A/2C receptors: mutual improvement of sleep, cognition and mood? Eur J Neurosci 2009;29(9): 1795–809.

29. Boutrel B, Franc B, Hen R, et al. Key role of 5-HT1B receptors in the regulation of paradoxical sleep as evidenced in 5-HT1B knock-out mice. J Neurosci 1999;19(8):3204–12.

30. Boutrel B, Monaca C, Hen R, et al. Involvement of 5-HT1A receptors in homeostatic and stress- induced adaptive regulations of paradoxical sleep: studies in 5-HT1A knock-out mice. J Neurosci 2002;22(11): 4686–92.

31. Frank MG, Stryker MP, Tecott LH. Sleep and sleep homeostasis in mice lacking the 5-HT2c re- ceptor. Neuropsychopharmacology 2002;27(5):869–73.

32. Popa D, Léna C, Fabre V, et al. Contribution of 5-HT2 receptor subtypes to sleep-wakefulness and respiratory control, and functional adaptations in knock out mice lacking 5-HT2A receptors. J Neurosci 2005;25(49):11231–8.

33. Monti JM. Serotonin control of sleep-wake behavior. Sleep Med Rev 2011;15(4):269–81.

34. Miyazaki KW, Miyazaki K, Tanaka KF, et al. Optogenetic activation of dorsal raphe serotonin neurons enhances patience for future rewards. Curr Biol 2014;24(17):2033–40.

35. Cho JR, Treweek JB, Robinson JE, et al. Dorsal raphe dopamine neurons modulate arousal and pro mote wakefulness by salient stimuli. Neuron 2017;94(6):1205–19. e8.

36. Sherin JE, Elmquist JK, Torrealba F, et al. Innervation of histaminergic tuberomammillary neurons by GABAergic and galaninergic neurons in the ventrolateral preoptic nucleus of the rat. J Neurosci 1998;18(12):4705–21.

37. Williams RH, Chee MJS, Kroeger D, et al. Optogenetic-mediated release of histamine re- veals distal and autoregulatory mechanisms for controlling arousal. J Neurosci 2014;34(17):6023–9.

38. Holst SC, Valomon A, Landolt HP. Sleep pharmacogenetics: personalized sleep-wake therapy. Annu Rev Pharmacol Toxicol 2016;56:577–603.

39. Dahan L, Astier B, Vautrelle N, et al. Prominent burst firing of dopaminergic neurons in the ventral tegmental area during paradoxical sleep. Neuropsychopharmacology 2007;32(6):1232–41.

40. Lena I, Parrot S, Deschaux O, et al. Variations in extracellular levels of dopamine, noradrenaline, glutamate, and aspartate across the sleep-wake cy- cle in the medial prefrontal cortex and nucleus ac- cumbens of freely moving rats. J Neurosci Res 2005;81(6):891–9.

41. Holst SC, Landolt HP. Sleep homeostasis, meta bo- lism, and adenosine. Curr Sleep Med Rep 2015; 1(1):27–37.

42. Lazarus M, Huang Z-L, Lu J, et al. How do the basal ganglia regulate sleep wake behavior? Trends Neurosci 2012;35(12):723–32.

43. Monti JM, Monti D. The involvement of dopamine in the modulation of sleep and waking. Sleep Med Rev 2007;11(2):113–33.

44. Qiu MH, Yao QL, Vetrivelan R, et al. Nigrostriatal dopamine acting on globus pallidus regulates sleep. Cereb Cortex 2016;26(4):1430–9.

45. Burbach JPH. Neuropeptides from concept to online database. Eur J Pharmacol 2010;626(1):27–48. Available at. www.neuropeptides.nl.

46. Richter C, Woods IG, Schier AF. Neuropeptidergic control of sleep and wakefulness. Annu Rev Neurosci 2014;37(1):503–31.

47. Monti JM, Torterolo P, Lagos P. Melanin-concentrating hormone control of sleep-wake behavior. Sleep Med Rev 2013;17(4):293–8.

48. BY Mileykovskiy, Kiyashchenko LI, Siegel JM. Behavioral correlates of activity in identified hypocretin/orexin neurons. Neuron 2005;46(5):787–98.

49. España RA, Scammell TE. Sleep neurobiology from a clinical perspective. Sleep 2011;34(7):845–58.

50. Mochizuki T, Crocker A, McCormack S, et al. Behavioral state instability in orexin knock-out mice. J Neurosci 2004;24(28):6291–300.

51. Adamantidis AR, Zhang F, Aravanis AM, et al. Neural substrates of awakening probed with optogenetic control of hypocretin neurons. Nature 2007; 450(7168):420–4.

52. Carter ME, Adamantidis A, Ohtsu H, et al. Sleep homeostasis modulates hypocretin-mediated sleep-to-wake transitions. J Neurosci 2009;29(35):10939–49.

53. Kilduff TS, De Lecea L. Mapping of the mRNAs for the hypocretin/orexin and melanin-concentrating hormone receptors: networks of overlapping peptide systems. J Comp Neurol 2001;435(1):1–5.

54. Konadhode RR, Pelluru D, Shiromani PJ. Neurons containing orexin or melanin concentrating hormone reciprocally regulate wake and sleep. Front Syst Neurosci 2015;8. https://doi.org/10.3389/fnsys.2014.00244. Available at.

55. Willie JT, Sinton CM, Maratos-Flier E, et al. Abnormal response of melanin-concentrating hormone deficient mice to fasting: hyperactivity and rapid eye movement sleep suppression. Neuroscience 2008; 156(4):819–29.

56. Jego S, Glasgow SD, Herrera CG, et al. Optogenetic identification of a rapid eye movement sleep modulatory circuit in the hypothalamus. Nat Neurosci 2013;16(11):1637–43.

57. Tsunematsu T, Ueno T, Tabuchi S, et al. Optogenetic manipulation of activity and temporally controlled cell-specific ablation reveal a role for MCH neurons in sleep/wake regulation. J Neurosci 2014;34(20):6896–909.

58. Konadhode RR, Pelluru D, Blanco-Centurion C, et al. Optogenetic stimulation of MCH neurons increases sleep. J Neurosci 2013;33(25):10257–63.

59. Bodenmann S, Hohoff C, Freitag C, et al. Polymorphisms of ADORA2A modulate psychomotor vigilance and the effects of caffeine on neurobehavioural perfor mance and sleep EEG after sleep deprivation. Br J Pharmacol 2012;165(6):1904–13.

60. Huang Z-L, Qu W-M, Eguchi N, et al. Adenosine A2A, but not A1, receptors mediate the arousal effect of caffeine. Nat Neurosci 2005;8(7):858–9.

61. Lazarus M, Oishi Y, Bjorness TE, et al. Gating and the need for sleep: dissociable effects of adenosine A1 and A2A receptors. Front Neurosci 2019; 13:740.

62. Rétey JV, Adam M, Khatami R, et al. A genetic vari ation in the adenosine A2A receptor gene (ADORA2A) contributes to individual sensitivity to caffeine effects on sleep. Clin Pharmacol Ther 2007;81(5):692–8.

63. Sebastião AM, Ribeiro JA. Adenosine receptors and the central nervous system. Handb Exp Pharmacol 2009;471–534. https://doi.org/10.1007/978-3-540-89615-9_16. Available at.

64. Jagannath A, Varga N, Dallmann R, et al. Adenosine integrates light and sleep signalling for the regulation of circadian timing in mice. Nat Commun 2021;12(1):2113.

65. Virus RM, Djuricic-Nedelson M, Radulovacki M, et al. The effects of adenosine and 2'-deoxycoformycin on sleep and wakefulness in rats. Neuropharmacology 1983;22(12 PART 2):1401–4.

66. Porkka-Heiskanen T, Strecker RE, McCarley RW. Brain site-specificity of extracellular adenosine con- centration changes during sleep deprivation and spontaneous sleep: an in vivo microdialysis study. Neuroscience 2000;99(3):507–17.

67. Porkka-Heiskanen T, Strecker RE, Thakkar M, et al. Adenosine: a mediator of the sleep-inducing effects of prolonged wakefulness. Science 1997;276(5316):1265–7.

68. Blanco-Centurion C, Xu M, Murillo-Rodriguez E, et al. Adenosine and sleep homeostasis in the basal forebrain. J Neurosci 2006;26(31):8092–100.

69. Sherin JE, Shiromani PJ, McCarley RW, et al. Activa tion of ventrolateral preoptic neurons during sleep. Science 1996;271(5246):216–9.

70. Suntsova N, Szymusiak R, Alam MN, et al. Sleep-waking discharge patterns of median preoptic nucleus neurons in rats. J Physiol 2002;543(2):665–77.

71. McGinty DJ, Sterman MB. Sleep suppression after basal forebrain lesions in the cat. Science 1968; 160(3833):1253–5.

72. Saito YC, Tsujino N, Hasegawa E, et al. GABAergic neurons in the preoptic area send direct inhibitory projections to orexin neurons. Front Neural Circuits

2013;7. https://doi.org/10.3389/fncir.2013.00192. Available at.

73. Rudolph U, Möhler H. GABA-based therapeutic approaches: GABAA receptor subtype functions. Curr Opin Pharmacol 2006;6:18–23.

74. Gachon F, Nagoshi E, Brown SA, et al. The mammalian circadian timing system: from gene expression to physiology. Chromosoma 2004;113(3):103–12.

75. Berson DM, Dunn FA, Takao M. Phototransduction by retinal ganglion cells that set the circadian clock. Science 2002;295(5557):1070–3.

76. Gooley JJ, Lu J, Chou TC, et al. Melanopsin in cells of origin of the retinohypothalamic tract. Nat Neurosci 2001;4(12):1165.

77. Blake MJF. Relationship between circadian rhythm of body temperature and introversion-extraversion. Nature 1967;215(5103):896–7.

78. Richter CP. A behavioristic study of the activity of the rat. Comp Psychol Monogr 1922;1(2):1–54.

79. Colwell CS. Linking neural activity and molecular oscillations in the SCN. Nat Rev Neurosci 2011;12(10):553–69.

80. Chou TC, Scammell TE, Gooley JJ, et al. Critical role of dorsomedial hypothalamic nucleus in a wide range of behavioral circadian rhythms. J Neurosci 2003;23(33):10691–702.

81. Fuller PM, Gooley JJ, Saper CB. Neurobiology of the sleep-wake cycle: sleep architecture, circadian regulation, and regulatory feedback. J Biol Rhythms 2006;482–93. https://doi.org/10.1177/0748730406294627. Available at.

82. Hardeland R, Cardinali DP, Srinivasan V, et al. Melatonin-A pleiotropic, orchestrating regulator molecule. Prog Neurobiol 2011;350–84. https://doi.org/10.1016/j.pneurobio.2010.12.004. Available at.

83. De Berardis D, Fornaro M, Serroni N, et al. Agomelatine beyond borders: current evidences of its efficacy in disorders other than major depression. Int J Mol Sci 2015;1111–30. https://doi.org/10.3390/ijms16011111. Available at.

84. Gandhi AV, Mosser EA, Oikonomou G, et al. Melatonin is required for the circadian regulation of sleep. Neuron 2015;85(6):1193–9.

85. Fuller P, Sherman D, Pedersen NP, et al. Reassessment of the structural basis of the ascending arousal system. J Comp Neurol 2011;519(5):933–56.

86. Anaclet C, Lin J-S, Vetrivelan R, et al. Identification and characterization of a sleep-active cell group in the rostral medullary brainstem. J Neurosci 2012;32(50):17970–6.

87. Dang-Vu TT, Schabus M, Desseilles M, et al. Functional neuroimaging insights into the physiology of human sleep. Sleep 2010;33(12):1589–603.

88. Dang-Vu TT, Schabus M, Desseilles M, et al. Spontaneous neural activity during human slow wave sleep. Proc Natl Acad Sci U S A 2008;105(39):15160–5.

89. Dittrich L, Morairty SR, Warrier DR, et al. Homeostatic sleep pressure is the primary factor for activation of cortical nNOS/NK1 neurons. Neuropsychopharmacology 2015;40(3):632–9.

90. Holst SC, Sousek A, Hefti K, et al. Cerebral mGluR5 availability contributes to elevated sleep need and behavioral adjustment after sleep deprivation. Elife 2017;6. https://doi.org/10.7554/eLife.28751. Available at.

91. Maquet P, Degueldre C, Delfiore G, et al. Functional neuroanatomy of human slow wave sleep. J Neurosci 1997;17(8):2807–12.

92. Murphy M, Riedner BA, Huber R, et al. Source modeling sleep slow waves. Proc Natl Acad Sci U S A 2009;106(5):1608–13.

Sleep in Normal Aging

Junxin Li, PhD[a],*, Michael V. Vitiello, PhD[b], Nalaka S. Gooneratne, MD, MSc[c]

KEYWORDS

- Sleep architecture • Circadian rhythm • Sleep homeostasis • Hormone • Normal aging

KEY POINTS

- Age-related changes in sleep include advanced sleep timing, shortened nocturnal sleep duration, increased frequency of daytime naps, increased nocturnal awakenings and time spent awake, and decreased slow-wave sleep.
- Most age-related changes in sleep are stable after 60 years of age among older adults with excellent health.
- Aging is associated with less robust circadian rhythms and sleep homeostasis, which contribute to sleep changes in aging.
- Age-related changes in neuroendocrine functions contribute to or correlate with alterations of sleep quality and architecture in normal aging.
- Multiple factors, including medical comorbidities and psychiatric illness, primary sleep disorders, and changes in social engagement, lifestyle, and environment contribute to sleep disturbances in older adults.

INTRODUCTION

Sleep has received increasing attention within the context of geriatric research based on a growing body of evidence that links poor sleep with many adverse health outcomes, especially decline in cognition, in older adults. Along with many other physiologic alterations in normal aging, sleep patterns change with aging, independent of many factors, including medical comorbidity and medications.[1] Total sleep time (TST), sleep efficiency, and deep sleep (slow-wave sleep) decrease with aging, and the number of nocturnal awakenings and time spent awake during the night increase with aging.[2] These age-related changes in sleep are associated not only with changes in the circadian and homeostatic processes but also with some normal physiologic and psychosocial changes in aging. This article describes age-related changes in sleep, circadian rhythms, and sleep-related hormones. We focus on changes associated with normal aging rather than changes that accompany common pathologic processes in older adults, which are discussed in detail elsewhere.

AGE-RELATED CHANGES IN SLEEP

There is no doubt that sleep changes as a function of age.[3] Aging is associated with decreased ability to maintain sleep (increased number of awakenings and prolonged nocturnal awakenings), reduced nocturnal sleep duration, and decreased deep sleep (slow-wave sleep).[4] Herein we discuss in detail age-related changes in sleep duration, sleep initiation, sleep efficiency, sleep maintenance, sleep stages, daytime sleep behaviors, and self-reported sleep quality. An important aspect of this discussion is to differentiate changes in sleep that occur from childhood to age 60 years (or 65 years), versus those that occur after this point. Ohayon and colleagues[2] comprehensively reviewed the normative sleep changes from childhood to old age using meta-analysis results from 65 studies (polysomnography or actigraphy) representing 3577 healthy subjects aged

[a] School of Nursing, Johns Hopkins University, 525 North Wolfe Street, Baltimore, MD 21205, USA; [b] Center for Sleep and Circadian Neurobiology, Perelman School of Medicine, University of Pennsylvania, 3624 Market Street, Philadelphia, PA 19104, USA; [c] Department of Psychiatry and Behavioral Sciences, University of Washington, Box 356560, Seattle, WA 98195-6560, USA
* Corresponding author.
E-mail address: junxin.li@jhu.edu

Sleep Med Clin 17 (2022) 161–171
https://doi.org/10.1016/j.jsmc.2022.02.007

between 5 and 102 years, and this work informs many of the insights discussed in this review. Older subjects (defined as age >60 years) in this analysis were more representative of older adults with excellent health and who were optimally aging, rather than the general older adult population.[4]

Sleep Duration

The current literature supports that, in general, the TST decreases with age (from pediatric to older adulthood). However, further age-associated decreases in TST have not been observed consistently after entering older age brackets. Campbell and colleagues[5] in 2007 conducted a laboratory study with 50 healthy adults aged between 19 and 81 years to evaluate the spontaneous sleep across the 24-h day among young, middle-aged, and older adults. Compared with young adults (10.5 hours), middle-aged (9.1 hours) and older adults (8.1 hours) had significantly shorter average nighttime sleep duration. Data from 160 healthy adults (without sleep complaints) aged between 20 and 90 years from the SIESTA database showed that TST decreased about 8 minutes per decade in men and 10 minutes per decade in women.[6] Similarly, 3 meta-analysis reviews reported that age was linearly associated with decreased TST, with an approximately 10- to 12-min reduction per decade of age in the adult population.[2,7,8] This association was stronger when comparing young adults with middle-aged or older adults, but vanished within older subjects who were 60 years of age and older. These findings indicate that TST plateaued after 60 years of age. Also, the association was stronger in women than men.[2]

Sleep Initiation

People commonly assume that the ability to initiate sleep decreases significantly with age. However, current evidence does not support this assumption but suggests that both sleep latency and the ability to fall back to sleep after nocturnal awakenings demonstrate minimal increases after the age of 60 years. Results from 2 meta-analyses, for example, suggest that sleep latency does increase with age. However, the magnitude of change is very modest.[2,8] In these studies, sleep latency holds constant from childhood to adolescence. The significant age-related increase in sleep latency was only found between very young adults and older adults. A mathematical modeling, which was conducted using data from 7 laboratory sleep studies (258 subjects aged 17–91 years), suggested that sleep latency increased between the late teens and 20s, remains constant from age

30 years until approximate age 50 years, and then increased steadily after age 50 years.[9] However, the amount or magnitude of changes were not reported. In addition, even though more frequent arousals were found in healthy older adults than young people, older adults maintained their ability to reinitiate sleep and fell back to sleep as rapidly as younger adults.[3,10]

Sleep Efficiency

Sleep efficiency remains largely unchanged from childhood to adolescence and significantly decreases with age in adulthood. Different from all other sleep parameters that hold steady after 60 years of age, sleep efficiency continues to decline very slowly with advancing age.[2]

Sleep Maintenance

Aging from birth to older adulthood is associated with a decreased ability to maintain sleep, which presents as the increased number of arousals (arousal index) and longer duration of wake after sleep onset (WASO), but also tends to plateau after age 60 years.[2,8] In the meta-analysis performed by Ohayon and colleagues,[2] age-related changes in WASO achieved the largest effect size among all sleep parameters, which yielded a steady 10 minutes increase of WASO per decade of age from 30 to 60 years. WASO remained mostly unchanged after age 60 years.

Sleep Stages

In general, deep sleep (slow-wave sleep) decreases with age in the adult population. During nocturnal sleep, the proportion of nonrapid eye movement sleep stage 1 and stage 2 increases with age, and the proportion of slow-wave sleep and rapid eye movement (REM) sleep decreases with age[2,11] (**Fig. 1**). These changes were not significant among healthy older adults aged more than 60 years.[2] Also, the association between age and decreased REM latency was minimal.[2] Floyd and colleague's[7] meta-analysis reported a linear decrease in the proportion of REM with a small rate of 0.6% per decade from age 19 until 75 years, then small increases were found in the proportion of REM between 75 and 85 years of age.

There may be gender differences in age-related changes in sleep stages. The meta-analysis conducted by Ohayon and colleagues suggested that the age effect on the percentage of stage 1 sleep was stronger in women, and women had less percentage of stage 2 sleep and a greater percentage of slow-wave sleep than age-matched men. The SIESTA study found that women had

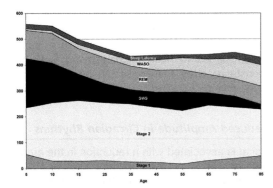

Fig. 1. Age-related changes in sleep architecture. SWS, slow-wave sleep. (*From* Ohayon MM, Carskadon MA, Guilleminault C, et al. Meta-analysis of quantitative sleep parameters from childhood to old age in healthy individuals: developing normative sleep values across the human lifespan. Sleep 2004;27(7):1255–73.)

no change in slow-wave sleep with age, in contrast with men, who had a 1.7% decrease in slow-wave sleep per decade of age. In addition, women had a smaller rate of increase in stage 1 sleep, a greater rate of increase in stage 2 sleep, and a greater rate of decline in REM, in comparison with men.[6] These results indicate that men may be more prone to age-related decline in slow-wave sleep than women.

Daytime Napping and Daytime Sleepiness

Daytime napping is a daily routine for many people across their lifespan. Results from epidemiology studies suggest that daytime napping is more prevalent in older adults than that seen in younger adults.[12–15] Several studies have found that older adults nap more frequently than younger and middle-aged adults,[14,16,17] this is also true when comparing healthy older adults with younger individuals.[18] Within the older population, 1 study found that nap frequency increased with age.[19] A recent study using 7664 people, aged 20 to 99 years, from a national representative sample in Japan, found that a higher proportion of older adults (27.4%) take frequent naps (>4 d/wk) than young (11.9%) and middle-aged (14.4%) adults.[14] However, no clear evidence supports that nap duration is different between older adults and other adult populations.[5,19] A laboratory study by Campbell and colleagues[5] in 2007 showed that nap durations were not different among the young, middle-aged, and older adults, but that the number of daytime naps increased with age. Yoon and colleagues[18] reported that older adults tended to nap at a different time than younger adults, where older adults were more likely to nap in the

early evening, whereas younger adults were more likely to nap in the afternoon.[20]

People choose to take a nap for many reasons, such as to compensate for nighttime sleep loss, to restore energy and reduce daytime sleepiness, or just to relax.[20] Cultural background also has a considerable influence on nap habits. For example, midday naps are a common practice of people from China, Mediterranean, and several Latin American countries.[21] Older adults may nap more frequently due to both biological changes, but also to lifestyle changes that accompany aging. For example, older adults may spend less time on work and physical and social activities, and thus have more opportunities to nap than young and middle-aged adults during the day. Also, Foley and colleagues[22] found that frequent napping was associated with excessive daytime sleepiness (EDS), depression, pain, and nocturia in a US nationally representative poll of older adults.

Epidemiologic studies indicated that up to 20% of older adults reported EDS.[23–26] EDS usually coexists with multiple adverse health conditions, including cognitive impairment, cardiovascular events, and increased mortality risk.[27,28] Certainly, EDS is not a part of normal aging but may be a signal or symptom of certain diseases. An epidemiologic study found a linear decline in the prevalence of EDS with age between 30 and 75 years. In addition, the prevalence of EDS decreased at a greater rate after the age of 75 years.[29] Daytime napping could be a practice to reduce daytime sleepiness[15]; however, some older adults may experience daytime sleepiness but do not fall asleep during the day.[26]

Self-Reported Sleep Quality

People may expect that older adults complain more about their sleep than younger-aged adults because most objectively measured sleep parameters decrease with age. However, this may not be the case; there can be significant differences between objective and self-reported perceptions of sleep, and comorbidities can play a major role. For example, although some epidemiologic studies found that up to 50% of older adults have self-reported poor sleep,[30,31] a large proportion of these complaints are attributable to older adults' poor health status and disease burden.[30,32] Evidence shows that older adults were less likely to self-report poor sleep than younger individuals, especially after controlling for comorbidities and health.[33] Vitiello and colleagues[30] examined objectively measured sleep among 150 healthy older adults who reported no sleep problems and found that significant proportions of them (33% of women and 16% of men) had impaired objectively measured sleep. Healthy older adults may be prone to perceive good sleep quality.[34] In addition, older adults may expect their sleep will be less consolidated as they age, and they may accept some noticeable sleep changes as a part of normal aging owing to an adjustment of their perception of "acceptable" health with aging.[33,35]

As described, many sleep characteristics change with age in adulthood. For example, nocturnal sleep duration, sleep efficiency, slow-wave sleep, and self-reported poor sleep decrease with age; in contrast, the number of awakenings, WASO, and daytime napping frequency increase with age. However, most of these changes stop at approximately 60 years of age. After that age, most sleep variables seem to remain largely unchanged within the older adult population.

AGE-RELATED CHANGES IN CIRCADIAN RHYTHMS

The circadian system regulates several human physiologic functions, including body temperature, heart rate, blood pressure, release of certain hormones, bone remodeling, sleep-wake rhythm, and rest-activity pattern.[36] It is well-documented in the literature that circadian rhythms become less robust with aging, which typically presents as an advance in circadian timing, a decrease in circadian amplitude, and a reduced ability to adjust to phase shifting (changes in the phase of circadian rhythms). The suprachiasmatic nucleus is the central endogenous circadian pacemaker that regulates 24-h circadian rhythms. The disruption of circadian rhythms with advancing age may be associated with a progressive decline in the function of the suprachiasmatic nucleus.[37]

Phase Advance

The timing and structure of sleep are mainly regulated by the circadian system and homeostatic sleep regulation.[38] Older adults commonly experience an advance of sleep schedule to earlier hours. They tend to have sleepiness earlier in the evening and wake up earlier in the morning than desired.[36] This earlier sleep timing in older adults may be due to the age-related phase advance in their circadian rhythm. This phase advance is seen not only in the sleep-wake cycle, but also in the body temperature rhythm, and in the timing of secretion of melatonin and cortisol,[39–41] all of which are about 1 hour advanced in older people compared with young adults.[42] **Fig. 2** compares the circadian phase between older and younger

adults. However, Duffy and colleagues[43] found that the phase advance in sleep timing was greater than phase advance in other circadian clocks, which suggested that a mechanism (eg, sleep homeostasis) other than circadian phase advance alone may be involved in older adult's early sleep timing.

Reduced Amplitude in Circadian Rhythms

Aging is associated with a reduction in the amplitude of several circadian rhythms in older adults, including core body temperature, melatonin and cortisol secretion, activity, and sleep.[44–47] The age-related reduction in circadian amplitude may be related to sleep disruption in older adults.[48] It was reported that, compared with young adults, older adults were more likely to wake up close to the timing when body temperature reached nadir.[49] This finding indicated that the biological clock (eg, body temperature) in older adults might also regulate their awakening time, which may result in even earlier awakenings in older adults.[36,49] Also, the reduced amplitude of daytime activity may result in daytime napping, which may further reduce the amplitude of the sleep-wake rhythm. Age-related decreases in the amplitude of melatonin secretion may also play a role in sleep problems in older adults[50,51] (as described elsewhere in this article).

Decreased Ability Adjusting to Phase Shifting

The ability to phase shift decreases with aging.[52] Older adults are subject to more difficulties in adjusting to phase shifts, such as shift work and jet lag.[4,52] Monk and colleagues[53] found that older adults needed more time to recover from phase shifting, and experienced a longer period of sleep disruption and daytime dysfunction. The age-related loss of rhythmic function within the suprachiasmatic nucleus may partially explain this impaired ability in phase shifting.[54]

Changes in Sleep Homeostasis

Some research indicates that the earlier sleep timing and less consolidated sleep in older adults may be attributable to the interaction between the circadian system and homeostatic regulation, rather than simply resulting from an age-related phase advance in circadian rhythm.[6,55] Sleep homeostasis regulates wake and sleep and generates sleep pressure as a function of time of being awake. Sleep pressure increases during waking and sleep deprivation, and decreases during sleep.[56] Sleep homeostasis declines with aging. The age-related decrease in TST and sleep efficiency may be partially due to the reduced

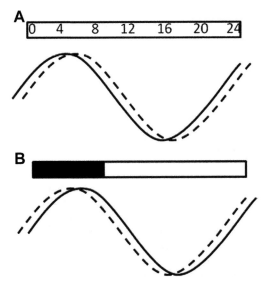

Fig. 2. Circadian phase in older adults. The solid line represents older adults' body temperature and plasma melatonin circadian profile. The dashed line represents young adults' body temperature and plasma melatonin circadian profile. The bar across the top of (*A*) represents the clock time. The horizontal black bar denotes the sleep or dark period. The horizontal white bar denotes wake or light period. (*A*) When compared with clock time, the phase of both core body temperature and plasma melatonin is earlier in older adults (*solid line*) than it is in young adults (*dashed line*). (*B*) When compared with their usual sleep-wake and dark-light timing, the phase of both core body temperature and plasma melatonin is later with respect to sleep/darkness in older adults (*solid line*) than it is in young adults (*dashed line*). (*From Duffy JF, Zitting KM, Chinoy ED. Aging and circadian rhythms. Sleep Med Clin 2015;10(4):423-34*).

homeostatic sleep pressure with aging.[57–59] Also, this reduced homeostatic sleep pressure contributes to an increased number of nocturnal awakenings and reduced daytime sleepiness.[58,59] For example, 1 study that forced desynchronized circadian cycles found that older adults had 2.7 times more nocturnal awakenings than young individuals at most circadian phases.[10]

SLEEP-RELATED HORMONES, AGING, AND SLEEP

Age-related changes in neuroendocrine function are associated with alterations in sleep quality and sleep architecture with normal aging. We briefly review changes of several sleep-related hormones with normal aging and their associations with sleep. Most studies in this area group older adults into a single age category as compared with young or middle-aged adults, and few data exist related to hormonal changes with advancing age within the older adult age group per se.

Growth Hormone

Growth hormone (GH) secretion and slow-wave sleep impact each other.[60,61] GH secretion mainly pulses during nocturnal sleep (no matter whether the sleep is advanced, delayed, or fragmented) at about 1 hour after sleep onset and decreases at transient awakenings.[62] On the other hand, the inhibition of GH-releasing hormone suppresses GH secretion, promotes corticotrophin-releasing hormone, and reduces slow-wave sleep.[62,63]

Furthermore, there is an age-related decrease in the secretion of GH.[64,65] GH secretion reaches its peak during adolescence, rapidly decreases in an exponential manner between young adulthood and middle age, and then decreases slowly between middle age and old age. This phenomenon is similar to the detected age-related decrease of slow-wave sleep.[66] The decrease in nocturnal GH with aging may have a direct or indirect impact on slow-wave sleep, and may be partially responsible for the observed reduction of slow-wave sleep in aging.

Cortisol

Cortisol secretion has a clear circadian pattern that peaks shortly after the morning awakening, gradually declines throughout the day, and reaches its nadir in the late evening, and then increases toward the morning peak.[66] Sleep, particularly slow-wave sleep, inhibits cortisol secretion.[67,68] The increase in cortisol secretion during sleep could lead to awakenings.[68,69] The circadian rhythm of cortisol changes with aging, as manifested by a decreased circadian amplitude, an increased nocturnal cortisol level, and likely a phase-advanced rhythm.[63,70,71] The increased nocturnal cortisol level may contribute to decreased slow-wave sleep and frequent awakenings during nocturnal sleep in older adults.[70]

Prolactin

No clear evidence shows that the secretion of prolactin affects sleep. However, sleep has an influence on prolactin secretion.[70] Sleep onset is associated with an increased secretion of prolactin, regardless of day or night sleep.[66] Also, decreased slow-wave sleep or fragmented sleep may be associated with a reduced elevation of prolactin during nocturnal sleep.[66] Studies show increased prolactin secretion during slow-wave sleep or by enhancing slow-wave sleep, and decreased prolactin secretion in prolonged awakening during the sleep period.[72,73] Prolactin secretion during sleep may decrease with aging because of the lighter and more fragmented sleep in older adults. Studies suggest that nocturnal prolactin in healthy older adults was significantly lower than that in young adults.[65,74]

Thyroid-Stimulating Hormone

Thyroid-stimulating hormone (TSH) secretion has a circadian pattern, which maintains a stable low level during the daytime, starts increasing in the late afternoon, peaks around sleep onset, and then gradually decreases through the night, returning to its daytime level after morning awakenings.[66,75] Studies have shown that slow-wave sleep was associated with inhibited nocturnal TSH secretion, and awakenings were associated with increased nocturnal TSH secretion.[76–78] The circadian release of TSH (with regard to acrophase and nadir) is maintained with aging.[70] However, research suggests that the overall 24-h TSH secretion is decreased in older adults.[79]

Melatonin

The 24-h profile of plasma melatonin is primarily regulated by the light-dark circle and the sleep-wake cycle.[66] Melatonin normally remains stable at a low level during the daytime, starts to increase progressively in the evening (2 hours before habitual bedtime) and remains elevated during the middle of the sleep period, and then decreases gradually to its daytime level in the morning (8–9 AM).[66] The onset of evening sleepiness correlates with the increase in evening melatonin secretion. Overall melatonin secretion decreases with aging, but daytime melatonin (which is already at a low basal level) may remain unchanged with aging. The increase in nocturnal melatonin in older adults was significantly reduced when compared with young adults.[50,80] Studies suggest that the age-related decreases in melatonin secretion contribute to the increased sleep disruption in older adults.[50]

Sex Hormones

Changes in gonadotropins and sex steroids with aging are associated with sleep changes in older adults. In men, testosterone levels decrease progressively with aging after 30 years of age.[81,82] Older men may also lose the diurnal testosterone pattern.[83] The decreased testosterone with aging may relate to the increased sleep fragmentation in older adults.[70] In women, estradiol levels decrease and follicle-stimulating hormone levels increase significantly during the menopause transition and after menopause. These changes in reproductive hormones have been associated with increased complaints of difficulty falling asleep and staying asleep.[70] Also, the decreased levels of endogenous estrogen and progesterone may have a negative impact on the upper airway, thereby increasing the incidence of sleep-disordered breathing after menopause.[84]

RISK FACTORS FOR SLEEP DISTURBANCES IN OLDER ADULTS

As reviewed, most sleep parameters decrease with age until the age of 60 years, but remain generally unchanged after 60 years of age. Also, older adults are less likely to complain of sleep problems and tend to accept some noticeable sleep alterations as normal changes with aging. The age-associated sleep changes discussed herein are mostly relevant to older adults who have excellent health and are aging successfully. In the real world, medical comorbidities and psychiatric illness, primary sleep disorders, and changes in social engagement, lifestyle, and environment commonly accompany aging. These factors contribute to sleep disturbances in older adults. Indeed, up to 50% to 60% of older adults reported poor sleep quality.[4,52] Therefore, sleep problems reported in older adults are usually multifactorial and are not necessarily be explained by age alone.

Medical Comorbidities and Psychiatric Illness

Approximately 67% of older adults have multiple comorbidities.[85] Osteoarthritis, cardiovascular disease, lung disease, gastroesophageal reflux, cancer, and diabetes are the most commonly reported medical comorbidities in older adults.[4,86] About 90% of adults aged 65 years and older take prescription drugs to treat their chronic medical conditions. More than one-third of them routinely take more than 5 medications.[87,88] The discomfort and emotional distress from medical conditions contribute to an increased number of nocturnal awakenings and EDS in older adults. Also, chronic medical conditions are positively associated with the diagnosis or prevalence of sleep disorders, including insomnia, sleep apnea, and restless legs syndrome.[89] Of note, not only do these medical conditions cause sleep disturbances in older adults, but these sleep disturbances can also have a negative impact on medical illnesses and their associated symptoms. Evidence also shows that the multiple medications that older adults take can result in EDS, worsen primary sleep disorders, and contribute to comorbid insomnia.[89,90]

Depression and anxiety, prevalent psychiatric problems among older adults, commonly coexist with insomnia in older adults. Epidemiologic studies reported that more than 50% of older adults with depression have insomnia. Furthermore, longitudinal studies have found that insomnia may increase the risk of depression in older adults. In addition, depression has been positively associated with EDS and the diagnosis and severity of obstructive sleep apnea.[90]

Primary Sleep Disorders

Several primary sleep disorders that are common in older adults contribute to poor sleep in older adults. These sleep disorders include insomnia, sleep-disordered breathing, periodic limb movements in sleep, restless legs syndrome, and REM sleep behavior disorder. Epidemiologic studies found that the prevalence of these primary sleep disorders is considerably higher in older adults than that in younger adults.[91,92] Medical and psychological comorbidities of aging contribute to the increased rebalance of insomnia symptoms (approximately 50%) in older adults. Interestingly, the prevalence of insomnia in older adults with excellent health is similar to that of younger adults.[93] The increase in sleep-disordered breathing frequency in older adults may partially be due to an age-related reduction in pharyngeal muscle function and an increase in comorbidities in older adults.[94] The presentation of these primary sleep disorders contributes to poor sleep in older adults, in terms of difficulties in falling asleep, increased number of nocturnal awakenings, EDS, and complaints of nonrestorative sleep.[91]

Social, Lifestyle, and Environmental Factors

Many social and lifestyle changes with aging contribute to sleep problems in older adults. Retired older adults have more flexible sleep schedules (which can be irregular), have more opportunities to nap during the day, are more sedentary, and are less involved in social activity than they used to be.[95,96] These factors affect both sleep homeostasis and circadian regulation, thus contributing to sleep disturbances. In addition, the loss of loved ones can produce emotional distress and loneliness, which are known to contribute to sleep disturbance.[4] Environmentally, many older adults, especially those who have multiple morbidities, lose independence in activities of daily living, and may move to new homes or long-term care facilities. This transition can be a major life event in later life and create several physical and psychological stressors. Sleep problems can be heightened or get worse during and after this transition. Finally, other environmental factors, such as temperature, noise, and light exposure, are also associated with sleep quality in older adults.[97,98]

SUMMARY

Sleep changes with normal aging. In general, aging is associated with advanced sleep timing, decreased nocturnal sleep time and sleep efficiency, increased frequency of daytime naps, increased nocturnal awakenings, and decreased slow-wave sleep. Most sleep parameters remain unchanged after 60 years of age in healthy older adults. Circadian system and sleep homeostasis become less robust with normal aging. The amount and pattern of sleep-related hormone secretion change in normal aging. All these changes contribute to or correlate with age-related changes in sleep. Poor sleep quality and sleep disturbances are not necessarily due to aging alone, even though sleep schedule, sleep quantity, and sleep architecture change with age. Multiple factors that accompany the aging process, including medical and psychiatric conditions, and environmental, social, and lifestyle changes, can contribute to sleep problems in older adults.

CLINICS CARE POINTS

- Primary care providers need to routinely assess sleep health in older adults needs to be accessed routinely in clinical practice and refer older adults with disrupted sleep to a sleep specialist for further assessment.
- Disturbed sleep commonly coexists with other chronic conditions, such as depression, anxiety, and cognitive impairment in older adults. Treating disturbed sleep may help other coexisting conditions and vice versa.
- Physical and social activities are essential for maintaining healthy sleep in older adults.

DISCLOSURE

This work is supported by National Institute of Nursing Research R00NR016484.

REFERENCES

1. Foley D, Ancoli-Israel S, Britz P, et al. Sleep distur bances and chronic disease in older adults: results

of the 2003 National Sleep Foundation Sleep in America Survey. J Psychosomatic Res 2004;56(5): 497–502.

2. Ohayon MM, Carskadon MA, Guilleminault C, et al. Meta-analysis of quantitative sleep parameters from childhood to old age in healthy individuals: developing normative sleep values across the human lifespan. Sleep 2004;27(7):1255–73.

3. Espiritu JR. Aging-related sleep changes. Clin Geriatr Med 2008;24(1):1–14, v.

4. Vitiello MV. Sleep in normal aging. Sleep Med Clin 2006;1(2):171–6.

5. Campbell SS, Murphy PJ. The nature of spontaneous sleep across adulthood. J Sleep Res 2007; 16(1):24–32.

6. Dorffner G, Vitr M, Anderer P. The effects of aging on sleep architecture in healthy subjects. Adv Exp Med Biol 2015;821:93–100.

7. Floyd JA, Janisse JJ, Jenuwine ES, et al. Changes in REM-sleep percentage over the adult lifespan. SLEEP 2007;30(7):829.

8. Floyd JA, Medler SM, Ager JW, et al. Age-related changes in initiation and maintenance of sleep: a meta-analysis. Res Nurs Health 2000;23(2): 106–17.

9. Floyd JA, Janisse JJ, Marshall Medler S, et al. Nonlinear components of age-related change in sleep initiation. Nurs Res 2000;49(5):290–4.

10. Klerman EB, Davis JB, Duffy JF, et al. Older people awaken more frequently but fall back asleep at the same rate as younger people. Sleep 2004;27(4): 793–8.

11. Potari A, Ujma PP, Konrad BN, et al. Age-related changes in sleep EEG are attenuated in highly intelligent individuals. Neuroimage 2017;146:554–60.

12. Fang W, Li Z, Wu L, et al. Longer habitual afternoon napping is associated with a higher risk for impaired fasting plasma glucose and diabetes mellitus in older adults: results from the Dongfeng-Tongji cohort of retired workers. Sleep Med 2013;14(10):950–4.

13. Cao Z, Shen L, Wu J, et al. The effects of midday nap duration on the risk of hypertension in a middle-aged and older Chinese population: a preliminary evidence from the Tongji-Dongfeng cohort study, China. J Hypertens 2014;32(10):1993–8 [discussion: 1998].

14. Furihata R, Kaneita Y, Jike M, et al. Napping and associated factors: a Japanese nationwide general population survey. Sleep Med 2016;20:72–9.

15. Milner CE, Cote KA. Benefits of napping in healthy adults: impact of nap length, time of day, age, and experience with napping. J Sleep Res 2009;18(2): 272–81.

16. Buysse DJ, Browman KE, Monk TH, et al. Napping and 24-hour sleep/wake patterns in healthy elderly and young adults. J Am Geriatr Soc 1992;40(8): 779–86.

17. Ficca G, Axelsson J, Mollicone DJ, et al. Naps, cognition and performance. Sleep Med Rev 2010; 14(4):249–58.

18. Yoon IY, Kripke DF, Youngstedt SD, et al. Actigraphy suggests age-related differences in napping and nocturnal sleep. J Sleep Res 2003;12(2):87–93.

19. Beh HC. A survey of daytime napping in an elderly Australian population. Aust J Psychol 1994;46(2): 100–6.

20. Stong KL, Ancoli-Israel S. Napping in older adults. In: Avidan AY, Alessi C, editors. Geriatric sleep medicine. 1st edition. New York: Informa Healthcare USA, Inc; 2008. p. 227–40.

21. Naska A, Oikonomou E, Trichopoulou A, et al. Siesta in healthy adults and coronary mortality in the general population. Arch Intern Med 2007;167(3): 296–301.

22. Foley DJ, Vitiello MV, Bliwise DL, et al. Frequent napping is associated with excessive daytime sleepiness, depression, pain, and nocturia in older adults: findings from the National Sleep Foundation '2003 Sleep in America' Poll. Am J Geriatr Psychiatry 2007;15(4):344–50.

23. Chasens ER, Sereika SM, Weaver TE, et al. Daytime sleepiness, exercise, and physical function in older adults. J Sleep Res 2007;16(1):60–5.

24. Jaussent I, Bouyer J, Ancelin ML, et al. Excessive sleepiness is predictive of cognitive decline in the elderly. Sleep 2012;35(9):1201–7.

25. Empana JP, Dauvilliers Y, Dartigues JF, et al. Excessive daytime sleepiness is an independent risk indicator for cardiovascular mortality in community-dwelling elderly: the Three City Study. Stroke 2009; 40(4):1219–24.

26. Whitney CW, EnrightPL, Newman AB, et al. Correlates of daytime sleepiness in 4578 elderly persons: the car diovascular health study. Sleep 1998;21(1): 27–36.

27. Lopes JM, Dantas FG, Medeiros JL. Excessive day time sleepiness in the elderly: association with car diovascular risk, obesity and depression. Rev Bras Epidemiol 2013;16(4):872–9.

28. Blachier M, Dauvilliers Y, Jaussent I, et al. Excessive daytime sleepiness and vascular events: the Three City Study. Ann Neurol 2012;71(5):661–7.

29. Bixler E, Vgontzas A, Lin HM, et al. Excessive day time sleepiness in a general population sample: the role of sleep apnea, age, obesity, diabetes, and depression. J Clin Endocrinol Metab 2005; 90(8):4510–5.

30. Vitiello MV, Larsen LH, Moe KE. Age-related sleep change: gender and estrogen effects on the subjective-objective sleep quality relationships of healthy, noncomplaining older men and women. J Psychosom Res 2004;56(5):503–10.

31. Luo J, Zhu G, Zhao Q, et al. Prevalence and risk factors of poor sleep quality among Chinese elderly in

an urban community: results from the Shanghai ag
ing study. PLoS One 2013;8(11):e81261.

32. Foley DJ, Monjan A, Simonsick EM, et al. Incidence
    and remission of insomnia among elderly adults: an
    epidemiologic study of 6,800 persons over three
    years. Sleep 1999;22(Suppl 2):S366–72.

33. Gooneratne NS, Vitiello MV. Sleep in older adults:
    normative changes, sleep disorders, and treatment
    options. Clin Geriatr Med 2014;30(3):591–627.

34. Gooneratne NS, Bellamy SL, Pack F, et al. Case-
    control study of subjective and objective differences
    in sleep patterns in older adults with insomnia symp
    toms. J Sleep Res 2011;20(3):434–44.

35. Brouwer WB, van Exel NJ, Stolk EA. Acceptability of
    less than perfect health states. Soc Sci Med 2005;
    60(2):237–46.

36. Wright KP, Frey DF. Age related changes in sleep
    and circadian physiology: from brain mechanisms
    to sleep behavior. In: Avidan AY, Alessi C, editors.
    Geriatric sleep medicine. 1st edition. New York:
    CRC Press; 2008. p. 1–18.

37. Mattis J, Sehgal A. Circadian rhythms, sleep, and
    disorders of aging. Trends Endocrinol Metab 2016;
    27(4):192–203.

38. Schmidt C, Peigneux P, Cajochen C. Age-related
    changes in sleep and circadian rhythms: impact
    on cognitive performance and underlying neuroana-
    tomical networks. Front Neurol 2012;3:118.

39. Kripke DF, Elliott JA, Youngstedt SD, et al. Circa-
    dian phase response curves to light in older and
    young women and men. J Circadian Rhythms
    2007;5(1):1.

40. Kim SJ, Benloucif S, Reid KJ, et al. Phase shifting
    response to light in older adults. J Physiol 2014;
    592(1):189–202.

41. Duffy JF, Zitting KM, Chinoy ED. Aging and circa
    dian rhythms. Sleep Med Clin 2015;10(4):423–34.

42. Tranah GJ, Stone KL, Ancoli-Israel S. Circadian
    rhythms in older adults. In: Kryger MH, Roth T,
    Dement WC, editors. Principles and practice of
    sleep medicine. 6th edition. Philadelphia: Elsevier;
    2017. p. 1510–5.

43. Duffy JF, Zeitzer JM, Rimmer DW, et al. Peak of
    circadian melatonin rhythm occurs later within the
    sleep of older subjects. Am J Physiol Endocrinol
    Metab 2002;282(2):E297–303.

44. Czeisler CA, Dumont M, Duffy JF, et al. Association
    of sleep-wake habits in older people with changes
    in output of circadian pacemaker. Lancet 1992;
    340(8825):933–6.

45. Huang YL, Liu RY, Wang QS, et al. Age-associated
    difference in circadian sleep-wake and rest-activity
    rhythms. Physiol Behav 2002;76(4–5):597–603.

46. Dijk DJ, Duffy JF. Circadian regulation of human
    sleep and age-related changes in its timing, consol-
    idation and EEG characteristics. Ann Med 1999;
    31(2):130–40.

47. Carrier J, Monk TH, Buysse DJ, et al. Amplitude
    reduction of the circadian temperature and sleep
    rhythms in the elderly. Chronobiol Int 1996;13(5):
    373–86.

48. Van Someren EJ. More than a marker: interaction
    between the circadian regulation of temperature
    and sleep, age-related changes, and treatment
    pos sibilities. Chronobiol Int 2000;17(3):313–54.

49. Duffy JF, Dijk D-J, Klerman EB, et al. Later endoge-
    nous circadian temperature nadir relative to an
    earlier wake time in older people. Am J Physiol
    1998;275(5):R1478–87.

50. Pandi-Perumal S, Zisapel N, Srinivasan V, et al.
    Melatonin and sleep in aging population. Exp Ger
    Ontol 2005;40(12):911–25.

51. Kondratova AA, Kondratov RV. The circadian clock
    and pathology of the ageing brain. Nat Rev Neurosci
    2012;13(5):325–35.

52. Bliwise DL, Scullin MK. Normal aging. In:
    Kryger MH, Roth T, Dement WC, editors. Principles
    and practice of sleep medicine. 6th edition. Phila-
    delphia: Elsevier; 2017. p. 25–38.

53. Monk TH, Buysse DJ, Carrier J, et al. Inducing jet lag
    in older people: directional asymmetry. J Sleep Res
    2000;9(2):101–16.

54. Farajnia S, Deboer T, Rohling JH, et al. Aging of the
    suprachiasmatic clock. Neuroscientist 2014;20(1):
    44–55.

55. Dijk D-J, Duffy JF, Czeisler CA. Contribution of circa-
    dian physiology and sleep homeostasis to age-
    related changes in human sleep. Chronobiol Int
    2000;17(3):285–311.

56. Taillard J, Philip P, Coste O, et al. The circadian
    and homeostatic modulation of sleep pressure
    during wakefulness differs between morning and
    evening chronotypes. J Sleep Res 2003;12(4):
    275–82.

57. Dijk DJ, Duffy JF, Riel E, et al. Ageing and the circa-
    dian and homeostatic regulation of human sleep
    during forced desynchrony of rest, melatonin and
    tempera ture rhythms. J Physiol 1999;516(Pt 2):
    611–27.

58. Carrier J, Land S, Buysse DJ, et al. The effects of
    age and gender on sleep EEG power spectral den-
    sity in the middle years of life (ages 20-60 years old).
    Psychophysiology 2001;38(2):232–42.

59. Dijk DJ, Groeger JA, Stanley N, et al. Age-related
    reduction in daytime sleep propensity and nocturnal
    slow wave sleep. Sleep 2010;33(2):211–23.

60. Gronfier C, Luthringer R, Follenius M, et al.
    A quantitative evaluation of the relationships be-
    tween growth hormone secretion and delta wave
    electroencephalographic activity during normal
    sleep and after enrichment in delta waves. Sleep
    1996;19(10):817–24.

61. Holl RW, Hartman ML, Veldhuis JD, et al. Thirty-sec-
    ond sampling of plasma growth hormone in man:

correlation with sleep stages. J Clin Endocrinol Metab 1991;72(4):854–61.

62. Van Cauter E, Caufriez A, Kerkhofs M, et al. Sleep, awakenings, and insulin-like growth factor-I modulate the growth hormone (GH) secretory response to GH-releasing hormone. J Clin Endocrinol Metab 1992;74(6):1451–9.

63. Van Cauter E, Leproult R, Kupfer DJ. Effects of gender and age on the levels and circadian rhythmicity of plasma cortisol. J Clin Endocrinol Metab 1996;81(7):2468–73.

64. Van Cauter E, Leproult R, Plat L. Age-related changes in slow wave sleep and REM sleep and relationship with growth hormone and cortisol levels in healthy men. JAMA 2000;284(7):861–8.

65. van Coevorden A, Mockel J, Laurent E, et al. Neuroendocrine rhythms and sleep in aging men. Am J Physiol 1991;260(4 Pt 1):E651–61.

66. Copinschi G, Caufriez A. Sleep and hormonal changes in aging. Endocrinol Metab Clin North Am 2013;42(2):371–89.

67. Bierwolf C, Struve K, Marshall L, et al. Slow wave sleep drives inhibition of pituitary-adrenal secre- tion in humans. J Neuroendocrinol 1997;9(6):479–84.

68. Caufriez A, Moreno-Reyes R, Leproult R, et al. Immediate effects of an 8-h advance shift of the rest-activity cycle on 24-h profiles of cortisol. Am J Physiol Endocrinol Metab 2002;282(5):E1147–53.

69. Follenius M, Brandenberger G, Bandesapt JJ, et al. Nocturnal cortisol release in relation to sleep structure. Sleep 1992;15(1):21–7.

70. Buckley TM. Neuroendocrine and homeostatic changes in the elderly. In: Pandi-Perumal SR, Monti JM, Monjan AA, editors. Principles and practice of geriatric sleep medicine. 1st edition. New York: Cambridge University Press; 2010. p. 85–96.

71. Nater UM, Hoppmann CA, Scott SB. Diurnal profiles of salivary cortisol and alpha-amylase change across the adult lifespan: evidence from repeated daily life assessments. Psychoneuroendocrinology 2013;38(12):3167–71.

72. Spiegel K, Luthringer R, Follenius M, et al. Temporal relationship between prolactin secretion and slow-wave electroencephalic activity during sleep. Sleep 1995;18(7):543–8.

73. Blyton DM, Sullivan CE, Edwards N. Lactation is associated with an increase in slow-wave sleep in women. J Sleep Res 2002;11(4):297–303.

74. Greenspan SL, Klibanski A, Rowe JW, et al. Age alters pulsatile prolactin release: influence of dopaminergic inhibition. Am J Physiol 1990;258(5 Pt 1):E799–804.

75. Brabant G, Prank K, Ranft U, et al. Physiological regulation of circadian and pulsatile thyrotropin secretion in normal man and woman. J Clin Endocrinol Metab 1990;70(2):403–9.

76. Goichot B, Brandenberger G, Saini J, et al. Nocturnal plasma thyrotropin variations are related to slow-wave sleep. J Sleep Res 1992;1(3):1, 86 90 1 86—90.

77. Goichot B, Buguet A, Bogui P, et al. Twenty-four-hour profiles and sleep-related variations of cortisol, thyrotropin and plasma renin activity in healthy Afri- can melanoids. Eur J Appl Physiol Occup Physiol 1995;70(3):220–5.

78. Hirschfeld U, Moreno-Reyes R, Akseki E, et al. Pro gressive elevation of plasma thyrotropin during adaptation to simulated jet lag: effects of treatment with bright light or Zolpidem. J Clin Endocrinol Metab 1996;81(9):3270–7.

79. Van Coevorden A, Laurent E, Decoster C, et al. Decreased basal and stimulated thyrotropin secretion in healthy elderly men. J Clin Endocrinol Metab 1989;69(1):177–85.

80. Zeitzer JM, Duffy JF, Lockley SW, et al. Plasma mela tonin rhythms in young and older humans during sleep, sleep deprivation, and wake. Sleep 2007; 30(11):1437–43.

81. Shi Z, Araujo AB, Martin S, et al. Longitudinal changes in testosterone over five years in community-dwelling men. J Clin Endocrinol Metab 2013;98(8):3289–97.

82. Harman SM, Metter EJ, Tobin JD, et al. Baltimore Longitudinal Study of Aging. Longitudinal effects of aging on serum total and free testosterone levels in healthy men. Baltimore Longitudinal Study of Ag- ing. J Clin Endocrinol Metab 2001; 86(2):724–31.

83. Bremner WJ, Vitiello MV, Prinz PN. Loss of circadian rhythmicity in blood testosterone levels with aging in normal men. J Clin Endocrinol Metab 1983;56(6): 1278–81.

84. Lin CM, Davidson TM, Ancoli-Israel S. Gender differ ences in obstructive sleep apnea and treatment im plications. Sleep Med Rev 2008;12(6):481–96.

85. Salive ME. Multimorbidity in older adults. Epidemiol Rev 2013;35:75–83.

86. Fillenbaum GG, Pieper CF, Cohen HJ, et al. Comor bid- ity of five chronic health conditions in elderly commu- nity residents: determinants and impact on mortality. J Gerontol A Biol Sci Med Sci 2000; 55(2):M84–9.

87. Kaufman DW, Kelly JP, Rosenberg L, et al. Recent patterns of medication use in the ambulatory adult population of the United States: the Slone survey. JAMA 2002;287(3):337–44.

88. Linjakumpu T, Hartikainen S, Klaukka T, et al. Use of medications and polypharmacy are increasing among the elderly. J Clin Epidemiol 2002;55(8):809–17.

89. Barczi SR. Sleep and medical comorbidities. In: Avi dan AY, Alessi C, editors. Geriatric sleep medicine. 1st edition. New York: CRC Press; 2008. p. 19–36.

90. Boockvar KS. Reducing sedative-hypnotic medica-tion use in older adults with sleep problems. Clin Ther 2016;38(11):2330–1.

91. Crowley K. Sleep and sleep disorders in older adults. Neuropsychol Rev 2011;21(1): 41–53.

92. Rissling M, Ancoli-Israel S. Sleep in aging. In: Stickgold R, Walker MP, editors. Neuroscience of sleep. London, United Kingdom: Academic Press; 2009. p. 78–84.

93. Ohayon MM. Prevalence of DSM-IV diagnostic criteria of insomnia: distinguishing insomnia related to mental disorders from sleep disorders. J Psychiatr Res 1997;31(3):333–46.

94. McMillan A, Morrell MJ. Sleep disordered breathing at the extremes of age: the elderly. Breathe (Sheff) 2016;12(1):50–60.

95. Li J, Yang B, Varrasse M, et al. Sleep among long-term care residents in China a narrative review of literature. Clin Nurs Res 2018;27(1).

96. Zantinge EM, van den Berg M, Smit HA, et al. Retirement and a healthy lifestyle: opportunity or pitfall? a narrative review of the literature. Eur J Public Health 2014;24(3):433–9.

97. Li J, Grandner AM, Chang YP, et al. Person-centered dementia care and sleep in assisted living residents with dementia: a pilot study. Behav Sleep Med 2017; 15(2):97–113.

98. Hanford N, Figueiro M. Light therapy and Alzheimer's disease and related dementia: past, pre sent, and future. J Alzheimer's Dis 2013;33(4):913–22.

Epidemiology of Insomnia
Prevalence, Course, Risk Factors, and Public Health Burden

Charles M. Morin, PhD*, Denise C. Jarrin, PhD

KEYWORDS

- Insomnia • Sleep disorders • Epidemiology • Prevalence • Incidence • Risk factors

KEY POINTS

- The epidemiology of insomnia has received increased attention in the last decade, and investigators have moved from a purely cross-sectional approach to a more prospective and longitudinal approach.
- Progress on the epidemiology of insomnia has been hampered by important methodological shortcomings including, but not limited to, the lack of a consistent case definition and standardized assessment procedures across studies.
- Additional prospective and longitudinal studies are needed to identify early precursors of insomnia and factors moderating its trajectories over time.
- A better understanding of how insomnia evolves over time, and what factors trigger an episode or perpetuate it over time is critical for developing effective prevention and treatment programs.

INTRODUCTION

Insomnia is a significant public health problem, which affects large segments of the population at one point or another in life. The burden of chronic insomnia is also widespread both for the individual, in terms of reduced quality of life, and for society at large, in terms of work absenteeism, disability, and health care costs. Although significant advances have been made in therapeutics, there is more limited knowledge on its epidemiology, risk factors, long-term course, and prognosis. A better understanding of these critical issues would be informative to develop more effective therapies. This article summarizes the evidence on the epidemiology of insomnia, including its natural history, prevalence, incidence, and risk factors, as well as its long-term consequences and public health burden. In addition, some directions for future population-based research and for developing effective prevention programs are outlined.

NATURE OF INSOMNIA AND UPDATED DIAGNOSTIC CRITERIA

Insomnia is characterized by a spectrum of complaints reflecting dissatisfaction with the quality, duration, or continuity of sleep. The predominant nocturnal symptoms include difficulties falling asleep at bedtime, waking up in the middle of the night and having difficulty going back to sleep, or waking up too early in the morning with an inability to return to sleep.[1,2] These difficulties are not mutually exclusive, as a person may experience mixed problems initiating and maintaining sleep. In addition to nighttime sleep difficulties, daytime symptoms represent an integral component of insomnia. These symptoms include fatigue or decreased energy, cognitive impairments involving attention, concentration and memory, and mood disturbances (eg, irritability, dysphoria).[3–5] These latter symptoms contribute to significant role impairments[6] and are often the primary concern prompting patients to seek treatment.[7]

This article previously appeared in *Sleep Med Clin* 8 (2013) 281–297.

School of Psychology and Centre de Recherche CERVO, Université Laval, Québec G1V0A6, Canada

* Corresponding author. Université Laval, School of Psychology, Pavillon Félix-Antoine Savard, 2325, rue des Bibliothèques, Quebec, Quebec G1V0A6, Canada.

E-mail address: cmorin@psy.ulaval.ca

Sleep Med Clin 17 (2022) 173–191
https://doi.org/10.1016/j.jsmc.2022.03.003

Several important changes have been made to the diagnostic criteria of insomnia in the *Diagnostic and Statistical Manual of Mental Disorders, Fifth Edition* DSM-5[2] and in the *International Classification of Sleep Disorders, Third Edition* (ICSD-III).[8] For example, the symptom of nonrestorative sleep has been eliminated from the insomnia definition, mainly because this complaint is ill defined and not specific to insomnia. In the DSM-5,[2] the duration threshold for chronic insomnia has also been increased from 1 to 3 months, a change based on evidence that 3 months is a critical period, after which insomnia is more likely to persist[9] and its morbidity becomes more noticeable.[10] Likewise, a minimal frequency of 3 nights per week has been added to further operationalize the definition of clinical insomnia. More importantly, the DSM-V[2] no longer makes a distinction between primary insomnia and insomnia secondary to a psychiatric, medical, or another sleep disorder. This change was predicated on the evidence that when insomnia is comorbid with another disorder (eg, major depression), it is often difficult, if not impossible, to determine which disorder is the cause and which is the consequence. Historically, clinicians generally have assumed that insomnia was symptomatic of a more important disorder and that treating the underlying disorder (eg, depression, pain) would also improve sleep; as such, insomnia was often overlooked and undertreated. There is now solid evidence that insomnia is a prevalent residual symptom, even after successful treatment of depression,[11] and its persistence increases the risk of relapse of depression.[12] Furthermore, although insomnia has long been conceptualized as a symptom of another disorder, there is strong evidence showing that chronic insomnia is also a precursor or a risk factor for new-onset psychiatric disorders.[13] By moving away from the need to make a causal attribution between insomnia and coexisting disorders, it is hoped that clinicians will pay more attention to insomnia as a disorder on its own. Recent treatment studies have shown that when insomnia is comorbid with another psychiatric or medical disorder, treatment outcome is better when attending to both insomnia and the comorbid condition than when attending to the comorbid condition alone.[14,15]

PREVALENCE AND CORRELATES OF INSOMNIA
Prevalence

At least 50 epidemiologic studies on insomnia were published between the first population-based surveys by Karacan and colleagues[16] and Bixler and colleagues[17] in the 1970s and a landmark review paper in 2002 by Ohayon,[18] and since then, at least another 20 studies have been published. Prevalence estimates of insomnia vary widely across studies, partly because of differences in case definitions, assessment procedures, sample characteristics, and length of assessment intervals. With regard to the last point, most studies used point estimates (ie, past month), although some have relied on longer intervals (ie, past year or even lifetime). Depending on the specific definitions used (ie, insomnia symptoms vs disorder, sleep dissatisfaction), prevalence rates have varied from as low as 5% to as high as 50%.[18] In general, population-based data indicate that about one-third of adults (30%-36%) report at least one nocturnal insomnia symptom (ie, difficulty initiating or maintaining sleep, nonrestorative sleep), but this rate decreases to between 10% and 15% when daytime consequences (eg, fatigue) are added to the case definition. Rates of sleep dissatisfaction, without regard to specific sleep diagnosis, also vary widely (10%–25%) in the adult population. When using more stringent and operational DSM[2] or ICSD[1] diagnostic criteria, prevalence rates tend to cluster between 6% and 10%.[6,7,19–21] These highly variable estimates underscore the need to rely on operational definitions and standardized assessment procedures to derive accurate and comparable prevalence rates across studies.

Although the most common single symptom of insomnia is difficulty maintaining sleep, mixed difficulties in sleep onset and maintenance are more prevalent than any single complaint.[6,7,19,21] Among subtypes of sleep maintenance problems, both middle-of-the-night and early morning awakenings are equally prevalent, although the latter are more common among older adults.[21,22] Nonrestorative sleep is also a prevalent complaint, but less frequently as a single complaint; it is typically reported in association with other insomnia symptoms and also in association with several other sleep disorders. Its nonspecificity has led to its exclusion from the insomnia definition in both DSM-5[2] and ICSD-III.[8]

Insomnia is also highly prevalent in primary care medicine, usually the first entry point to access professional care for insomnia, with about 40% of patients reporting significant sleep disturbances.[23]

Patients with more severe and more chronic insomnia, more comorbid medical or psychiatric disorders, and those who are better educated are more likely to seek treatment of insomnia.[24]

Correlates of Insomnia

Insomnia is consistently more prevalent among women, middle-aged and older adults, shift workers, and patients with coexisting medical and psychiatric disorders. With regard to gender, a meta-analysis[25] revealed a risk ratio of 1.41 for women versus men. Although insomnia has a greater overall prevalence in middle-aged and older adults, the nature of insomnia interacts with age, such that sleep maintenance difficulties are more common among middle-aged and older adults, whereas sleep initiation difficulties are more frequent among younger adults.[6,18,21]

Strong associations (odds ratios = 4.0–6.0) have been reported between insomnia and poor mental and physical health, psychological distress, anxiety and depressive symptoms, as well as with somatic symptoms and poor self-rated physical health.[6,7,19,26,27] Insomnia has also been associated with lower socioeconomic status and with living alone (eg, single, separated, or widowed). Hormonal replacement therapy was found in one study to be a protective factor against insomnia in older adults.[22]

Prevalence Across Ethnicities and Cultures

In a nation-wide sleep survey in the United States, insomnia in adults was diagnosed in 10% of Whites, 7% of Hispanics, 4% of Asians, and 3% of African Americans.[28] Likewise, insomnia prevalence rates in European American, African American, and Mexican American adolescents were 5.3%, 5.2%, and 3.5%, respectively.[29] Comparative studies between immigrants and nonimmigrants have provided mixed results, with some research indicating immigrants report fewer,[30,31] more,[32] or similar numbers[33] of sleep complaints or insomnia symptoms compared with their nonimmigrant counterparts. These discrepancies may be attributed to the differences in sleep attitudes and beliefs reported across diverse ethnicities and cultures, including what individuals believe to be the causes and the consequences of sleep problems,[33] as well as the priority placed on obtaining adequate sleep within cultures.[31]

Although there are few direct cross-cultural comparisons of insomnia, a worldwide study found that the highest prevalence rates of insomnia were in Brazil (79.8%), followed by South Africa (45.3%), Eastern Europe (32%), Asia (28.3%), and Western Europe (23.2%).[34] In another cross-country survey, the highest prevalence rates of insomnia symptoms were reported in Western Europe (37.2%), followed by the United States (27%) and Japan (6.6%).[35] Prevalence rates of restless sleep (as opposed to insomnia) across 23 countries in Europe were less than 10% in Mediterranean and Nordic countries, ranged from 11% to 22% in Western European countries, and from 25% to 37% in Eastern

European countries among working-aged adults.[36] Likewise, the highest prevalence rates of sleep problems were found in the United States (56%), followed by Western Europe (31%) and Japan (23%).[37] Cross-cultural studies in pediatric samples suggest that toddlers and children from Asian cultures (eg, Hong Kong, India, Singapore) tend to go to bed at later times, wake up at earlier times, report shorter sleep durations, and are perceived by parents to show more sleep problems compared with children from White cultures (eg, Canada, United Kingdom, New Zealand).[38,39]

People from different cultures experience, perceive, and understand health problems differently, possibly as a result of religious beliefs, stigma, reasoning fallacy, differences in symptom presentation, processing, and expressing experiences.[40,41] These cultural differences can affect whether insomnia is perceived as normal (part of everyday life) or abnormal. For example, waking up in the middle of the night is sometimes seen as a gift for some religions, because it provides an additional opportunity to pray. Further qualitative research would be helpful to better understand cross-cultural and ethnic differences in the phenomenological experience and expression of insomnia, because this may help develop more targeted prevention and intervention strategies.

INCIDENCE AND RISK FACTORS
Incidence

There are few longitudinal incidence studies (**Table 1**) compared with the large number of cross-sectional prevalence studies. Nonetheless, incidence rates vary extensively across studies, depending on the case definition (eg, symptoms vs syndrome) and the interval used to track new onset. For instance, 4 population-based studies using the same 12-month interval between baseline and follow-up assessments revealed incidence rates of 2.8% in Sweden,[20] 6.0% in the United States,[26] 7.4% in Canada,[42] and 15% in the United Kingdom,[43] with the variability being partly accounted for by different case definitions across studies. For example, a Canadian study[42] found an incidence rate of 30.7% for insomnia symptoms compared with 7.4% for an insomnia syndrome. Another important variable explaining some of the variability is whether investigators make a distinction between incident cases of first episode (ie, no previous history of insomnia) and cases of recurrence (ie, with past insomnia episodes). For example, the 7.4% incidence rates in the LeBlanc and colleagues[42] study decreased almost by half (3.9%) when only individuals without previous lifetime episode of insomnia

Table 1
Summary of prevalence, incidence, and persistence rates of insomnia in population-based longitudinal, prospective studies

Author	Sample (Number, Age [y])	Follow-up Interval	Case Definition	Prevalence (%)	Incidence (%)	Persistence (%)
Ellis et al,[45] 2012	General population (1095, 32.72)	1 mo–3 mo	Acute insomnia: previous/ongoing problems with initiating/ maintaining sleep, early awakenings, feeling unrefreshed on waking (3 d–3 mo)	Acute insomnia: 7.9 First onset: 33.7 Recurrent: 48.8	Acute insomnia: 1 mo: 4.37 3 mo: 9.15 DSM-5: 1 mo: 3.4 3 mo: 7.8	—
			DSM-5 & prolonged sleep onset, wake after sleep onset, low quality of life	—	First onset: 1 mo: 61.1 3 mo: 4.4	—
			First onset: acute insomnia, no past sleep problem, no comorbidity	—	—	—
			Recurrent episode: first onset with previous sleep problem	—	—	—
LeBlanc et al,[42] 2009	General population (464 [good sleepers], >18)	6 mo–1 y	Symptoms: initial, maintenance, or late insomnia (≥3 nights/wk) or use of sleep-promoting medication	—	Overall symptoms (no previous insomnia): 30.7 (28.8) 6 mo: 14.4 (5.77)	—
			Syndrome: dissatisfied with sleep, initial, maintenance, or late insomnia (≥3 nights/wk) for at	—	1 y: 13.5 (6.82) Overall syndrome: 7.3 (3.9) 6 mo: 2.37 (1.57) 1 y: 4.52 (2.09)	—

least a month & daytime impairment or use of prescribed medication (≥3 nights/wk)

Study	Sample (n, age)	Time	Definition			
Ford & Kramer,[26] 1989	Community sample (7954, 18–>65)	1 y	Diagnostic interview (DSM-III) report difficulty initiating/ maintaining sleep or early awakening (≥2 wk) in past 6 mo	10.2	6	31
Roberts et al,[46] 1999	General population (2380, 50–102)	1y	Report difficulty initiating/ maintaining sleep in past 2 wk	23.4	9	13
Fok et al,[53] 2010	Community sample (656, ≥65)	1 y	Report trouble sleeping in past month	44.7	21.4	66.3
Jansson & Linton,[119] 2006	General population (1530, 20–60)	1 y	Report difficulty initiating/ maintaining sleep, early awakening, & daytime problems (>3 nights/wk) in past 3 mo	10	6	—
Morphy et al,[43] 2007	General population (2363, 18–98)	1 y	Symptoms: report difficulty initiating/ maintaining sleep, nocturnal awakenings (on most nights) in past month Syndrome: symptoms & waking up tired	Overall: 36.8 Symptoms: 30.4 Syndrome: 13.2	Overall: 14.6 Symptoms: 13.3 Syndrome: 6.8	Overall: 69.2 Symptoms: 67.9 Syndrome: 54.8

(continued on next page)

Table 1
(continued)

Author	Sample (Number, Age [y])	Follow-up Interval	Case Definition	Prevalence (%)	Incidence (%)	Persistence (%)
Jansson-Frojmark et al,[20] 2008	General population (1746, 20–60)	1 y	Report difficulty initiating/ maintaining sleep, early awakening, & daytime problems (>3 nights/wk) in past 3 mo	6.8–9.7	2.8	44.4
Jansson-Frojmark & Lindblom,[120] 2008	General population (1498, 20–60)	1 y	Report sleep problem & difficulty initiating/ maintaining sleep (3 nights/wk) in past 3 mo	15	—	14
Skapinakis et al,[121] 2012	Adults (2406, 16–74)	1.5 y	Report difficulty initiating/ maintaining sleep in past month	57.7	15.8	—
Kim et al,[54] 2009	Community sample (909, ≥65)	2 y	Report difficulty initiating/ maintaining sleep. Symptoms: 1–2 nights/wk over month. Syndrome: >3 nights/wk over month	Overall: 27 Symptoms: 32 Syndrome: 21	Overall: 23 Symptoms: 37 Syndrome: 20	Overall: 40 Symptoms: 38 Syndrome: 41
Komada et al,[122] 2012	General population (1434, ≥20)	2 y	Pittsburgh Sleep Quality Index cutoff score >5.5	30.7	12.9	18.7

Author	Sample (Number, Age [y])	Follow-up Interval	Case Definition	Prevalence (%)	Incidence (%)	Persistence (%)
Morin et al,[52] 2009	Population-based (388, M = 44.8 [13.9])	3 y	Symptoms: initial, maintenance, or late insomnia (>3 nights/wk) or use of sleep-promoting medication Syndrome: dissatisfied with sleep, initial, maintenance, or late insomnia (≥3 nights/wk) for at least a month & daytime impairment or use of prescribed medication (≥3 nights/wk)	—	—	Symptoms: 1 y: 23.4 2 y: 8.4 3 y: 37.2 ≥1 y: 69.0 Syndrome: 1 y: 11.3 2 y: 9.0 3 y: 66.1 ≥1 y: 86.4
Breslau et al,[44] 1996	HMO group (1007, 21–30)	3.5 y	Report difficulty initiating/maintaining sleep, early morning awakening (2 wk) Lifetime history of insomnia	Insomnia (no comorbidity): 16.6 Lifetime history: 24.6	Overall: 13.3 Lifetime history: 45 No lifetime: 8.7	—
Morgan & Clark,[55] 1997	Elderly adults (1042, ≥65)	4 y	Report sleep problem "often or all the time" in past week	—	3.1 (weighted)	36.1
Zhang et al,[27] 2012	Adults (2316, 46.3)	5.2 y	Report difficulty initiating/maintaining sleep, early morning awakening, daytime symptoms Symptoms: 3/wk over	Symptoms: 7.1 Syndrome: 4.8	Overall: 5.9 Symptoms: 3.6 Syndrome: 2.3	Overall: 36.5 Symptoms: 29.5 Syndrome: 47.0

(continued on next page)

Table 1
(continued)

Author	Sample (Number, Age [y])	Follow-up Interval	Case Definition	Prevalence (%)	Incidence (%)	Persistence (%)
			1 y Syndrome: symptoms & daytime symptoms			
Fernandez-Mendoza et al,[123] 2012	Random general population (1395, >20)	7.5 y	Poor sleep: moderate/severe difficulty initiating/ maintaining sleep, early final awakening, daytime symptoms Insomnia: insomnia complaint lasting >1y	Poor sleep: 32.3	Poor sleep: 18.4 Poor sleep to insomnia: 16.8	38.4
Vgontzas et al,[124] 2012	Random general population (1395, ≥20)	7.5 y	Insomnia compliant lasting >1y	11.9	—	43.6
Singareddy et al,[125] 2012	Random general population (1395, ≥20)	7.5 y	Chronic insomnia: "Do you feel you have insomnia with a duration of at least 1 y?"	10.6	9.3 (weighted)	—
Silversen et al,[68] 2012	Population-based (24,715; 19–80)	11 y	DSM-IV, onset, terminal, later insomnia, & daytime symptoms in past month	5.1	6.5	19.2
Buysse et al,[65] 2008	Population sample (278 [all 6 interviews], baseline age 20)	20 y	Based on symptom, duration, & frequency of episodes in past year 1 mo: sleep	Cumulative weighted 1 mo: 19.8 2–3 wk: 9.7 Recurrent brief: 20.6 Occasional brief: 17.5	—	At any future interview: 1 mo: 39 2–3 wk: 31 Recurrent brief: 40 Occasional brief: 30

difficulties for $\geq$ 1 mo & daytime impairments
2–3 wk: at least once over past year
Recurrent brief: <2 wk recurring at least monthly over past year
Occasional brief: <2 wk duration occurring less than monthly

Note: summary of results are presented from shortest to longest follow-up intervals.

were included in the case definition. A similar finding had also been reported (13.1% vs 8.7%) in a sample of young adults.[44]

Another variable that affects incidence rates is whether the reported rate includes all cumulative cases emerging between baseline and follow-up assessments (cumulative incidence) or only new cases present at the second assessment (point estimate). Because insomnia is a condition that often fluctuates over time, it is plausible that a new case might emerge after baseline assessment but remit by the follow-up assessment point. A recent study[45] examined the distribution of 3 subtypes of acute insomnia as a function of duration and found a significant difference between the 1-month (4.4%) and 3-month (9.2%) incidence rates; in addition, recurrent acute insomnia (3.8%) was more common than first episode of acute insomnia (2.6%) and comorbid acute insomnia (1.4%).

A related issue that may explain some of the variability in incidence rates is the time frame used to assess insomnia. In the LeBlanc and colleagues[42] study, assessment of insomnia at each time point was based on the previous month only, rather than the entire 6-month and 12-month intervals, which may have yielded more conservative rates because it did not capture those cases that developed insomnia and subsequently remitted within the follow-up intervals. Because insomnia is often waxing and waning, it is plausible that the incidence rates have been underestimated in some of these studies.

Risk Factors

Although several insomnia correlates have been identified reliably across studies, the data about risk factors predisposing to insomnia are more tentative. Nonetheless, the most commonly hypothesized factors predisposing to insomnia include demographic factors, such as female gender and older age, and a personal or familial history of insomnia. Women are at greater risk for insomnia, and perhaps more so during menopause, because of hormonal changes. The risk of insomnia also increases with aging, but this may be the result of increased health problems with aging rather than age per se.[46] The risk of insomnia is also higher among first-degree family members of individuals with insomnia than in the general population,[47,48] although it remains unclear whether this link is inherited through a genetic predisposition, learned by observations of parental models, or simply a by-product of another (eg, psychiatric) disorder. A past personal history of insomnia has also been identified as an important risk for future episodes of insomnia.[42]

Psychological and a biological predisposition are 2 additional factors that have been linked to greater risk to develop insomnia. The psychological vulnerability to insomnia is typically characterized by an anxiety-prone personality, with increased scores on measures of anxiety and depressive symptoms, worries, perfectionism, introversion, and lower abilities to cope with day-to-day stressful situations.[42] On the other hand, the biological vulnerability is characterized by indices of hyperarousability and increased hypothalamic–pituitary–adrenal axis activity.[49] Although this latter hypothesis has been around for some time,[50,51] it still remains unclear whether hyperarousal is a state that characterizes an individual's response to sleep difficulties or their apprehension or a more enduring trait that predisposes some individuals to develop insomnia under stressful circumstances.

COURSE OF INSOMNIA: PERSISTENCE, REMISSION, RELAPSE

The course of insomnia is of significant interest to both epidemiologists and clinicians. The extent to which insomnia is a transient, recurrent, or persistent condition has important implications in terms of whether and when to initiate treatment and long-term prognosis and morbidity.

Several longitudinal studies have documented the course of insomnia over various time intervals (see Table 1), but most of those have used only 2 assessment points. The evidence is clear that insomnia is often a persistent problem over time, with persistence rates varying as a function of the intervals between assessments. For example, data derived from some of the same longitudinal studies assessing incidence have produced persistence rates over a 1-year period of 31% in the United States,[26] 44.4% (syndrome like) in Sweden,[20] 69% (symptoms) in the United Kingdom,[43] and 74% (symptoms and syndromes combined) in Canada.[52] Studies conducted with cohorts of older adults have produced persistence rates of 66.3%[53] for 1-year period, 40% for a 2-year period,[54] and 36.1% for a 4-year period.[55] In a cohort of 4467 older adults involved in the Cardiovascular Health Study,[56] rates of persistent insomnia over a 1-year to 4-year period were 15.4% for trouble falling asleep and 22.7% for frequent awakenings, compared with 13.4% for excessive daytime sleepiness.

Factors associated with persistence of insomnia are often the same as those associated with its incidence (ie, female gender, older age, and presence of medical or mental health problems),[53] with depression and mental health problems presenting stronger associations than physical health problems. Insomnia can also be a persistent condition, independent of mental disorders.

As part of our ongoing longitudinal study,[52] we are following 4000 adults annually throughout Canada, and at each assessment these individuals are classified as good sleepers, individuals with insomnia symptoms, or individuals with an insomnia syndrome (disorder). Sleep status is based on information derived from standard assessment instruments (Insomnia Severity Index, Pittsburgh Sleep Quality Index) and is defined by an algorithm using a combination of insomnia diagnostic criteria (DSM and ICD) and the use of sleep-promoting medication.[42,52] For instance, individuals with an insomnia syndrome must report dissatisfaction with sleep; symptoms of initial, middle, or late insomnia at least 3 nights per week for a month; and significant distress or daytime impairments. Also included in this group are those taking prescribed sleep-promoting medication 3 nights or more per week for at least 1 month. Individuals classified with insomnia symptoms report some of these same symptoms but do not fulfill all diagnostic criteria for an insomnia syndrome. Individuals using prescribed medications fewer than 3 nights per week or over-the-counter medications for sleep at least 1 night per week are also classified in this group. Good sleepers do not report any sleep complaint and do not use medications to promote sleep.

Preliminary data from a subsample of 388 participants completing the first 3 annual follow-ups showed that 46% of individuals with insomnia (symptoms or syndrome) at baseline continued to report insomnia (symptoms or syndrome) at the 3-year follow-up, and for the remaining 54% who went into remission at some point in time, half of them eventually relapsed.[52] Different insomnia trajectories were observed across severity levels, with individuals presenting an insomnia syndrome at baseline showing a more persistent course over time, whereas individuals with subsyndromal insomnia had a more fluctuating trajectory, with a greater likelihood of remission status at a subsequent follow-up.

This study has also shown that insomnia status may change considerably even within a 12-month period. For example, an individual with insomnia at baseline may become a good sleeper 6 months later and again have insomnia 12 months later. This fluctuation over time underscores the need to adopt a more microscopic approach in longitudinal studies of insomnia. To examine this issue, we conducted monthly evaluations over a 12-month period with a subgroup of 100 individuals.[9] At baseline, 42 participants were classified as

good sleepers, 34 met criteria for insomnia symptoms, and 24 for an insomnia syndrome. There were significant fluctuations of insomnia over time, with 66% of the participants changing sleep status at least once over the 12 monthly assessments. Changes in sleep status were significantly more frequent among individuals with insomnia symptoms at baseline (M = 3.55) than among those initially classified as good sleepers (M = 2.14).

Among the subgroup with insomnia symptoms at baseline, 85.3% reported improved sleep (ie, became good sleepers) at least once over the 12 monthly assessments compared with 29.4% whose sleep worsened (ie, met criteria for an insomnia syndrome) during the same period. Among individuals classified as good sleepers at baseline, risks of developing insomnia symptoms and syndrome at least once over the subsequent months were respectively 14.4% and 3.2%. An interval of 6 months was found most reliable to estimate incidence rates, whereas an interval of 3 months proved the most reliable to estimate persistence rate. These results suggest significant sleep variability over a 12-month period and highlight the importance of conducting repeated assessment at a shorter than the typical yearly interval in order to reliably capture the natural course of insomnia over time.

CONSEQUENCES AND BURDEN OF INSOMNIA

Insomnia is associated with significant short-term and long-term consequences. Although the essential features of insomnia are nocturnal complaints, daytime impairments and distress over daytime functioning are also defining criteria of insomnia,[1,2] and this component has been identified as a research priority by insomnia expert panels.[57,58]

Short-Term Consequences of Insomnia

Short-term, daily consequences include physical discomfort on awakening, fatigue, tiredness, unpleasant body sensations (eg, heavy eyes), hypersensitivity to noise and light, and low energy/motivation throughout the day.[59] Insomnia is associated with mood disturbances (eg, irritability), heightened emotional reactiveness,[59,60] negative interactions with children[61] and partners,[62] reduced optimism and self-esteem,[63] as well as overall poor quality of life (eg, vitality).[60]

In a recent qualitative study, participants with insomnia symptoms reported feeling segregated and misunderstood by others (eg, friends, physicians); described daily life as an effort or struggle; and raised concerns over the cumulative and long-term impact of insomnia on physical and mental health, occupational and vocational functioning, as well as on social domains.[59] Although subjective complaints are not always corroborated with objective measurements, a recent meta-analysis[5] found subtle and selective, yet reliable deficits in studies using objective cognitive functioning measures. For instance, individuals with insomnia show deficits in cognitive performance, most notably in attention, concentration, and memory-related tasks, all of which can produce pervasive consequences in every aspect of daily life. Not surprisingly, daytime complaints are recognized as a primary determinant of help-seeking behaviors among individuals with insomnia.[7]

Long-Term Consequences of Insomnia

Psychological health

In addition to the strong association between insomnia and poor mental health derived from cross-sectional studies, prospective studies indicate that persistent insomnia is also a risk factor for worsening of mental health and the development of several psychiatric disorders.[27,44,64] Persistent insomnia is associated with 2 times higher likelihood of future anxiety[43] and 4 times greater likelihood of future depression in adults,[44,65] adolescents,[66] and children.[67] A meta-analysis summarizing the findings of 21 longitudinal studies found that participants with insomnia had a 2-fold greater risk for developing depression than participants without sleep complaints.[13] One putative mechanism hypothesized that the link between persistent insomnia and depression is the alteration of the arousal system and its subsequent impact on affective and cognitive systems.[64]

The relationship between insomnia and depression can be bidirectional, such that insomnia may be the cause or the result of depression and vice versa, and this relationship may change over time. In a prospective population-based study,[68] nondepressed participants with insomnia at baseline had a 6 times greater risk of developing depression at follow-up compared with counterparts without insomnia. Likewise, depressed participants without insomnia at baseline also had 6 times more risk of developing insomnia 11 years later compared with nondepressed participants. In addition, insomnia and sleep disturbances are associated with increased risk for suicide intentions, attempts, and successes in both clinical[69] and nonclinical samples.[70] In a longitudinal study conducted with 75,000 adults from Norway over a 20-year follow-up period, the age-adjusted and sex-adjusted hazard ratios for suicide were 1.9,

2.7, and 4.3 for reporting sleeping problems sometimes, often, or almost every night, respectively, compared with participants who reported no sleeping problems. Associations were stronger in younger (<50 years) participants, but even after adjusting for mental disorder and alcohol use at baseline, participants with the worst sleep patterns remained at a 2-fold increased risk of suicide.[71]

Physical health

In addition to its association with mental health problems, insomnia is linked with poor physical health as well. Evidence from cross-sectional studies indicates that various medical conditions (eg, hypertension, diabetes) are more common among individuals with insomnia relative to those without insomnia.[72] Individuals with chronic insomnia also show poorer immune functioning (eg, lower natural killer cell activity) compared with good sleepers.[73] Further, insomnia symptoms are linked with alterations in appetite-regulating hormones[74] and notably, the subsequent development of metabolic syndrome.[75] A recent longitudinal study showed that individuals with insomnia had a 40% to 60% increased risk of developing headaches such as migraines and tension-type headaches, respectively, over 11 years after adjusting for age, sex, and sleep medication.[76]

Chronic insomnia is associated with increased nocturnal systolic blood pressure and reduced day-to-night decrease of blood pressure.[77] Chronic insomnia is also considered a significant risk factor in the development of mild-to-moderate hypertension.[78,79] Yet, the insomnia–hypertension relationship remains equivocal; Phillips and colleagues[80] found that insomnia complaints (eg, difficulty initiating sleep) did not predict hypertension 6 years later and reduced the risk in an older cohort of non–African American men (average age of 73 years).

Additional evidence suggests that insomnia is a risk factor for future cardiac events, including acute myocardial infarction[81] and coronary heart disease,[82] even among individuals free of cardiovascular disease.[79] Individuals reporting multiple insomnia symptoms (ie, difficulties initiating/maintaining sleep, early morning awakening) at baseline showed increased incident rates of coronary heart disease compared with those with only one or without any symptoms at baseline.[83] In particular, frequent reports of difficulty initiating and maintaining sleep, as well as nonrestorative sleep, were associated with increased hazard ratios of 1.45, 1.30, and 1.27, respectively, for acute myocardial infarction.[81] Further, insomnia symptoms are significantly associated with cardiovascular and all-cause mortality up to 17 years after insomnia symptoms are detected.[84] This effect is most conspicuous among men with objectively determined short sleep duration.[85] A meta-analysis[86] found that those endorsing insomnia symptoms have a 45% increased risk of cardiovascular morbidity and mortality. However, other studies with shorter follow-up assessments (eg, 6 years) and additional covariates (eg, sleep duration, depression)[87,88] did not identify insomnia as a significant risk factor for future cardiovascular disease or all-cause mortality.[89]

Difficulties initiating or maintaining sleep are associated with 57% to 84% increased risk, respectively, for incident diabetes[90] up to 22 years later.[84] This finding is especially more pronounced among individuals with frequent reports of sleep disturbances[91]; however, this finding was not found in a study of older women[92] or in a more recent study of middle-aged Chinese adults.[27]

Occupational health

Insomnia is often associated with role impairments, particularly in the work environment. Workers with insomnia syndrome report reduced productivity, are absent 8.1 hours more per 3-month period,[93] and have a greater tendency to show up to work late than those without insomnia.[94] Insomnia is associated with a reduced likelihood of future professional advancements (eg, promotion, salary increase)[95–97] and an increased risk of permanent work disability, even after controlling for baseline exposure to disability, sick leave, sleep duration, and other possible confounders.[96,97] Compared with good sleepers, those with sleep disturbances report more intentions of switching occupations, have reduced job satisfaction, fewer adaptive coping skills, rely more on emotion-oriented coping strategies than problem-solving strategies, and report lower feelings of mastery.[98] Insomnia is thus recognized as a significant barrier in the achievement of career and life goals.

Insomnia is closely linked with greater cognitive failures in everyday activities[5] and thus, is also associated with an increased proneness for occupational mishaps, accidents, or errors.[99] Daley and colleagues[100] found that patients with insomnia syndrome were almost twice more likely to have experienced personal and work-related accidents than were good sleepers. Among the elderly, insomnia (and not hypnotic use) was shown to predict falls over a 5-month to 7-month observation period, with the highest risk noted among residents who remained untreated or remained unresponsive to treatment at follow-up.[101] Drivers reporting insomnia symptoms, poor sleep quality, prolonged wakefulness, or sleepiness also have an increased risk of being involved in nocturnal[102] and diurnal automobile accidents.[103]

ECONOMIC BURDEN OF INSOMNIA

Insomnia carries significant economic burden for the health care system. One study[104] projected that the costs for medical expenditures (ie, claims for inpatients/outpatients, pharmacy, emergency room services) were $934 more for young to middle-aged adults with insomnia (18–64 years) and $1143 more for older adults with insomnia (>65 years) compared with well-matched individuals without insomnia. Insomnia severity and frequency also show a dose-response effect with direct costs, such that annual health care costs among members of a health plan in the United States are estimated to be $1323 for those with moderate-to-severe insomnia, $907 for subthreshold insomnia, and $757 for good sleepers.[105] In a similar study,[106] participants with frequent complaints of insomnia symptoms reported higher annual medical costs ($2552) than did those with less frequent insomnia symptoms ($1510). In a population-based sample, Daley and colleagues[93] reported the annual per person insomnia-related direct costs were $293 for individuals with an insomnia syndrome, $160 for those with insomnia symptoms, and $45 for good sleepers. Cost-benefit analyses for insomnia treatment estimated lower monthly health care costs and increased quality-adjusted life year among remitted patients compared with their non-remitted counterparts.[107,108]

The indirect costs of insomnia can also add to the economic burden of society. Using an administrative database, annual mean incremental costs for sick leave, short-term and long-term disability, and workers' compensation was $567 more for employees with insomnia compared with employees without insomnia.[109] The estimated expenditures of employed health plan members because of absenteeism[104] and presenteeism (ie, attending work while ill, leading to low work performance) were significantly more among employees with insomnia than employees without insomnia.[110] Costs for reduced productivity were highest for employed health plan members with moderate-to-severe insomnia, followed by those with insomnia symptoms and those without insomnia.[105] Similar reports were documented in a population-based sample for overall indirect costs, with the highest cost per person for those with an insomnia syndrome estimated to be at $4717 annually, followed by those with insomnia symptoms at \$1271 and good sleepers at \$376.[93] The annual indirect costs for resources lost were nearly 10 times higher than the direct costs specific to treating insomnia.[93] Although insomnia carries a significant economic burden, it is difficult from the available evidence to separate expenses that are caused specifically by insomnia from those expenses driven by common co-occurring conditions such as depression and pain.

COMMUNITY/PUBLIC HEALTH EDUCATION AND PREVENTION OF INSOMNIA

Despite the considerable health, social, and economic burden of insomnia, it is often underrecognized and untreated in both pediatric[111] and adult populations. Although there is solid evidence showing the efficacy of insomnia therapies[112] and strong incentives for prevention strategies, methods for preventing insomnia remain underdeveloped.[113,114] As such, it is imperative to find appropriate strategies for the prevention of insomnia.

Although some risk factors are unmodifiable, (eg, age, sex, genetics), others are modifiable (eg, maladaptive sleep practices). Unmodifiable risk factors can be used to identify at-risk individuals, whereas education and behavioral interventions that are practical and easily sustainable[115] can be used to alter modifiable risk factors. For example, given the greater likelihood of insomnia within a family,[47,48] prevention approaches can be particularly helpful to alter lifestyle behaviors (eg, maintain a regular sleep schedule, reduced intake of stimulants) and sleeping environment (eg, reduced noise level), all of which may have a significant impact on the general population, but particularly among vulnerable populations.

From a public health perspective, an important step in insomnia prevention involves increasing awareness on the importance of adequate sleep and the debilitating effects of insomnia.[113,114] Some individuals hold misconceptions or lack knowledge about healthy sleep patterns and sleep disorders (eg, causes, consequences, treatment), which, in turn, can contribute to poor sleep practices. Public health education campaigns can prove beneficial to increase awareness about the importance of sleep and about behavioral practices to prevent sleep problems. Although it is recognized that health care professionals should routinely evaluate sleep and provide some sleep education as part of patient care, many professionals rate their own sleep knowledge as fair or poor.[116] Furthermore, during consultations, health care professionals do not typically initiate inquiries about their patient's sleep, unless the patient, a family member, or patient's caretaker presents sleep-related concerns.[111,116] Thus, an important step is increasing education and training on sleep for health care professionals.[113]

Sleep counseling may lead to changes in patients' attitudes, knowledge, and behaviors toward sleep. Borrowing successful strategies from other prevention programs may also lead to changes. For instance, providing accurate information about the importance of sleep and differences in sleep needs as a function of different age groups may bring people to make sleep more of a priority in their life. Likewise, making simple and specific behavioral recommendations (eg, reduce time spent awake in bed and get up at the same time every morning) can be effective to alleviate insomnia before it reaches clinical threshold. Although the relation between sleep knowledge and sleep practices is mixed, sleep education remains an essential step in promoting healthy sleep. In fact, general education interventions targeted at children[117] and parents[118] have yielded promising results.

Given the heavy burden that insomnia places on the individual and society, implementing prevention strategies at the community level is important. Recently, Kraus and Rabin[114] proposed launching a public-wide awareness campaign entitled *Sleep America*, with specific aims to (1) promote insomnia education using various mediums (eg, Web-based initiatives), (2) increase accessibility of insomnia treatments (eg, behavioral sleep medicine), and (3) monitor and potentially refute misleading claims about non–evidence-based insomnia treatments. Future research is needed to evaluate the cost-effectiveness of prevention strategies that focus on modifiable risk factors, emphasize knowledge translation on sleep education, and can be delivered at the individual and societal level. This research should be implemented, particularly, among at-risk populations for an effective campaign that improves public health.

KEY POINTS AND SUGGESTIONS FOR FUTURE EPIDEMIOLOGIC STUDIES

The epidemiology of insomnia has received increased attention in the last decade, and investigators have moved from a purely cross-sectional approach of estimating prevalence of insomnia and its correlates to a more prospective and longitudinal approach aimed at documenting its natural history, risk factors, and long-term consequences. There is now substantial evidence that insomnia is a highly prevalent and persistent condition, both as a symptom and as a syndrome. Its persistence is associated with increased risk for mental (eg, major depression), physical (eg, hypertension), and occupational health problems (eg, disability). At least half a dozen studies have documented the economic burden of insomnia, with the main finding being that insomnia is a costly health problem. Notably, treating insomnia (eg, professional consultations, medications, sleep-promoting aids) is far less costly compared with the loss of human resources (eg, absenteeism) due to insomnia.

Recent findings concerning the epidemiology of insomnia have direct implications for clinical studies, including (1) the need for large, population-based studies aimed at evaluating whether insomnia can be prevented in cohorts of at-risk individuals; (2) clinical studies that evaluate whether the morbidity associated with chronic insomnia can be reversed; and (3) prospective health economic evaluations (ie, cost-benefit, cost-usefulness, cost-effectiveness) of different therapeutic approaches and treatment delivery models (eg, individual vs group vs self-help therapies). Such studies might have the greatest impact on decision makers and the allocation of health care resources for insomnia.

Progress on the epidemiology of insomnia has been hampered by important methodological shortcomings, including, but not limited to, inconsistent case definitions and standardized assessment procedures across studies. These methodological problems have contributed to producing extensive variability in estimates of prevalence, incidence, and persistence rates of insomnia. It will be essential in future studies to rely on standard case definition and assessment procedures in order to derive more reliable estimates of insomnia. Given the recent efforts to harmonize insomnia diagnostic criteria between the DSM and ICSD nosology, it may be easier for investigators to follow this recommendation. Studies attempting to quantify the economic burden of insomnia have also produced variable and imprecise cost estimates because investigators have not separated the costs driven specifically by insomnia from those costs attributable to frequently comorbid psychiatric or medical disorders.

Although there is extensive evidence about the prevalence and incidence of insomnia, there is less information about its natural history and long-term course and prognosis. Also, little is known about moderating and mediating variables that modulate the course of insomnia (ie, remission, relapse). Additional prospective and longitudinal studies are especially important to identify early precursors and precipitating factors of insomnia. It is important to monitor these factors at regular intervals in relation to onset, remission, and relapse. Although there is evidence that insomnia is a condition that may wax and wane, it is difficult to predict whether an acute insomnia episode will be transient or develop a more chronic course. Previous studies have not examined course modifiers (eg, treatment initiation). Additional research is needed to achieve more precise identification of moderating and mediating factors likely to be associated with natural course changes. Information about life events, health status, treatment, and products used to alleviate sleep problems would help to characterize more precisely the natural history of insomnia and potential course modifiers. A better understanding of how insomnia evolves over time and what factors trigger an episode or perpetuate it over time is critical for developing effective prevention and treatment programs.

DISCLOSURE

Preparation of this article was supported by the Canadian Institutes of Health Research (MOP42504) and by the National Institutes of Health (MH078188 and MH60413).

REFERENCES

1. American Academy of Sleep Medicine. International classification of sleep disorders: diagnostic and coding manual. 2nd edition. Westchester (IL): American Academy of Sleep Medicine; 2005.
2. American Psychiatric Association. Diagnostic and statistical manual of mental disorders (DSM5). Washington, DC: American Psychiatric Association; 2013.
3. Buysse DJ, Thompson W, Scott J, et al. Daytime symptoms in primary insomnia: a prospective analysis using ecological momentary assessment. Sleep Med 2007;8:198–208.
4. Edinger JD, Bonnet MH, Bootzin RR, et al. Derivation of research diagnostic criteria for insomnia: report of an American Academy of Sleep Medicine work group. Sleep 2004;27:1567–96.
5. Fortier-Brochu E, Beaulieu-Bonneau S, IversH etal. Insomnia and daytime cognitive performance: a meta-analysis. Sleep Med Rev 2012;16:83–94.
6. Roth T, Jaeger S, Jin R, et al. Sleep problems, comorbid mental disorders, and role functioning in the national comorbidity survey replication. Biol Psychiatry 2006;60:1364–71.
7. Morin CM, LeBlanc M, Daley M, et al. Epidemiology of insomnia: prevalence, self-help treatments, consultations, and determinants of help-seeking behaviors. Sleep Med 2006;7:123–30.
8. Edinger J, Morin CM. Insomnia disorder: A unified approach. Paper presented at SLEEP 2013.

Proceedings of the 27th APSS, 2013 June 1-5; Baltimore, MD, USA.

9. Morin CM, LeBlanc M, Ivers H, et al. Monthly fluctuations of insomnia symptoms in a population-based sample. Sleep 2014;37:319–26.

10. Ohayon MM, Riemann D, Morin C, et al. Hierarchy of insomnia criteria based on daytime consequences. Sleep Med 2012;13:2–7.

11. Nierenberg AA, Keefe BR, Leslie VC, et al. Residual symptoms in depressed patients who respond acutely to fluoxetine. J Clin Psychiatry 1999;60: 221–5.

12. Perlis ML, Giles DE, Buysse DJ, et al. Self-reported sleep disturbance as a prodromal symptom in recurrent depression. J Affect Disord 1997;42: 209–12.

13. Baglioni C, Battagliese G, Feige B, et al. Insomnia as a predictor of depression: a meta analytic evaluation of longitudinal epidemiological studies. J Affect Disord 2011;135:10–9.

14. Fava M, McCall WV, Krystal A, et al. Eszopiclone co-administered with fluoxetine in patients with insomnia coexisting with major depressive disorder. Biol Psychiatry 2006;59:1052–60.

15. Manber R, Edinger JD, Gress JL, et al. Cognitive behavioral therapy for insomnia enhances depression outcome in patients with comorbid major depressive disorder and insomnia. Sleep 2008; 31:489–95.

16. Karacan I, Thornby JI, Anch M, et al. Prevalence of sleep disturbance in a primarily urban Florida County. Soc Sci Med 1976;10:239–44.

17. Bixler ED, Kales A, Soldatos CR, et al. Prevalence of sleep disorders in the Los Angeles metropolitan area. Am J Psychiatry 1979;136:1257–62.

18. Ohayon MM. Epidemiology of insomnia: what we know and what we still need to learn. Sleep Med Rev 2002;6:97–111.

19. Morin CM, LeBlanc M, Belanger L, et al. Epidemiology of insomnia in the adult Canadian population. Can J Psychiatry 2011;56:540–8.

20. Jansson-Frojmark M, Linton SJ. The course of insomnia over one year: a longitudinal study in the general population in Sweden. Sleep 2008;31: 881–6.

21. Ohayon MM, Reynolds CF 3rd. Epidemiological and clinical relevance of insomnia diagnosis algorithms according to the DSM-IV and the International Classification of Sleep Disorders (ICSD). Sleep Med 2009;10:952–60.

22. Jaussent I, Dauvilliers Y, Ancelin ML, et al. Insomnia symptoms in older adults: associated factors and gender differences. Am J Geriatr Psychiatry 2011;19:88–97.

23. Simon GE, VonKorff M. Prevalence, burden, and treatment of insomnia in primary care. Am J Psychiatry 1997;154:1417–23.

24. Aikens JE, Rouse ME. Help-seeking for insomnia among adult patients in primary care. J Am Board Fam Pract 2005;18:257–61.

25. Zhang B, Wing YK. Sex differences in insomnia: a meta-analysis. Sleep 2006;29:85–93.

26. Ford DE, Kamerow DB. Epidemiologic study of sleep disturbances and psychiatric disorders. An opportunity for prevention? J Am Med Assoc 1989;262:1479–84.

27. Zhang J, Lam SP, Li SX, et al. Long-term outcomes and predictors of chronic insomnia: a prospective study in Hong Kong Chinese adults. Sleep Med 2012;13:455–62.

28. National sleep Foundation (NSF) (n.d.). Sleep in America Poll. 2013. Available at: http://www. sleepfoundation.org/category/article-type/ sleepamerica-polls.

29. Roberts RE, Roberts CR, Chan W. Ethnic differences in symptoms of insomnia among adolescents. Sleep 2006;29:359–65.

30. Paine SJ, Gander PH, Harris R, et al. Who reports insomnia? Relationships with age, sex, ethnicity, and socioeconomic deprivation. Sleep 2004;27: 1163–9.

31. Seicean S, Neuhauser D, Strohl K, et al. An exploration of differences in sleep characteristics between Mexico-born US immigrants and other Americans to address the Hispanic paradox. Sleep 2011;34:1021–31.

32. Jean-Louis G, Magai CM, Cohen CI, et al. Ethnic differences in self-reported sleep problems in older adults. Sleep 2001;24:926–33.

33. Clever MN, Bruck D. Comparisons of the sleep quality, daytime sleepiness, and sleep cognitions of Caucasian Australians and Zimbabwean and Ghanaian black immigrants. S Afr J Psychol 2013;43:81–93.

34. Soldatos C, Allaert F, Ohta T, et al. How do individuals sleep around the world? Results from a single-day survey in ten countries. Sleep Med 2005;6: 5–13.

35. Leger D, Poursain B. An international survey of insomnia: under-recognition and under-treatment of a polysymptomatic condition. Curr Med Res Opin 2005;21:1785–92.

36. Dregan A, Armstrong D. Cross-country variation in sleep disturbance among working and older age groups: an analysis based on the European Social Survey. Int Psychogeriatr 2011;23:1413–20.

37. Leger D, Poursain B, Neubauer D, et al. An international survey of sleeping problems in the general population. Curr Med Res Opin 2008;24: 307–17.

38. Liu X, Liu L, Owens JA, et al. Sleep patterns and sleep problems among schoolchildren in the United States and China. Pediatrics 2005;115: 241–9.

39. Mindell J, Sadeh A, Wiegand B, et al. Cross- cultural differences in infant and toddler sleep. Sleep Med 2010;11:274–80.

40. Ban L, Kashima Y, Haslam N. Does understanding behaviour make it seem normal? Perceptions of abnormality among Euro-Australians and Chinese-Singaporeans. J Cross Cult Psychol 2012;43:286–98.

41. Sayar K, Kirmayer LJ, Taillefer SS. Predictors of somatic symptoms in depressive disorder. Gen Hosp Psychiatry 2003;25:108–14.

42. LeBlanc M, Mérette C, Savard J, et al. Incidence and risk factors of insomnia in a population- based sample. Sleep 2009;32:1027–37.

43. Morphy H, Dunn KM, Lewis M, et al. Epidemiology of insomnia: a longitudinal study in a UK population. Sleep 2007;30:274–80.

44. Breslau N, Roth T, Rosenthal L, et al. Sleep disturbance and psychiatric disorders: a longitudinal epidemiological study of young adults. Biol Psychiatry 1996;39:411–8.

45. Ellis JG, Perlis ML, Neale LF, et al. The natural history of insomnia: focus on prevalence and incidence of acute insomnia. J Psychiatr Res 2012;46:1278–85.

46. Roberts RE, Shema SJ, Kaplan GA. Prospective data on sleep complaints and associated risk factors in an older cohort. Psychosom Med 1999;61:188–96.

47. Dauvilliers Y, Morin CM, Cervena K, et al. Family studies in insomnia. J Psychosom Res 2005;58:271–8.

48. Beaulieu-Bonneau S, LeBlanc M, Merette C, et al. Family history of insomnia in a population-based sample. Sleep 2007;30:1739–45.

49. Vgontzas AN, Bixler EO, Lin HM, et al. Chronic insomnia is associated with nyctohemeral activation of the hypothalamic-pituitary-adrenal axis: clinical implications. J Clin Endocrinol Metab 2001;86:3787–94.

50. Riemann D, Spiegelhadler R, Feige B, et al. The hyperarousal model of insomnia: a review of the concept and its evidence. Sleep Med Rev 2010;14:19–31.

51. Bonnet MH, Arand DL. Hyperarousal and insomnia: state of the science. Sleep Med Rev 2010;14:9–15.

52. Morin CM, Bélanger L, LeBlanc M, et al. The Natural History of Insomnia: a population-based 3-year longitudinal study. Arch Intern Med 2009;169:447–53.

53. Fok M, Stewart R, Besset A, et al. Incidence and persistence of sleep complaints in a community older population. Int J Geriatr Psychiatry 2010;25:37–45.

54. Kim JM, Stewart R, Kim SW, et al. Insomnia, depression, and physical disorders in late life: a 2-year longitudinal community study in Koreans. Sleep 2009;32:1221–8.

55. Morgan K, Clarke D. Longitudinal trends in late-life insomnia: implications for prescribing. Age Ageing 1997;26:179–84.

56. Quan SF, Katz R, Olson J, et al. Factors associated with incidence and persistence of symptoms of disturbed sleep in an elderly cohort: the cardiovascular health study. Am J Med Sci 2005;329:163–72.

57. Buysse DJ, Ancoli-Israel S, Edinger JD, et al. Recommendations for a standard research assessment of insomnia. Sleep 2006;29:1155–73.

58. National Institutes of Health. National Institutes of Health State of the Science conference statement: manifestations and management of chronic insomnia in adults, June 13-15, 2005. Sleep 2005;28:1049–57.

59. Kyle SD, Espie CA, Morgan K. Not just a minor thing, it is something major, which stops you from functioning daily": quality of life and daytime functioning in insomnia. Behav Sleep Med 2010;8:123–40.

60. LeBlanc M, Beaulieu-Bonneau S, Mérette C, et al. Psychological and health-related quality of life factors associated with insomnia in a population-based sample. J Psychosom Res 2007;63:157–66.

61. Novak M, Mucsi I, Shapiro CM, et al. Increased utilization of health services by insomniacs-an epidemiological perspective. J Psychosom Res 2004;56:527–36.

62. Hasler PB, Troxel WM. Couples' nighttime sleep efficiency and concordance: evidence for bidirectional associations with daytime relationship functioning. Psychosom Med 2010;72:794–801.

63. Lemola S, Räikkönen K, Gomez V, et al. Optimism and self-esteem are related to sleep. Results from a large community-based sample. Int J Behav Med 2012. https://doi.org/10.1007/s12529-012-9272-z.

64. Baglioni C, Riemann D. Is chronic insomnia a precursor to major depression? Epidemiological and biological findings. Curr Psychiatry Rep 2012;14:511–8.

65. Buysse DJ, Angst J, Gamma A, et al. Prevalence, course, and comorbidity of insomnia and depression in young adults. Sleep 2008;31:473–80.

66. Roberts RE, Duong HT. Depression and insomnia among adolescents: a prospective perspective. J Affect Disord 2012;148:66–71.

67. Gregory AM, Rijsdijk FV, Lau JY, et al. The direction of longitudinal associations between sleep problems and depression symptoms: a study of twins aged 8 and 10 years. Sleep 2009;32:189–99.

68. Sivertsen B, Salo P, Mykletun A. The bidirectional association between depression and insomnia: the HUNT study. Psychosom Med 2012;74:758–65.

69. Krakow B, Ribeiro JD, Ulibarri VA, et al. Sleep disturbances and suicidal ideation in sleep medical center patients. J Affect Disord 2011;131:422–7.

70. Carli V, Roy A, Bevilacqua L, et al. Insomnia and suicidal behaviour in prisoners. Psychiatry Res 2011;185:141–4.

71. Bjørngaard JH, Bjerkeset O, Romundstad P, et al. Sleeping problems and suicide in 75,000 Norwegian adults: a 20 year follow-up of the HUNT I Study. Sleep 2011;34:1155–9.

72. Pearson NJ, Johnson L, Nahin RL. Insomnia, trouble sleeping, and complementary and alternative medicine: analysis of the 2002 National Health Interview Survey Data. Arch Intern Med 2006;166: 1775–82.

73. Savard J, Laroche L, Simard S, et al. Chronic insomnia and immune functioning. Psychosom Med 2003;65:211–21.

74. Motivala SJ, Tomiyama AJ, Ziegler M, et al. Nocturnal levels of ghrelin and leptin and sleep in chronic insomnia. Psychoneuroendocrinology 2009;34:540–5.

75. Troxel WM, Buysse DJ, Matthews KA, et al. Sleep symptoms predict the development of the metabolic syndrome. Sleep 2010;33:1633–40.

76. Odegård SS, Sand T, Engstrøm M, et al. The long-term effect of insomnia on primary headaches. A prospective population-based cohort study (HUNT-2 and HUNT-3). Headache 2011;51:570–80.

77. Lanfranchi PA, Pennestri MH, Fradette L, et al. Nighttime blood pressure in normotensive subjects with chronic insomnia: implications for cardiovascular risk. Sleep 2009;32:760–6.

78. Suka M, Yoshida K, Sugimori H. Persistent insomnia is a predictor of hypertension in Japanese male workers. J Occup Health 2003;45: 344–50.

79. Phillips B, Mannino DM. Do insomnia complaints cause hypertension or cardiovascular disease? J Clin Sleep Med 2007;3:489–94.

80. Phillips B, Bůzková P, Enright P. Insomnia did not predict incident hypertension in older adults in the cardiovascular health study. Sleep 2009;32: 65–72.

81. Laugsand LE, Vatten LJ, Platou C, et al. Insomnia and the risk of acute myocardial infarction. Circulation 2011;124:2073–81.

82. Chandola T, Ferrie JE, Perski A, et al. The effect of short sleep duration on coronary heart disease risk is greatest among those with sleep disturbance: a prospective study from the Whitehall II cohort. Sleep 2010;33:739–44.

83. Loponen M, Hublin C, Kalimo R, et al. Joint effect of self-reported sleep problems and three components of the metabolic syndrome on risk of coronary heart disease. J Psychosom Res 2010;68: 149–58.

84. Nilsson PM, Roost M, Engstrom G, et al. Incidence of diabetes in middle-aged men is related to sleep disturbances. Diabetes Care 2004;27:2464–9.

85. VgontzasAN, Liao D, Pejovic S, et al. Insomnia with short sleep duration and mortality: the Penn State Cohort. Sleep 2010;33:1159–64.

86. Sofi F, Cesari F, Casini A, et al. Insomnia and risk of cardiovascular disease: a meta-analysis. Eur J Prev Cardiol 2012. https://doi.org/10.1177/2047487312460020.

87. Kripke DF, Garfinkel L, Wingard DL, et al. Mortality associated with sleep duration and insomnia. Arch Gen Psychiatry 2002;59:131–6.

88. Phillips BA, Mannino DM. Does insomnia kill? Sleep 2005;28:965–71.

89. Schwartz SW, Cornoni-Huntley J, Cole SR, et al. Are sleep complaints an independent risk factor for myocardial infarction? Ann Epidemiol 1998;8: 384–92.

90. Cappuccio FP, D'Elia L, Strazzullo P, et al. Quantity and quality of sleep and incidence of type 2 diabetes: a systematic review and meta-analysis. Diabetes Care 2010;33:414–20.

91. Kawakami N, Takatsuka N, Shimizu H. Sleep disturbance and onset of type 2 diabetes. Diabetes Care 2004;27:282–3.

92. Bjorkelund C, Bondyr-Carlsson D, Lapidus L, et al. Sleep disturbances in midlife unrelated to 32-year diabetes incidence: the prospective population study of women in Gothenburg. Diabetes Care 2005;28:2739–44.

93. Daley M, Morin CM, LeBlanc M, et al. The economic burden of insomnia: direct and indirect costs for individuals with insomnia syndrome, insomnia symptoms, and good sleepers. Sleep 2009;32: 55–64.

94. David B, Morgan K. Workplace performance, but not punctuality, is consistently impaired among people with insomnia. Proceedings of the 19th Congress of the European Sleep Research Society, Glasgow. J Sleep Res 2008;17:193.

95. Johnson LC, Spinweber C. Quality of sleep and performance in the navy: a longitudinal study of good and poor sleepers. In: Guilleminault C, Lugaresi E, editors. Sleep/wake disorders. New York: Raven Press; 1983. p. 13–28.

96. Sivertsen B, Overland S, Pallesen S, et al. Insomnia and long sleep duration are risk factors for later work disability. Hordaland Health Study J Sleep Res 2009;18:122–8.

97. Sivertsen B, Overland S, Neckelmann D, et al. The long-term effect of insomnia on work disability: the HUNT-2 historical cohort study. Am J Epidemiol 2006;163:1018–24.

98. Morin CM, Rodrigues S, Ivers H. Role of stress, arousal, and coping skills in primary insomnia. Psychosom Med 2003;65:259–67.

99. Shahly V, Berglund PA, Coulouvrat C, et al. The associations of insomnia with costly workplace accidents and errors: results from the America

Insomnia Survey. Arch Gen Psychiatry 2012;69: 1054–63.

100. Daley M, Morin CM, LeBlanc M, et al. Insomnia and its relationship to health-care utilization, work absenteeism, productivity and accidents. Sleep Med 2009;10:427–38.

101. Avidan AY, Fries BE, James ML, et al. Insomnia and hypnotic use, recorded in the minimum data set, as predictors of falls and hip fractures in Michigan nursing homes. J Am Geriatr Soc 2005;53:955–62.

102. Philip P, Sagaspe P, Lagarde E, et al. Sleep disorders and accidental risk in a large group of regular registered highway drivers. Sleep Med 2010;11: 973–9.

103. Lucidi F, Mallia L, Violani C, et al. The contributions of sleep-related risk factors to diurnal car accidents. Accid Anal Prev 2013;51:135–40.

104. Ozminkowski RJ, Wang S, Walsh JK. The direct and indirect costs of untreated insomnia in adults in the United States. Sleep 2007;30:263–73.

105. Sarsour K, Kalsekar A, Swindle R, et al. The association between insomnia severity and healthcare and productivity costs in a health plan sample. Sleep 2011;34:443–50.

106. Foley KA, Sarsour K, Kalsekar A, et al. Subtypes of sleep disturbance: associations among symptoms, comorbidities, treatment, and medical costs. BeHav Sleep Med 2010;8:90–104.

107. Botteman M. Health economics of insomnia therapy: implications for policy. Sleep Med 2009;10: S22–5.

108. Morgan K, Dixon S, Mathers N, et al. Psychological treatment for insomnia in the regulation of long-term hypnotic drug use. Health Technol Assess 2004;8:1–68.

109. Kleinman NL, Brook RA, Doan JF, et al. Health benefit costs and absenteeism due to insomnia from the employer's perspective: a retrospective, case-control, database study. J Clin Psychiatry 2009;70:1098–104.

110. Kessler RC, Berglund PA, Coulouvrat C, et al. Insomnia and the performance of US workers: results from the America Insomnia Survey. Sleep 2011;34:1161–71.

111. Owens JA. The practice of pediatric sleep medicine: results of a community survey. Pediatrics 2001;108:E51.

112. Morin CM, Benca R. Chronic insomnia. Lancet 2012;379:1129–41.

113. Institute of Medicine of the National Academies (IMNA). Sleep disorders and sleep deprivation. Washington, DC: The National Academies Press; 2006.

114. Kraus SS, Rabin LA. Sleep America: managing the crisis of adult chronic insomnia and associated conditions. J Affect Disord 2012;138:192–212.

115. Pawson R, Owen L, Wong G. Legislating for health: locating the evidence. J Public Health Policy 2010; 31:164–77.

116. Rosen RC, Zozula R, Jahn EG, et al. Low rates of recognition of sleep disorders in primary care: comparison of a community-based versus clinical academic setting. Sleep Med 2001;2:47–55.

117. Sousa IC, Araújo JF, Azevedo CV. The effect of a sleep hygiene education program on the sleep-wake cycle of Brazilian adolescent students. Sleep Biol Rhythms 2007;5:251–8.

118. Jones CH, Owens JA, Pham B. Can a brief educational intervention improve parents' knowledge of healthy children's sleep? A pilot test. Health Educ J 2012. https://doi.org/10.1177/0017896912452073.

119. Jansson M, Linton SJ. Psychosocial work stressors in the development and maintenance of insomnia: a prospective study. J Occup Health Psychol 2006;11:241–8.

120. Jansson-Fröjmark M, Lindblom K. A bidirectional relationship between anxiety and depression, and insomnia? A prospective study in the general population. J Psychosom Res 2008;64:443–9.

121. Skapinakis P, Rai D, Anagnostopoulos F, et al. Sleep disturbances and depressive symptoms: an investigation of their longitudinal association in a representative sample of the UK general population. Psychol Med 2013;43:329–39.

122. Komada Y, Nomura T, Kusumi M, et al. A two-year follow-up study on the symptoms of sleep disturbances/insomnia and their effects on daytime functioning. Sleep Med 2012;13:1115–21.

123. Fernandez-Mendoza J, Vgontzas AN, Bixler EO, et al. Clinical and polysomnographic predictors of the natural history of poor sleep in the general population. Sleep 2012;35:689–97.

124. Vgontzas AN, Fernandez-Mendoza J, Bixler EO, et al. Persistent insomnia: the role of objective short sleep duration and mental health. Sleep 2012;35: 61–8.

125. Singareddy R, Vgontzas AN, Fernandez-Mendoza J, et al. Risk factors for incident chronic insomnia: a general population prospective study. Sleep Med 2012;3:346–53.

The Effects of Insomnia and Sleep Loss on Cardiovascular Disease

Meena S. Khan, MD[a,b,*], Rita Aouad, MD[a]

KEYWORDS

- Short sleep duration • Insomnia • Hypertension • Diabetes • Prediabetes • Cardiovascular disease

KEY POINTS

- Chronic insomnia is a pervasive issue in the general population. It is associated with poor quality of life, increased use of heath care resources, and poor mood.
- Those who are sleep deprived or have insomnia have elevated cortisol levels, increased markers of sympathetic system activity, increased metabolic rate, and endothelial dysfunction; all of which are correlated with increased risk of cardiovascular disease and risk factors.
- Both short sleep duration and insomnia are linked to the development of diabetes and hypertension.
- Insomnia is associated with increased risk of cardiovascular disease and mortality although not all studies show consistent findings of a positive association.
- Evaluation of sleep health may be an important part of the management of those with cardiovascular disease.

INTRODUCTION

Sleep and its impact on health have been increasingly explored over the past few decades. Sleep loss has negative impacts on quality of life, mood, cognitive function, and health. Insomnia and difficulty sleeping are also prevalent issues, affecting up to 35% of the population at some point in their lives. Insomnia is linked to poor mood, increased use of health care resources and decreased quality of life as well as possibly cardiovascular risk factors and disease. Studies have shown increased cortisol levels, decreased immunity, and increased markers of sympathetic activity in sleep-deprived healthy subjects and those with chronic insomnia. The literature also shows that subjective complaints consistent with chronic insomnia and shortened sleep time, both independently and in combination, can be associated with the development of diabetes, hypertension, and cardiovascular disease. This article explores the relationship and strength of association between insufficient sleep and insomnia with these health conditions.

SLEEP AND HEALTH

Various sleep disorders, such as obstructive sleep apnea and insomnia, have been associated with a variety of health problems and impaired quality of life. Chronic sleep loss can lead to impaired vigilance and performance, slowing of cognitive processes, depressed mood, and poor attention.[1,2] Sleep quality and duration can affect cellular immunity and cytokine levels, such that a person's immunity can be impaired with even mild sleep loss.[3,4] Impaired sleep is also linked to changes in metabolism, increased caloric intake, and

Sleep Med Clin 12 (2017) 167-177 http://dx.doi.org/10.1016/j.jsmc.2017.01.0051556-407X/17/© 2017 Elsevier Inc. All rights reserved.
[a] Division of Pulmonary, Critical Care, and Sleep Medicine, Department of Internal Medicine, The Ohio State University, Columbus, OH, USA; [b] Department of Neurology, The Ohio State University, Columbus, OH, USA
* Corresponding author. Division of Pulmonary, Critical Care, and Sleep Medicine, Department of Internal Medicine, The Ohio State University, 201 DHLRI, 473 West 12th Avenue, Columbus, OH 43210.
E-mail address: Meena.Khan@osumc.edu

Sleep Med Clin 17 (2022) 193–203
https://doi.org/10.1016/j.jsmc.2022.02.008
1556-407X/22/© 2022 Elsevier Inc. All rights reserved.

obesity.[5,6] Short sleep duration is associated with deleterious effects on health, such as increased incidence of all-cause mortality, coronary artery disease, type 2 diabetes mellitus, obesity, and hypertension.[7–11] Short sleep duration has multiple causes, including behavior-induced sleep deprivation, obstructive sleep apnea, shift work syndrome, and insomnia.

Insomnia is a sleep disorder plaguing an estimated 15% of the population[12] and often goes untreated. Chronic insomnia is defined by the *International Classification of Sleep Disorders–Third Edition* as a patient or caregiver, describing difficulty falling asleep, maintaining sleep, waking up earlier than desired, resistance to going to bed on an appropriate schedule, or difficulty sleeping without a parent or caregiver intervention, associated with at least one symptom that is a consequence of insomnia, for 3 months or more. The 2005 US National Health and Wellness Survey showed that insomnia is associated with a subjective feeling of decreased quality of life and increased mental health symptoms as well as increased absenteeism from work and decreased work productivity.[13] Insomnia is associated with increased reports of heart disease, high blood pressure, chronic pain, and development of depression and anxiety[14–16] as well as increased use of medical resources and economic burden.[17] Subjective complaints of insomnia and increased sleeping pill use are associated with increased mortality.[18,19] Although the link to mortality has not been demonstrated in all studies,[20–22] this possible association emphasizes the importance of sleep on health.

SLEEP AND ITS EFFECTS ON IMMUNITY AND METABOLIC ACTIVITY

Sleep can influence measures of immunity as well as metabolism and inflammation. There are several possible mechanisms of how insomnia and sleep loss may lead to cardiovascular disease and associated risk factors. Immunity can be divided into adaptive and innate immunity, both of which are regulated by circadian rhythms and sleep. Adaptive immunity refers to immunity that is acquired against a live pathogen to which the organism was previously exposed. Innate immunity refers to defense mechanisms against any foreign body that develops within hours of exposure. The distribution of immune cells is circadian related. Leukocytes, granulocytes, monocytes, and major lymphocytes reach peak levels in the early evening and decline throughout the night.[23] Alternatively, the immune cells responsible for the adaptive immune system are regulated by sleep, during which

the levels of interleukin (IL)-2, interferon-», and IL-12[24–26] increase. Nocturnal sleep also regulates innate immunity by increasing natural killer cells during sleep and increasing levels the further the night progresses.[27] Sleep loss leads to a decrease in IL-2,[23] and chronic insomnia is associated with a decrease in CD3, CD4, and CD8 counts.[28] A loss of natural killer cells and an increase in proinflammatory cytokines, such as IL-6, are also seen during nocturnal sleep.[29] Clinically, sleep loss is associated with decreased immune response to vaccinations and increased susceptibility to infections, such as pneumonia, herpes zoster, and the common cold.[30–34]

The sympathetic nervous system and endocrine system are also affected by sleep. Experimental sleep loss has been demonstrated to lead to alterations in these systems, reflecting a proinflammatory state that can lead to obesity and cardiovascular risk. Sleep fragmentation for 5 months in mice models was shown to cause vascular endothelial dysfunction and increased blood pressure changes.[35] Norepinephrine and epinephrine are normally decreased during sleep although the degree of change across stages is not definable due to conflicting data.[36–38] Partial sleep deprivation is associated with increased sympathetic activity; a study looking at sleep loss of 3 hours for one night only showed increased norepinephrine and epinephrine levels during sleep.[39] Restricting sleep in healthy individuals can increase hunger, impair glucose tolerance, decrease insulin sensitivity, increase cortisol levels, and increase sympathetic system activity.[40–43] Reducing slow-wave sleep, in particular, can result in reduced insulin sensitivity and increased glucose tolerance, even if the total sleep time remains the same.[44] A randomized crossover study by Rao and colleagues[45] compared five nights of normal sleep with five nights of partial sleep deprivation (4 hours in bed) in 14 healthy subjects and found the partial sleep deprivation group had signs of decreased insulin sensitivity, increased cortisol, and increased catecholamine levels, all of which are indicators of increased stress.[45] The increased hunger, impaired glucose tolerance, and other metabolic changes that occur as a result of sleep restriction may lead to an increased risk of obesity, diabetes, and other cardiovascular risk factors.[43]

The consequences of sleep deprivation to the sympathetic and endocrine systems have been demonstrated in insomnia subjects as well. Chronic insomniacs have higher evening corticotropin and cortisol levels compared with age-matched and body mass index (BMI)-matched healthy controls.[46] Increased arousals during sleep are associated with elevated evening cortisol levels in both chronic insomniacs and age-matched and gender-matched healthy controls.[47] Increased wake time is correlated with increased 24-h cortisol levels, whereas increased catecholamine levels are associated with increased stage 1 and decreased stage 3 sleep in chronic insomniacs.[48] Insomniacs also have an increased metabolic rate, defined as increased whole-body oxygen consumption, compared with age-matched, gender-matched, and weight-matched controls,[49] as well as increased heart rate.[50] These observed metabolic changes may be an underlying mechanism for increased cardiovascular risk factors and disease.

SLEEP LOSS, INSOMNIA, AND DIABETES

Diabetes mellitus is a disease characterized by hyperglycemia that is due to defects in insulin secretion, insulin activity, or both.[51] Chronically elevated blood glucose leads to end-organ damage in several organ systems, including the heart and blood vessels, making it a risk factor for cardiovascular disease. Type 2 diabetes mellitus, the most prevalent form of diabetes,[51] is characterized by insulin resistance and inadequate insulin secretion. Glucose intolerance predates diabetes, and if not managed, advances to full-blown type 2 diabetes mellitus. Sleep loss and insomnia are associated with increased prevalence and incidence of both glucose intolerance and type 2 diabetes mellitus. Experimental sleep deprivation on healthy subjects has demonstrated the development of insulin resistance and decreased insulin sensitivity, which are early indicators of developing glucose intolerance and diabetes. Insulin resistance has been induced after just 1 week of partial sleep deprivation in healthy subjects.[52] This has been demonstrated by serum measures of insulin resistance as well as in metabolic markers in the actual adipocyte tissue.[53] Using the hyperinsulinemic-euglycemic clamp, an increase in endogenous glucose production and a decrease in glucose disposal rate, indicating increased insulin resistance, was demonstrated by Donga and colleagues[54] when comparing one night of partial sleep deprivation of 4 hours to normal sleep duration in healthy men and women. Even one night of partial sleep deprivation can result in a decrease in insulin sensitivity when measured by the homeostasis model assessment (HOMA) index.[55]

The consequences of poor sleep on glucose metabolism have also been demonstrated in clinical studies analyzing the prevalence and incidence of prediabetes and diabetes in those with insufficient or disturbed sleep. Cross-sectional studies reveal an association between decreased sleep time and increased prevalence of diabetes. A cross-sectional analysis of the Sleep Heart Health Study cohort indicated that short sleep time of less than 6 hours, with or without subjective complaints of insomnia, was significantly associated with the increased prevalence of diabetes or glucose intolerance.[56] Another cross-sectional study by Chao and colleagues[57] found that short sleep duration of less than 6 hours is independently associated with increased prevalence of type 2 diabetes mellitus, even after controlling for other risk factors, such as age, gender, obesity, family history of diabetes, tobacco use, and alcohol consumption. No significant association was found with prediabetes in this study. Prospective studies also support a possible association between short sleep time and the development of new-onset diabetes and prediabetes. A study by Rafalson and colleagues[58] that followed subjects over a 6-year period found a significant association between the development of impaired fasting glucose and short sleep duration of less than 5 hours a night, even after accounting for other confounding factors. Yaggi and colleagues[59] analyzed the Massachusetts Male Aging Study and found a significant association between sleep duration of less than 6 hours a night and the onset of diabetes, independent of other risk factors. A similar study by Beihl and colleagues[60] also revealed a link between the onset of diabetes and average sleep time of 7 hours or less. Large population-based studies, such as the Nurses' Health Study and the Whitehall II study, reinforce this positive association. Published prospective findings from the Nurses' Health Study indicate that subjective reports of sleep duration less than or equal to 5 hours is associated with an incident diagnosis of self-reported symptomatic diabetes over 10 years, even after adjusting for age and BMI.[61] Another subjective survey conducted on men in Sweden found those with complaints of short sleep duration and difficulties maintaining sleep had an increased incidence of reporting new-onset diabetes over a 12-year period, even after adjusting for age, hypertension, snoring, BMI, and depression.[62] Similarly, the Whitehall II study cohort conducted over a 5-year period found those with persistent short sleep of less than 5.5 hours a night had increased incidence of type 2 diabetes mellitus even after adjusting for confounding factors.[63] Although this association was weakened when BMI was accounted for, it maintained a trend for a positive association. Although these studies show comparable results of an independent association between short sleep duration and diabetes, the individual study designs vary in their population composition (one study had an all-male cohort, whereas another an all-female cohort) and amount of sleep loss (one study looked at sleep duration of less than 5 hours, whereas another looked at <7 hours). These differences in individual study construct become inconsequential, however, when considering the association between short sleep duration and incident diabetes is retained in large metaanalysis studies. These study results show that sleep duration of less than 6 hours and even 7 hours is associated with an increased risk of incident type 2 diabetes mellitus.[64,65]

Although the results of these studies on sleep duration are compelling, other questions that can be raised, specifically, are whether this association is also found in those with insomnia and whether these findings are limited to those with behaviorally induced insufficient sleep. Cross-sectional data show that subjective reports of difficulty maintaining sleep and waking up early are associated with clinically identified prediabetes in some but not all studies.[66,67] Chronic self-reported near-nightly sleep disturbance has been shown associated with the incidence of diabetes.[67] Hung and colleagues[68] evaluated sleep quality as measured by the Pittsburg Sleep Quality Index (PSQI) versus purely subjective complaints of poor sleep and diabetes and found that both impaired glucose tolerance and diabetes were associated with higher PSQI scores, reflecting poorer sleep quality. This finding remained significant even after adjusting for age, gender, alcohol use, smoking, exercise, BMI, blood pressure, and lipid levels. Likewise, results from prospective studies illustrate that subjective reports of difficulty initiating and maintaining sleep on a chronic basis are associated with incident diabetes. Some studies, however, support sleep initiation as the perpetrator, some support sleep maintenance, and some support both. Nilsson and colleagues[69] published prospective findings indicating subjective reports of difficulty initiating sleep and regular use of hypnotics were associated with incident diabetes, over 12 years, after adjusting for confounding factors. Another survey of Japanese men showed an association between subjective reports of difficulty initiating and maintaining sleep, often or almost every day, and incidence of type 2 diabetes mellitus, after controlling for other risk factors.[70] In Germany, complaints of difficulty maintaining sleep are associated with a higher risk of developing type 2 diabetes over 7.5 years, after adjusting for confounding factors.[71] A meta-analysis looking at the longitudinal study data on sleep disturbance and incidence of type 2 diabetes mellitus revealed that difficulty initiating and

maintaining sleep was associated with the development of type 2 diabetes mellitus,[10] suggesting that both aspects of insomnia are implicated in this risk. Vgontzas and colleagues[72] used polysomnography as an objective measure of sleep duration in combination with subjective insomnia and found that insomnia with an objective sleep duration of less than 5 hours is associated with a 300% higher odds for type 2 diabetes mellitus compared with those who did not have sleep complaints and slept at least 6 hours a night. Furthermore, Vgontzas and colleagues[72] found that neither insomnia alone nor short sleep duration alone without subjective sleep complaints was associated with an increased odd of diabetes. Not only may insomnia be a risk for the development of diabetes but also it may worsen glycemic control in diabetics. Knut-son and colleagues[73] used actigraphy and subjective reports to assess the association between insomnia and glycemic control in both diabetics and nondiabetics as part of the Coronary Artery Risk Development in Young Adults study. This study found that sleep fragmentation in diabetics is associated with a 23% higher fasting glucose level, 48% higher fasting insulin level, and 82% higher HOMA. There was no association found between these measured sleep parameters and glucose levels in nondiabetics. The literature mainly supports a positive association between insufficient sleep resulting from insomnia and the prevalence and incidence of type 2 diabetes mellitus; this association may also hold for prediabetes and impaired glycemic control in diabetics. Given the ubiquitous nature of diabetes, and its consequences of end-organ damage and cardiovascular disease, screening for sleep disturbances/insufficient sleep should be considered an essential part of the management of type 2 diabetes mellitus.

SLEEP AND HYPERTENSION

Hypertension is a well-known major risk factor for cardiovascular disease. The prevalence of hypertension worldwide ranges from 5% to 71%, with a prevalence of 29% in the United States.[74,75] Early identification and reduction of risk factors are important parts of health maintenance. A potential association of sleep disorders and poor sleep with hypertension is well documented.[76] Home measurements of blood pressure and heart rate are more variable, day to day and morning to evening, in those with insomnia than those without.[77] Normotensive subjects with chronic insomnia have increased nighttime systolic blood pressure (SBP) and blunting of the normal dip in nocturnal blood pressure compared with age-matched and gender-matched controls without insomnia.[78] A meta-analysis looking at cross-sectional and longitudinal study data on sleep duration found that short sleep duration is associated with an increased risk of hypertension with an odds ratio of 1.21 (95% confidence interval [CI], 1.09–1.34) and relative risk ratio of 1.23 (95% CI, 1.06–1.42), respectively.[79] The Sleep Heart Health Study conducted a cross-sectional analysis of sleep duration (measured by the subjective report and polysomnography) and prevalence of hypertension, defined as SBP 140 mm Hg, diastolic blood pressure (DBP) > 90 mm Hg, or use of medication to treat hypertension. Those with a subjective report of less than 7 hours of sleep per night had a higher odds ratio for hypertension.[80] This persisted even after adjustments for age, gender, race, BMI, and apnea–hypopnea index. The presence of insomnia also did not significantly affect this association, and the study found that subjects slept less than what they reported when their subjective report was compared with their polysomnography data. A review of cross-sectional studies on insomnia and hypertension reveals conflicting results. A cross-sectional study exploring hypertension (defined as SBP >140 mm Hg, DBP >90 mm Hg, or use of antihypertensive medications) in chronic insomnia for more than a year (reported as difficulty initiating and maintaining early morning awakening or nonrefreshing sleep for at least a year) and normal sleepers (those without any of these sleep complaints) used polysomnography to objectively measure sleep duration and found those with complaints of insomnia had a significantly increased risk for hypertension, as did those with sleep duration of less than or equal to 5 hours. The association was much stronger for insomnia than short sleep duration and persisted even after adjusting for confounding factors. The risk of hypertension was additive in those with insomnia and short sleep duration with a 500% increased risk of hypertension.[81] In contrast, Vozoris'[82] cross-sectional analysis of the US National Health and Nutrition Examination Survey, a survey that obtains data annually from a nationally representative sample of the population, did not reveal an association between insomnia and hypertension. The study analyzed the association among insomnia, short sleep duration of less than 6 hours, and hypertension and found that subjective insomnia complaints alone did not correlate with the presence of hypertension, whereas insomnia with short sleep duration was associated with a subjective report of hypertension but not with objective measures of hypertension.[82] Another multiyear cross-sectional analysis of this same cohort by Vozoris[83]

investigated whether a correlation exists between the frequency of insomnia symptoms and the presence of hypertension. On initial analysis, results revealed that an increasing frequency of insomnia (measured at 1–15 times in the past 1 month) was correlated with an increased risk of physician-diagnosed hypertension and use of antihypertensive medications, but the significance was lost after controlling for confounding factors. A similar trend was observed even after short sleep duration of less than 6 hours was accounted for.[83] Across-sectional analysis by Cheng and colleagues[84] looking at two separate time points on the Evolution of Pathways to Insomnia Cohort followed those with hypertension at the first time point and found that neither increased sleep-onset latency nor increased wake time after sleep onset was correlated with the presence of hypertension. Those who had increased wake time after sleep onset of greater than 30 minutes, however, had an increased risk for developing hypertension at the 1-year follow-up, even after accounting for age, gender, race, risk for obstructive sleep apnea, sleep duration, and length of insomnia.[84] This association did not hold for those with an increased sleep onset time of more than 30 minutes.

Longitudinal studies of insomnia and hypertension also have conflicting results. A prospective analysis of a health examination database in Japanese office workers looked at subjective sleep and development of hypertension (defined as SBP >140 mm Hg and/or DBP >90 mm Hg or initiating antihypertensive medication) over 4 years. This study found that those reporting always or sometimes having difficulty initiating or maintaining sleep had a higher incidence of hypertension than those without those complaints, even after adjusting for age, BMI, stress, alcohol, and smoking.[85] Another prospective study on insomnia, objective sleep duration, and incidence of hypertension over 7.5 years found that chronic insomnia for more than a year was statistically associated with an increased risk of developing hypertension even after controlling for confounding factors. A synergistic effect was observed with a short sleep duration of less than 6 hours, and the combination increased the risk of developing hypertension by fourfold compared with normal sleepers.[86] In contrast, Phillips and Mannino's[87] analysis of a cohort from the Atherosclerosis Risk in Communities study, looking at the development of incident hypertension over 6 years in those with chronic insomnia, found that subjective complaints of insomnia (difficulty falling asleep, staying asleep, and nonrestorative sleep) are not associated with an increased risk of hypertension.[87] Another analysis of the Cardiovascular Health Study cohort looked at several parameters of subjective sleep complaints (difficulty falling asleep, several awakenings a night, and early morning awakenings), separately and cohesively to examine if an association exists with the development of hypertension over a 6-year time frame. This study did not find a significant association between insomnia complaints and the development of hypertension.[88] Some of the discrepancies in results can be attributed to different methods of assessing subjective insomnia complaints, varying durations of what is considered short sleep, and varying longitudinal timelines of symptom logging. A meta-analysis looking at prospective studies on incident hypertension and presence of insomnia symptoms of at least 1 year found that short sleep duration, complaints of difficulty maintaining sleep, and early morning awakenings, individually and in combination, is associated with an increased risk of developing hypertension.[89] A recent review looking at cross-sectional and longitudinal data concluded that persistent insomnia was associated with increased blood pressure and hypertension risk after controlling for other risk factors in the middle-aged subjects.[90] Overall, the published data on the association of insomnia and hypertension are conflicting although meta-analysis studies suggest there is a positive association between chronic insomnia and development of hypertension. Before recommendations can be made for sleep screenings as a potential risk modifier for hypertension, more studies are needed to establish a definite association.

SLEEP AND CARDIOVASCULAR DISEASE

Cardiovascular disease is a widespread public health issue in the United States, with an estimated 2200 Americans dying daily from cardiovascular-related events and an estimated 785,000 Americans believed to have a new coronary attack each year.[91] This phenomenon is due to the high prevalence of risk factors, such as 33.5% of adults with hypertension, 20.7% of adults using tobacco, 15% with hyperlipidemia, and 67% of adults classified as overweight, of whom nearly 34% are obese.[91] In addition to these well-known risk factors, subjective complaints of trouble sleeping have been associated with coronary heart disease and incident myocardial infarction, even after excluding obstructive sleep apnea and controlling for other traditional cardiovascular risk factors.[92–94] A large 6-year prospective study of men in the United States revealed an increased risk of mortality after controlling for age, lifestyle, excessive daytime sleepiness, tranquilizer use, and chronic conditions in those with subjective

sleep disturbances.[95] In particular, difficulty initiating sleep and nonrestorative sleep had a significantly increased risk of cardiovascular mortality compared with those without such symptoms, and this association remained significant even after excluding patients with cardiovascular disease and depression and controlling for other risk factors.[95] Underlying mechanisms possibly linking these two conditions are increased sympathetic activity and vascular endothelial dysfunction, which have been found in chronic insomniacs and sleep-deprived healthy subjects.[35,46–48] Insomnia is also associated with higher nighttime SBP and blunted dipping of nocturnal blood pressure, which could place those patients at risk for cardiovascular disease.[78] Subjective complaints of regular disturbed sleep have been associated with a higher risk of developing hypertension and dyslipidemia, which further elevate risk for cardiovascular disease.[96]

Studies looking at insomnia and sleep duration and their associations with cardiovascular disease and mortality have revealed positive associations with various types of sleep complaints. There are also conflicting results, however, with some trends to association but without statistical significance and some negative results. The studies are heterogeneous in their construct, specifically in terms of questions asked to assess sleep quality, varying length of sleep duration, and varying populations studied, which may account for the differences in results. When looking at insomnia, an analysis of the Atherosclerosis Risk in Communities study cohort spanning 6 years found that having a combination of sleep complaints (trouble falling asleep, staying asleep, and awakening unrefreshed) had a slightly increased risk of developing cardiovascular disease.[87] Mallon and colleagues[97] found a significant risk of cardiovascular mortality in men, but not women, with insomnia. They conducted a prospective 12-year study that revealed insomnia (defined as trouble initiating sleep and habitual sleeping pill use) was independently associated with increased all-cause mortality in women but not cardiovascular mortality. In men, however, trouble falling asleep was independently associated with cardiovascular morality.[97] Prospective data from another study with a longer follow-up of 16 years showed that subjective reports of habitual insomnia were independently associated with all-cause mortality and a trend of an increased number of cardiovascular events although this was not statistically significant.[98] A prospective analysis of the Whitehall II cohort, however, looking at sleep in fatal and nonfatal cardiovascular events over a 15-year follow-up period, found that subjectively disturbed sleep had a statistically significant increased hazard ratio of cardiovascular events after adjusting for confounding factors. Sleep duration of less than 6 hours also shows a significantly increased risk when combined with insomnia but not when looked at alone.[99] Data from the Nurses' Health Study also support a possible link between short sleep duration and cardiovascular disease and found that when subjects were followed for 10 years, sleep duration of less than or equal to 5 hours was associated with fatal and nonfatal coronary artery disease-related events even after adjusting for factors, such as age, BMI, smoking, diabetes, and hypertension.[100] Both the Whitehall II cohort and the Nurses' Health Study support that sleep duration may be associated with cardiovascular disease. The studies looking specifically at insomnia are, however, conflicting. First-time myocardial infarction risk has been correlated to insomnia in two studies although there are some gender differences between male and female risk. Laugsand and colleagues[101] found that regular difficulties with initiating sleep, maintaining sleep, and having nonrestorative sleep were associated with a significant risk of having first-time acute myocardial infarction after controlling for confounding factors, such as BMI, cholesterol, blood pressure, and smoking.[101] Women were found to have a slightly higher relative risk compared with men. When looked at individually, each sleep complaint also carried a significant risk, with trouble initiating sleep having the strongest association. Meisinger and colleagues[102] also found that in a 10-year prospective cohort, difficulty maintaining sleep was associated with an increased risk of incident myocardial infarction in women that weakened but still demonstrated a positive association after controlling for confounding factors. This was not found in the male subjects, and this same trend was seen for a short sleep duration of less than 6 hours.

The data on insomnia, sleep duration, and fatal/nonfatal cardiovascular events are conflicting. This can be partly attributed to the heterogeneous nature of the studies, as discussed previously. A recent meta-analysis found that symptoms of difficulty initiating sleep and maintaining sleep and early morning awakenings are associated with an increased risk of cardiovascular mortality, with hazard ratios of 1.45, 1.03, and 1.00, respectively,[95] suggesting that poor sleep may be associated with cardiovascular health and should be considered in the management of cardiovascular disease. Depression has also been associated with an increased risk of coronary artery disease and myocardial infarction. In some studies, when depression was accounted for, sleep complaints

as a risk factor for cardiovascular disease became less significant.[93] Accounting for depression, along with a more uniform approach of quantifying insomnia, would be helpful in future studies to elucidate the independent role that sleep loss may play in cardiovascular health.

SUMMARY

Sleep deprivation and insomnia have a variety of health implications. They affect cognition, mood, and health. Insomnia is a global public health issue that affects more than a quarter of the US population at any point in time and is associated with decreased quality of life and increased economic burden. This article examines the literature on poor sleep and insomnia and their associations with diabetes, hypertension, and cardiovascular disease. Although some studies produced conflicting results, overall the literature supports a possible association that warrants further investigation. Differing study constructs and methods, such as varying methods of quantifying insomnia and inconsistencies, in screening for other confounding sleep disorders, such as obstructive sleep apnea, may explain the conflicting results. Despite these discrepancies, however, there is value in the screening of patients with cardiovascular disease or risk factors for sleep disturbances, especially with regard to improving their health outcomes and quality of life.

DISCLOSURE

The authors have nothing to disclose.

REFERENCES

1. Cohen DA, Wang W, Wyatt JK, et al. Uncovering residual effects of chronic sleep loss on human performance. Sci Transl Med 2010;2(14):14ra3.
2. Banks S, Dinges DF. Behavioral and physiological consequences of sleep restriction. J Clin Sleep Med 2007;3(5):519–28.
3. Irwin M. Effects of sleep and sleep loss on immunity and cytokines. Brain Behav Immun 2002; 16(5):503–12.
4. Spiegel K, Sheridan JF, Van Cauter E. Effect of sleep deprivation on response to immunization. JAMA 2002;288(12):1471–2.
5. Broussard JL, Van Cauter E. Disturbances of sleep and circadian rhythms: novel risk factors for obesity. Curr Opin Endocrinol Diabetes Obes 2016;23(5):353–9.
6. Nedeltcheva AV, Kilkus JM, Imperial J, et al. Sleep curtailment is accompanied by increased intake of calories from snacks. Am J Clin Nutr 2009;89(1): 126–33.

7. Cappuccio FP, Stranges S, Kandala NB, et al. Gender-specific associations of short sleep duration with prevalent and incident hypertension: the White hall II study. Hypertension 2007;50(4): 693–700.

8. Gangwisch JE, Heymsfield SB, Boden-Albala B, et al. Short sleep duration as a risk factor for hypertension: analyses of the first national health and nutrition examination survey. Hypertension 2006; 47(5):833–9.

9. Cappuccio FP, D'Elia L, Strazzullo P, et al. Sleep duration and all-cause mortality: a systematic review and meta-analysis of prospective studies. Sleep 2010;33(5):585–92.

10. Cappuccio FP, D'Elia L, Strazzullo P, et al. Quantity and quality of sleep and incidence of type 2 diabetes: a systematic review and meta-analysis. Diabetes Care 2010;33(2):414–20.

11. Tobaldini E, Costantino G, Solbiati M, et al. Sleep, sleep deprivation, autonomic nervous system and cardiovascular diseases. Neurosci Biobehav Rev 2017;74(Pt B):321–9.

12. Chung KF, Yeung WF, Ho FY, et al. Cross-cultural and comparative epidemiology of insomnia: the Diagnostic and statistical manual (DSM), International classification of diseases (ICD) and International classification of sleep disorders (ICSD). Sleep Med 2015;16(4):477–82.

13. Bolge SC, Doan JF, Kannan H, et al. Association of insomnia with quality of life, work productivity, and activity impairment. Qual Life Res 2009;18(4): 415–22.

14. Taylor DJ, Mallory LJ, Lichstein KL, et al. Comorbidity of chronic insomnia with medical problems. Sleep 2007;30(2):213–8.

15. Neckelmann D, Mykletun A, Dahl AA. Chronic insomnia as a risk factor for developing anxiety and depression. Sleep 2007;30(7):873–80.

16. Riemann D, Voderholzer U. Primary insomnia: a risk factor to develop depression? J Affect Disord 2003;76(1–3):255–9.

17. Ozminkowski RJ, Wang S, Walsh JK. The direct and indirect costs of untreated insomnia in adults in the United States. Sleep 2007;30(3):263–73.

18. Pollak CP, Perlick D, Linsner JP, et al. Sleep problems in the community elderly as predictors of death and nursing home placement. J Community Health 1990;15(2):123–35.

19. Kripke DF, Garfinkel L, Wingard DL, et al. Mortality associated with sleep duration and insomnia. Arch Gen Psychiatry 2002;59(2):131–6.

20. Althuis MD, Fredman L, Langenberg PW, et al. The relationship between insomnia and mortality among community-dwelling older women. J Am Geriatr Soc 1998;46(10):1270–3.

21. Foley DJ, Monjan AA, Brown SL, et al. Sleep complaints among elderly persons: an epidemiologic study of three communities. Sleep 1995;18(6): 425–32.

22. Phillips B, Mannino DM. Does insomnia kill? Sleep 2005;28(8):965–71.

23. Born J, Lange T, Hansen K, et al. Effects of sleep and circadian rhythm on human circulating immune cells. J Immunol 1997;158(9):4454–64.

24. Lange T, Dimitrov S, Fehm HL, et al. Shift of monocyte function toward cellular immunity during sleep. Arch Intern Med 2006;166(16): 1695–700.

25. Lissoni P, Rovelli F, Brivio F, et al. Circadian secretions of IL-2, IL-12, IL-6 and IL-10 in relation to the light/dark rhythm of the pineal hormone melatonin in healthy humans. Nat Immun 1998;16(1):1–5.

26. Petrovsky N, McNair P, Harrison LC. Diurnal rhythms of pro-inflammatory cytokines: regulation by plasma cortisol and therapeutic implications. Cytokine 1998;10(4):307–12.

27. Kronfol Z, Nair M, Zhang Q, et al. Circadian immune measures in healthy volunteers: relationship to hypothalamic-pituitary-adrenal axis hormones and sympathetic neurotransmitters. Psychosom Med 1997;59(1):42–50.

28. Savard J, Laroche L, Simard S, et al. Chronic insomnia and immune functioning. Psychosom Med 2003;65(2):211–21.

29. Irwin MR. Why sleep is important for health: a psychoneuroimmunology perspective. Annu Rev Psyhol 2015;66:143–72.

30. Cohen S, Doyle WJ, Alper CM, et al. Sleep habits and susceptibility to the common cold. Arch Intern Med 2009;169(1):62–7.

31. Patel SR, Malhotra A, Gao X, et al. A prospective study of sleep duration and pneumonia risk in women. Sleep 2012;35(1):97–101.

32. Miller GE, Cohen S, Pressman S, et al. Psychological stress and antibody response to influenza vaccination: when is the critical period for stress, and how does it get inside the body? Psychosom Med 2004;66(2):215–23.

33. Prather AA, Hall M, Fury JM, et al. Sleep and antibody response to hepatitis B vaccination. Sleep 2012;35(8):1063–9.

34. Pressman SD, Cohen S, Miller GE, et al. Loneliness, social network size, and immune response to influenza vaccination in college freshmen. Health Psychol 2005;24(3):297–306.

35. Carreras A, Zhang SX, Peris E, et al. Chronic sleep fragmentation induces endothelial dysfunction and structural vascular changes in mice. Sleep 2014; 37(11):1817–24.

36. Somers VK, Dyken ME, Mark AL, et al. Sympathetic-nerve activity during sleep in normal subjects. N Engl J Med 1993;328(5):303–7.

37. Esler M, Jennings G, Lambert G, et al. Overflow of catecholamine neurotransmitters to the circulation:

source, fate, and functions. Physiol Rev 1990; 70(4):963–85.

38. Wallin BG. Relationship between sympathetic nerve traffic and plasma concentrations of noradrenaline in man. Pharmacol Toxicol 1988; 63(Suppl 1):9–11.

39. Irwin M, Thompson J, Miller C, et al. Effects of sleep and sleep deprivation on catecholamine and interleukin-2 levels in humans: clinical implications. J Clin Endocrinol Metab 1999;84(6):1979–85.

40. Spiegel K, Leproult R, Van Cauter E. Impact of sleep debt on metabolic and endocrine function. Lancet 1999;354(9188):1435–9.

41. Leproult R, Copinschi G, Buxton O, et al. Sleep loss results in an elevation of cortisol levels the next evening. Sleep 1997;20(10):865–70.

42. Stamatakis KA, Punjabi NM. Effects of sleep fragmentation on glucose metabolism in normal subjects. Chest 2010;137(1):95–101.

43. Van Cauter E, Holmback U, Knutson K, et al. Impact of sleep and sleep loss on neuroendocrine and metabolic function. Horm Res 2007;67(Suppl-I V O Q I):2–9.

44. Tasali E, Leproult R, Ehrmann DA, et al. Slow-wave sleep and the risk of type 2 diabetes in humans. Proc Natl Acad Sci USA 2008;105(3): 1044–9.

45. Rao MN, Neylan TC, Grunfeld C, et al. Subchronic sleep restriction causes tissue-specific insulin resistance. J Clin Endocrinol Metab 2015;100(4): 1664–71.

46. Vgontzas AN, Bixler EO, Lin HM, et al. Chronic insomnia is associated with nyctohemeral activation of the hypothalamic-pituitary-adrenal axis: clinical implications. J Clin Endocrinol Metab 2001; 86(8):3787–94.

47. Rodenbeck A, Huether G, Rüther E, et al. Interactions between evening and nocturnal cortisol secretion and sleep parameters in patients with severe chronic primary insomnia. Neurosci Lett 2002; 324(2):159–63.

48. Vgontzas AN, Tsigos C, Bixler EO, et al. Chronic insomnia and activity of the stress system: a preliminary study. J Psychosom Res 1998;45(1): 21–31.

49. Bonnet MH, Arand DL. 24-Hour metabolic rate in insomniacs and matched normal sleepers. Sleep 1995;18(7):581–8.

50. Bonnet MH, Arand DL. Heart rate variability in insomniacs and matched normal sleepers. Psychosom Med 1998;60(5):610–5.

51. Report of the expert committee on the diagnosis and classification of diabetes mellitus. Diabetes Care 1997;20(7):1183–97.

52. Buxton OM, Pavlova M, Reid EW, et al. Sleep restriction for 1 week reduces insulin sensitivity in healthy men. Diabetes 2010;59(9):2126–33.

53. Broussard JL, Ehrmann DA, Van Cauter E, et al. Impaired insulin signaling in human adipocytes after experimental sleep restriction: a randomized, crossover study. Ann Intern Med 2012;157(8): 549–57.

54. Donga E, van Dijk M, van Dijk JG, et al. A single night of partial sleep deprivation induces insulin resistance in multiple metabolic pathways in healthy subjects. J Clin Endocrinol Metab 2010; 95(6):2963–8.

55. Cedernaes J, Osler ME, Voisin S, et al. Acute sleep loss induces tissue-specific epigenetic and transcriptional alterations to circadian clock genes in men. J Clin Endocrinol Metab 2015;100(9): E1255–61.

56. Gottlieb DJ, Punjabi NM, Newman AB, et al. Association of sleep time with diabetes mellitus and impaired glucose tolerance. Arch Intern Med 2005;165(8):863–7.

57. Chao CY, Wu JS, Yang YC, et al. Sleep duration is a potential risk factor for newly diagnosed type 2 diabetes mellitus. Metabolism 2011;60(6): 799–804.

58. Rafalson L, Donahue RP, Stranges S, et al. Short sleep duration is associated with the development of impaired fasting glucose: the Western New York health study. Ann Epidemiol 2010;20(12):883–9.

59. Yaggi HK, Araujo AB, McKinlay JB. Sleep duration as a risk factor for the development of type 2 diabetes. Diabetes Care 2006;29(3):657–61.

60. Beihl DA, Liese AD, Haffner SM. Sleep duration as a risk factor for incident type 2 diabetes in a multiethnic cohort. Ann Epidemiol 2009;19(5):351–7.

61. Ayas NT, White DP, Al-Delaimy WK, et al. A prospective study of self-reported sleep duration and incident diabetes in women. Diabetes Care 2003;26(2):380–4.

62. Mallon L, Broman JE, Hetta J. High incidence of diabetes in men with sleep complaints or short sleep duration: a 12-year follow-up study of a middle-aged population. Diabetes Care 2005; 28(11):2762–7.

63. Ferrie JE, Kivimäki M, Akbaraly TN, et al. Change in sleep duration and type 2 diabetes: the Whitehall II study. Diabetes Care 2015;38(8):1467–72.

64. Holliday EG, Magee CA, Kritharides L, et al. Short sleep duration is associated with risk of future diabetes but not cardiovascular disease: a prospective study and meta-analysis. PLoS One 2013; 8(11):e82305.

65. Shan Z, Ma H, Xie M, et al. Sleep duration and risk of type 2 diabetes: a meta-analysis of prospective studies. Diabetes Care 2015;38(3):529–37.

66. Engeda J, Mezuk B, Ratliff S, et al. Association between duration and quality of sleep and the risk of pre-diabetes: evidence from NHANES. Diabet Med 2013;30(6):676–80.

67. Kowall B, Lehnich AT, Strucksberg KH, et al. Associations among sleep disturbances, nocturnal sleep duration, daytime napping, and incident pre- diabetes and type 2 diabetes: the Heinz Nixdorf Recall Study. Sleep Med 2016;21:35–41.

68. Hung H, Yang Y, Ou H, et al. The association between impaired glucose tolerance and self- reported sleep quality in a Chinese population. Can J Diabetes 2012;36:95–9.

69. Nilsson PM, Rööst M, Engström G, et al. Incidence of diabetes in middle-aged men is related to sleep disturbances. Diabetes Care 2004; 27(10):2464–9.

70. Kawakami N, Takatsuka N, Shimizu H. Sleep disturbance and onset of type 2 diabetes. Diabetes Care 2004;27(1):282–3.

71. Meisinger C, Heier M, Loewel H, et al. MONICA/ KORA Augsburg Cohort Study. Sleep disturbance as a predictor of type 2 diabetes mellitus in men and women from the general population. Diabetologia 2005;48(2):235–41.

72. Vgontzas AN, Liao D, Pejovic S, et al. Insomnia with objective short sleep duration is associated with type 2 diabetes: a population-based study. Dia betes Care 2009;32(11):1980–5.

73. Knutson KL, Van Cauter E, Zee P, et al. Cross-sectional associations between measures of sleep and markers of glucose metabolism among sub jects with and without diabetes: the Coronary Artery Risk Development in Young Adults (CARDIA) Sleep Study. Diabetes Care 2011;34(5):1171–6.

74. Kearney PM, Whelton M, Reynolds K, et al. Worldwide prevalence of hypertension: a systematic review. J Hypertens 2004;22(1):11–9.

75. Ong KL, Cheung BM, Man YB, et al. Prevalence, awareness, treatment, and control of hypertension among United States adults 1999-2004. Hypertension 2007;49(1):69–75.

76. Bansil P, Kuklina EV, Merritt RK, et al. Associations between sleep disorders, sleep duration, quality of sleep, and hypertension: results from the National Health and Nutrition Examination Survey, 2005 to 2008. J Clin Hypertens (Greenwich) 2011;13(10): 739–43.

77. Johansson JK, Kronholm E, Jula AM. Variability in home-measured blood pressure and heart rate: associations with self-reported insomnia and sleep duration. J Hypertens 2011;29(10): 1897–905.

78. Lanfranchi PA, Pennestri MH, Fradette L, et al. Nighttime blood pressure in normotensive subjects with chronic insomnia: implications for cardiovascular risk. Sleep 2009;32(6):760–6.

79. Guo X, Zheng L, Wang J, et al. Epidemiological evidence for the link between sleep duration and high blood pressure: a systematic review and metaanalysis. Sleep Med 2013;14(4):324–32.

80. Gottlieb DJ, Redline S, Nieto FJ, et al. Association of usual sleep duration with hypertension: the sleep heart health study. Sleep 2006;29(8): 1009–14.

81. Vgontzas AN, Liao D, Bixler EO, et al. Insomnia with objective short sleep duration is associated with a high risk for hypertension. Sleep 2009; 32(4):491–7.

82. Vozoris NT. The relationship between insomnia symptoms and hypertension using United States population-level data. J Hypertens 2013;31(4): 663–71.

83. Vozoris NT. Insomnia symptom frequency and hypertension risk: a population-based study. J Clin Psychiatry 2014;75(6):616–23.

84. Cheng P, Pillai V, Mengel H, et al. Sleep maintenance difficulties in insomnia are associated with increased incidence of hypertension. Sleep Health 2015;1:50–4.

85. Suka M, Yoshida K, Sugimori H. Persistent insomnia is a predictor of hypertension in Japanese male workers. J Occup Health 2003;45(6): 344–50.

86. Fernandez-Mendoza J, Vgontzas AN, Liao D, et al. Insomnia with objective short sleep duration and incident hypertension: the Penn state cohort. Hypertension 2012;60(4):929–35.

87. Phillips B, Mannino DM. Do insomnia complaints cause hypertension or cardiovascular disease? J Clin Sleep Med 2007;3(5):489–94.

88. Phillips B, Bůzková P, Enright P, et al, Cardiovascular Health Study Research Group. Insomnia did not predict incident hypertension in older adults in the cardiovascular health study. Sleep 2009;32(1): 65–72.

89. Meng L, Zheng Y, Hui R. The relationship of sleep duration and insomnia to risk of hypertension incidence: a meta-analysis of prospective cohort studies. Hypertens Res 2013;36(11):985–95.

90. Palagini L, Bruno RM, Gemignani A, et al. Sleep loss and hypertension: a systematic review. Curr Pharm Des 2013;19(13):2409–19.

91. Roger VL, Go AS, Lloyd-Jones DM, et al. Heart disease and stroke statistics-2012 update: a report from the American Heart Association. Circulation 2012;125(1):e2–220.

92. Schwartz S, McDowell Anderson W, Cole SR, et al. Insomnia and heart disease: a review of epidemiologic studies. J Psychosom Res 1999;47(4): 313–33.

93. Schwartz SW, Cornoni-Huntley J, Cole SR, et al. Are sleep complaints an independent risk factor for myocardial infarction? Ann Epidemiol 1998; 8(6):384–92.

94. Eaker ED, Pinsky J, Castelli WP. Myocardial infarction and coronary death among women: psychosocial predictors from a 20-year follow-up of women

in the Framingham Study. Am J Epidemiol 1992; 135(8):854–64.

95. Li Y, Zhang X, Winkelman JW, et al. Association between insomnia symptoms and mortality: a prospective study of U.S. men. Circulation 2014; 129(7):737–46.

96. Clark AJ, Salo P, Lange T, et al. Onset of impaired sleep and cardiovascular disease risk factors: a longitudinal study. Sleep 2016;39(9):1709–18.

97. Mallon L, Broman JE, Hetta J. Sleep complaints predict coronary artery disease mortality in males: a 12-year follow-up study of a middle-aged Swedish population. J Intern Med 2002;251(3):207–16.

98. Chien KL, Chen PC, Hsu HC, et al. Habitual sleep duration and insomnia and the risk of cardiovascular events and all-cause death: report from a community-based cohort. Sleep 2010;33(2): 177–84.

99. Chandola T, Ferrie JE, Perski A, et al. The effect of short sleep duration on coronary heart disease risk is greatest among those with sleep disturbance: a prospective study from the Whitehall II cohort. Sleep 2010;33(6):739–44.

100. Ayas NT, White DP, Manson JE, et al. A prospective study of sleep duration and coronary heart disease in women. Arch Intern Med 2003;163(2):205–9.

101. Laugsand LE, Vatten LJ, Platou C, et al. Insomnia and the risk of acute myocardial infarction: a population study. Circulation 2011;124(19):2073–81.

102. Meisinger C, Heier M, Löwel H, et al. Sleep duration and sleep complaints and risk of myocardial infarction in middle-aged men and women from the general population: the MONICA/KORA Augsburg cohort study. Sleep 2007;30(9):1121–7.

Sleep and Cognition
A Narrative Review Focused on Older Adults

Joseph M. Dzierzewski, PhD[a],*, Elliottnell Perez, MS[b], Scott G. Ravyts, MS[b],
Natalie Dautovich, PhD[c]

KEYWORDS

• Sleep • Insomnia • Sleep apnea • Cognition • Cognitive function • Age • Aging

KEY POINTS

• Sleep and cognitive functioning show negative changes with advanced age.
• Although the associations are varied, sleep seems to be related to cognitive functioning within good-sleeping older adults, older adults with insomnia, and older adults with sleep-disordered breathing.
• Both insomnia and sleep apnea may be associated with cognitive decline and dementia.
• Treatment of sleep disorders may provide cognitive benefits in late life. Additional research is warranted.
• Examination of sex-differences in the sleep–cognition association may address unanswered questions.

INTRODUCTION

This article reviews the growing literature examining sleep and cognitive functioning in older adults. The main focus is on normal, age-related cognitive changes, as opposed to neurodegenerative disease processes; however, those are reviewed as appropriate. Age-related cognitive changes are the result of developmental maturation. These cumulative, long-term processes are universal or nearly universal, and are resistant to efforts to reverse the change.[1,2] Investigation into cognitive aging has found a general cognitive decline experienced with increasing age,[3–5] which has been shown to be pervasive, affecting many subdomains of cognition, including

• Reaction time
• Sensory processing
• Attention
• Memory
• Reasoning
• Executive functioning

Although much is known regarding developmental changes in cognitive functioning, comparatively little is known regarding sleep's association with the traditional developmental course of late-life cognitive functioning.

Sleep represents an intriguing individual difference variable because it may relate to late-life cognitive functioning. Sleep has shown consistent age-related changes as a result of developmental maturation. Many of these developmental changes parallel the age-related changes observed in cognitive functioning. For example, slow wave sleep (stage N3) and rapid eye movement sleep decrease with advanced age.[6] In addition to these normal, developmentally appropriate changes in sleep, older adults also experience an

Published: December 07, 2017 DOI: https://doi.org/10.1016/j.jsmc.2017.09.009

[a] Department of Psychology, Virginia Commonwealth University, 806 West Franklin Street, Room 306, Box 842018, Richmond, VA 23284-2018, USA; [b] Department of Psychology, Virginia Commonwealth University, Box 842018, Richmond, VA 23284-2018, USA; [c] Department of Psychology, Virginia Commonwealth University, 800 West Franklin Street, Room 203, Box 842018, Richmond, VA 23284-2018, USA
* Corresponding author.
E-mail address: dzierzewski@vcu.edu

Sleep Med Clin 17 (2022) 205–222
https://doi.org/10.1016/j.jsmc.2022.02.001

increased prevalence of insomnia and sleep-disordered breathing (SDB).[7–9] **Fig. 1** shows general age-related changes in cognitive functioning and general age-related changes in sleep. The parallel changes in sleep and cognition with age, coupled with anecdotal reports of disturbed cognitive abilities following poor sleep, have resulted in research efforts focused on examining sleep and cognition in older adults. This article summarizes the literature for normal-sleeping older adults, older adults with insomnia, and older adults with SDB.

SLEEP AND COGNITION IN NORMAL-SLEEPING OLDER ADULTS WITHOUT DEMENTIA
Self-Reported Sleep Duration and Cognition

Several large-scale epidemiologic studies have garnered information regarding habitual sleep duration and/or difficulty and cognitive functioning in older adults. In a study of more than 3000 older adults, long sleep duration was associated with worse overall/global cognitive functioning, whereas no association with short sleep duration and cognitive functioning was observed.[10] In a similar study of more than 5000 adults, sleep duration was associated with verbal fluency and list memory, such that long and short sleep durations were associated with poorer performance.[11] In a sample of community-dwelling older women, sleeping less than 5 hours per night was associated with poorer global cognition and poorer performance across many of the individual indicators of cognitive functioning (ie, verbal memory, verbal fluency, working memory) compared with women sleeping 7 hours or more per night.[12] The investigators of these studies suggest that sleep duration may be related to cognitive functioning through changes in sleep architecture, fragmentation, quality, and neurologic conditions.[10,11]

In addition to individual large epidemiologic studies, the association between sleep duration measured via self-reported retrospective recall and cognitive functioning has been corroborated by a meta-analysis showing deleterious effects in long and short sleepers on multiple domains of cognitive functioning in older adults.[13] Similarly, a review by Devore and colleagues[14] examined cross-sectional and longitudinal studies of sleep duration and cognitive function in older adults. Although actigraphy, polysomnography (PSG), and self-reported sleep duration were included in the review, the authors found that all significant associations between sleep duration and cognitive function were from studies using self-reported sleep duration. The review reported 5 of 27 cross-sectional studies and four of seven longitudinal studies found an association between short sleep duration and worse cognitive function, whereas 9 of 27 cross-sectional studies and three of seven prospective studies found an association between long sleep duration and worse cognitive function. Moreover, shifting to short sleep duration and longer sleep duration from a normal duration of sleep was also associated with poorer cognitive function.

In addition to nocturnal sleep duration, additional cross-sectional and longitudinal evidence suggests sleep duration during the day, or napping, may be associated with cognitive performance in older adults.[15] Older adults who slept longer during the day demonstrated significantly poorer visuospatial ability and slower processing speed than those who slept less during the day. Moreover, sleep during the day was associated with greater decline in visuospatial reasoning and processing speed 6 years later and remained after controlling for significant health covariates. However, sleep during the day was not significantly associated with verbal memory ability.

Polysomnography-Measured Sleep and Cognition

Investigation into the relationship between PSG-assessed sleep and waking cognitive functioning has provided mixed results. It has been reported that longer sleep-onset latency is related to poorer verbal memory and executive functioning, whereas greater total wake time is related to lower psychomotor speed and memory in normal-sleeping older adults.[13] However, in another investigation, slow wave sleep was unrelated to performance on a simple reaction time task, continuous performance task, and attention test in good-sleeping older adults.[16] Djonlagic and colleagues[17] examined macro and micro sleep architecture and cognitive functioning in two large samples of older adults. Increased rapid eye movement duration, sleep efficiency, sleep maintenance efficiency, and reduced slow wave oscillation were associated with better cognitive processing speed and executive functioning in older adults. An additional study from Cox and colleagues[15] found no evidence supporting an association between sleep duration and cognitive abilities. These findings are consistent with null findings reported in an earlier systematic review.[14] As such, it seems that additional research is need to further explicate the relationship between PSG-measured sleep and cognitive functioning in older adults without a sleep complaint.

Dzierzewski et al

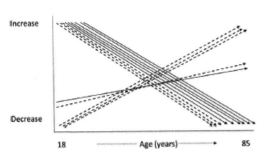

Fig. 1. Normative changes with age in cognitive functioning and sleep. *Solid arrows* represent general cognitive changes. *Dashed arrows* represent general sleep changes. Cognitive abilities that decline with age include processing speed, working memory, long-term memory, attention, reasoning, and executive control. Sleep characteristics that decline with age include total sleep time, slow wave sleep, and rapid eye movement sleep. Sleep characteristics that increase with age include wake time after sleep onset, and light sleep (stages N1 and N2). Crystalized intelligence and sleep-onset latency showed slight increases with advancing age.

Actigraphy-Measured Sleep and Cognition

There is some research supporting an association between objective sleep measured with actigraphy and cognitive performance. In a study of nearly 3000 older community-dwelling women, actigraphy-measured sleep (sleep efficiency, sleep-onset latency, wake after sleep onset, and napping) was associated with an increased risk of poorer general cognition and executive performance.[18] However, total sleep time was not related to cognitive functioning, which led the investigators to conclude that "it is disturbance of sleep rather than quantity that affects cognition."[18] This conclusion is supported by preliminary evidence showing sleep disruption (the number of wake bouts) is significantly associated with cognitive decline 5 years later. Furthermore, the association was moderated by sex, with greater wake bouts increasing the odds of cognitive decline for men but decreasing the odds of cognitive decline for women.[19]

In a different but complementary vein, 7 nights of actigraphy were used to compute sleep/wake patterns in 144 community-dwelling older adults. Older adults who displayed many shifts from rest to activity performed worse on composites of executive functioning, memory, and speed than elderly with more consistent rest-activity patterns.[20] Despite some evidence for actigraphy-

measured sleep and cognition in late-life, discrepant findings from the systematic review performed by Devore and colleagues[14] suggest there may be additional nuance to this association with older adults. The scarcity of research examining actigraphy-measured sleep and cognition in older adults precludes any definitive conclusions being drawn.

Sleep Deprivation and Cognition

Short-term total sleep deprivation has a significant deleterious effect across most cognitive domains, including attention, working memory, processing speed, short-term memory, and reasoning, with smaller effects being observed for tasks of greater complexity.[21] Webb and Levy[22] and Webb[23] conducted experiments to examine potential age differences in cognitive response to sleep deprivation. In both experiments, older adults' and younger adults' performance on a variety of cognitive tasks were compared following 2 nights of sleep deprivation. Older adults showed greater deterioration following sleep deprivation than did the younger adults in vigilance, visual search, reaction times, word detection, addition, anagrams, and objects uses.[22,23] A similar study was conducted by Pasula and colleagues[24] comparing younger and older adults on visuospatial and verbal working memory abilities following a night of normal sleep and 32 hours of sleep deprivation. Although young adults outperformed older on encoding and displacement process for verbal and visuospatial working memory, older adults showed significantly less decline than younger adults in verbal encoding and visuospatial displacement processes. Following sleep deprivation older adults did not show significant changes in visuospatial working memory, but did demonstrate verbal working memory displacement deficits. Jones and Harrison[25] summarized the extant sleep deprivation work by stating that, "neurocognitive studies present many inconsistencies, task classification is often ambiguous and, in the absence of any unifying explanation at the level of cognitive mechanisms, the overall picture is one of a disparate range of impairment following sleep loss."[25]

Sleep Restriction and Cognition

The experimental evidence regarding the sleep-cognition relationship garnered through studies using sleep restriction methodology have consistently yielded results indicating an impact on vigilance, which may be reduced in older adults.[26] Similarly, moderation analyses from a meta-analytic review indicated a differential impact of sleep restriction on cognitive function across the lifespan.[27] Although the association between sleep restriction and global cognition function strengthened with age, the association was not significant in older adults. The authors recommended cautious interpretation of the findings because of limited studies in the review examining sleep restriction and cognitive function in older adults. However, they suggested older adults may be more resilient than other age groups to the effects of sleep loss. Relatedly, Bliese and colleagues[26] examined age-related changes in reaction time/attention after modest sleep restriction. Older adults showed less pronounced effects of sleep restriction on their reaction times than younger adults. However, the oldest adult included in the study was 62 years old, so aging effects must be interpreted cautiously. Nevertheless, the investigators suggest that older adults may have "expended more effort across days"[21] resulting in blunted differences.[26] Regarding potential mechanisms underlying the relationship between sleep restriction and cognitive functioning, Banks and Dinges[28] summarized the evidence by suggesting that there is no "definitive evidence of what is accumulating and destabilizing cognitive functions over time when sleep is regularly restricted."[28]

Sleep and Learning

As opposed to examination of the negative consequences of poor sleep (or sleep loss), some researchers have investigated the potential benefits of sleep gained. In this line of research, participants are allowed to sleep while manipulating the timing of cognitive testing/training to either allow sleep to occur following testing or not to examine any effects of posttraining sleep on subsequent testing. Most of this research has been conducted with younger adults with findings indicating optimized performance following sleep. Tucker and colleagues[29] trained 16 healthy older adults in a finger tapping sequencing task and found that older adults performed significantly better following sleep than 12 hours of not sleeping, suggesting sleep-dependent motor skill performance in the elderly. Older adults showed similar rates of improvement as were found in younger samples; however, specific sleep characteristics did not correlate with the next day's performance (in contrast, stage 2 sleep and sleep spindle activity does correlate in younger adults). The investigators concluded that sleep in the elderly does optimize motor skill learning; however, it may do so differently than in younger adults.[29]

SLEEP AND COGNITION IN OLDER ADULTS WITH INSOMNIA

Older adults are at an increased risk for insomnia and experiencing negative changes in cognitive functioning. Given the comorbidity of insomnia and cognitive dysfunction in older adults, researchers have attempted to understand the role of insomnia in predicting cognitive functioning in a variety of samples (eg, cognitively intact older adults and older adults experiencing cognitive decline or dementia). Furthermore, a small number of studies have examined the effect of behavioral interventions for insomnia on cognitive outcomes. A sample of representative studies is presented later that illustrates these different approaches.

Insomnia Status and Normal Cognitive Aging

The association between insomnia and cognitive performance in younger and middle-aged adults is well-established, with impairments in working memory, episodic memory, and some aspects of executive functioning.[30] However, less is known about the association between insomnia diagnosis and cognitive performance in cognitively healthy older adults who are not experiencing cognitive decline or dementia. To date, insomnia and cognitive functioning have been examined in older adults with insomnia through cross-sectional designs with matched healthy control subjects[31,32] or using comparisons across insomnia subtypes.[33]

Overall, in contrast with healthy control subjects, insomnia status was associated with worse performance on a subset of cognitive tasks. Specifically, participants with insomnia performed significantly worse on memory span, integration of visual and semantic dimensions, and executive functioning tasks.[32] The insomnia groups performed better than healthy control subjects on the simple attending task.[31] The better attentional performance on simple attending did not persist for complex attending, perhaps reflecting the higher arousal that is characteristic of individuals diagnosed with insomnia.[34] This higher arousal may be beneficial for unambiguous stimuli but a hindrance for complex tasks requiring more cognitive resources.[31] In addition to differences in cognitive performance dependent on the presence or absence of insomnia, performance also seems to differ depending on the type of insomnia complaint. Specifically, Ling and colleagues[33] found that only early morning awakening was associated with significantly worse cognitive performance in the executive functioning domain. No association was found between difficulty initiating sleep or difficulty maintaining sleep across

Table 1
Differences in performance across cognitive task group by insomnia status

Cognitive Task	Better Performance by Insomnia Group	Better Performance by Healthy Control Group	No Group Difference
Sustained attention	X (simple tasks)[31]	X (simple tasks,[32] complex tasks[31])	X (complex tasks)[32]
Naming	—	—	X[32]
Psychomotor skills	—	—	X[32]
Memory span	—	X[32]	—
Integration of 2 dimensions (visual and semantic)	—	X[32]	—
Time estimation	—	X[32]	—
Executive functioning	—	X[32]	—

the following cognitive domains: attention, verbal memory, visuospatial ability, and executive functioning. **Table 1** lists the differences in cognitive functioning between older adults with and without insomnia.

Overall, across the reviewed studies examining cognitive performance in cognitively intact older adults with insomnia, insomnia status and specific characteristics of insomnia (eg, early morning awakening) seem to be associated with worse cognitive performance. However, the poorer performance of the individuals with insomnia is not consistent across all cognitive domains or across all tasks within cognitive domains. Consequently, despite a trend toward worse cognitive performance associated with insomnia status, the existing body of evidence is too small and inconsistent to arrive at a broad conclusion.

Insomnia and Cognitive Decline/Dementia Diagnoses

Compared with research that has examined insomnia and cognitive performance in cognitively healthy older adults, more work has been done to explore the role of insomnia in predicting cognitive decline or dementia status. Despite the greater breadth of research with cognitively impaired older adults, the association between insomnia and cognitive decline and/or dementia status remains unclear.

A minority of studies identified an association between insomnia and cognitive decline or dementia.[35–37] A meta-analysis reported that older adults with insomnia or insomnia complaints had significantly higher risk for incidence of all-cause dementia than those without insomnia at 9 years follow-up.[38] Older adults with long-term insomnia and long-term use of hypnotics had a two-fold risk of developing dementia during a 3-year

follow-up period compared with healthy control subjects.[35] Controlling for hypnotic use, similar results were found with long-term insomnia predicting an increased risk for cognitive decline at a 3-year follow-up for older adults with insomnia compared with healthy controls.[36] These results point to the importance of considering the duration of the insomnia complaint as a predictor of cognitive function, because long-term/chronic insomnia, rather than concurrent or acute insomnia, has been more consistently associated with cognitive decline.[36]

In contrast, another set of studies found a positive association between insomnia symptoms and cognitive performance.[39,40] Using a longitudinal design, Jaussent and colleagues[39] found that complaints of awakenings during the night and total number of insomnia complaints at baseline predicted a decreased risk for cognitive decline during an 8-year follow-up period. In addition, a cross-sectional approach with older adults with dementia residing in assisted living facilities showed that individuals with insomnia symptoms performed significantly better on the Mini-Mental State Examination than those without insomnia symptoms.[40] Of note, neither of these studies assessed the duration of the insomnia complaint.

A large proportion of studies investigating insomnia and cognitive decline or dementia have failed to report significant associations. Using longitudinal and cross-sectional designs, with and without comparison groups, and various approaches to insomnia and cognitive evaluations, insomnia was not associated with cognitive decline[41–43] or dementia status.[44] Given these discrepant findings, it could be concluded that insomnia status does not predict cognitive decline in older adults. However, it is more likely that the equivocal findings result from methodologic differences in research approaches. For example, one study examined the moderating role of insomnia symptoms in the association between elevated amyloid-β and cognitive decline among older adults without dementia.[45] A preliminary analyses revealed that elevated amyloid-β predicted faster cognitive decline in all cognitive domains 8 years later, but insomnia was not an independent predictor of cognitive decline. However, older adults with elevated amyloid-β and insomnia exhibited greater rates of decline in memory, executive function, and language compared with those with only elevated amyloid-β or only insomnia or neither.[45] **Table 2** provides a summary of the associations between insomnia and cognitive decline/dementia status in older adults.

Insomnia Treatment and Cognitive Functioning

In addition to examining cross-sectional and longitudinal associations between insomnia and cognitive outcomes, a small number of studies have investigated whether the treatment of insomnia leads to an improvement in cognitive performance (**Table 3**).[31,46] In one such study, an insomnia intervention was used with community-dwelling older adults with insomnia.[31] The insomnia intervention consisted of sleep restriction, cognitive restructuring, sleep hygiene, bright light exposure, body temperature manipulations, and structured physical activity. Following treatment, sleep-onset latency and sleep efficiency were significantly improved in the treatment group compared with the waitlist group. Treatment was also associated with improved performance on complex vigilance tasks and worsened performance on simple vigilance tasks compared with the waitlist control group. A possible explanation for the performance differences on simple versus complex tasks following treatment is that improved sleep results in a reduction of arousal levels to normal,[31] resulting in slower performance on simpler tasks.

Two studies used a brief behavioral treatment of insomnia approach with a sample of community-dwelling older adults who were cognitively intact and diagnosed with insomnia.[46,47] One study found individuals in the treatment group showed a significantly greater decrease in wake time after sleep onset following treatment compared with the information-only control group. However, the treatment group did not show significantly better improvement in cognitive performance across three cognitive domains (episodic memory, working memory, abstract reasoning) compared with the control group. The investigators posited that the null findings might be caused by the short follow-up period (4 weeks after the start of the intervention). Allowing more time postintervention for the sleep treatment to take effect might have enabled detection of effects on cognitive performance.[46] Similarly, the second study found significant improvement in actigraphy-measured wake after sleep onset and sleep diary–measured wake time after sleep onset, sleep-onset latency, sleep efficiency, and sleep quality. However, no significant improvement was found following the intervention for global cognitive functioning, attention, language, memory, or executive functioning.[47]

Building on this work, McCrae and colleagues[48] examined the patterns of association between nighttime sleep and next-day cognitive performance among older adults following brief behavioral treatment of insomnia.[48] At posttreatment, total sleep time, sleep-onset latency, and sleep efficiency were not associated with sustained attention and processing speed. However, greater wake after sleep onset was associated with better next day sustained attention and processing speed. At posttreatment, longer total sleep time was associated with better next-day inductive reasoning performance, but no significant relationships were found between inductive reasoning and sleep-onset latency, wake after sleep onset, and sleep efficiency.[48]

SLEEP AND COGNITION IN OLDER ADULTS WITH SLEEP-DISORDERED BREATHING

The estimated prevalence of SDB and cognitive impairment increases with age.[49,50] Moreover, individuals with SDB show cognitive changes similar to those associated with aging.[51] Recent research has posited that SDB and advanced age act independently to impair cognitive functioning, with the combination of SDB and advanced age leading to cognitive impairments greater than either factor alone.[51]

Although some studies have found an association between SDB and impairments in global cognitive functioning,[52,53] not all cognitive domains seem to be equally affected. Instead, the domains of vigilance, executive function, and memory are particularly implicated.[54] The impact of SDB on all three of these cognitive domains has been observed among community-based and clinic-based populations with different neuropsychological tests (**Table 4**). SDB in older adults has been found to impair

- Vigilance[55,56]
- Attention[57–60]
- Reaction time[61]
- Executive functioning[58,62–64]

Table 2
Insomnia status and cognitive decline or dementia diagnosis

Insomnia Measure	Cognitive Measure	Results	Study
Negative Associations			
ICD-9 codes	ICD-9 codes	Patients with insomnia diagnosis and prescribed hypnotics, > risk for dementia during the 3-y follow-up compared with control subjects	35
Interview indicating either problem most of the time: trouble falling asleep or waking up too early and not falling asleep again	Pfeiffer SPMSQ, >2 errors on the SPMSQ classified as cognitive decline	Insomnia associated with increased risk of cognitive decline for men, independent of depression and comorbid with depression Insomnia associated with increased risk of cognitive decline for women when insomnia was comorbid with depression	36
Positive Associations			
Interview and questionnaire: difficulty initiating sleep, awakenings during the night, early morning awakening, insomnia severity	Incident cognitive impairment defined as 4-point reduction in MMSE, 4-point reduction in BVRT, and 14-point reduction in the IST scores	Number of insomnia complaints and difficulty with awakenings during the night were negatively associated with MMSE cognitive decline during follow-up No associations found for BVRT or IST	39
Johns Hopkins Alzheimer's Disease Research Center questionnaire	Severity of dementia was classified based on MMSE scores (mild = MMSE >20; moderate = MMSE 11–19; severe = MMSE <10)	Participants diagnosed with insomnia performed better on the MMSE than those without sleep disturbance or those with insomnia and daytime sleepiness	40
Adapted Brief Insomnia Questionnaire	A composite score was produced based on a global test that included several cognitive	Time-varying insomnia symptoms associated with MCI and dementia after controlling for	37

(continued on next page)

Table 2
(continued)

Insomnia Measure	Cognitive Measure	Results	Study
	domains; scores range from 0 to 35 0–6: dementia 7–11: cognitively impaired with no dementia (MCI) 12–27: not cognitively impaired	covariates including age, race, gender, education, BMI, smoking status, drinking, and chronic disease[37]	
No Associations			
Self-report questionnaire assessing "Usually having trouble falling asleep or waking up far too early and not going back to sleep"	CASI; cognitive decline was defined as a >9-point decrease in the CASI	Insomnia not associated with greater risk for dementia diagnosis or cognitive decline	41
Interview assessing difficulty falling asleep, staying asleep, or both	Incident cognitive impairment defined as an MMSE <21	No sleep problems associated with increased risk for incident cognitive impairment at 2- and 10-y follow-ups	42
Clinical interview: at least 1 symptom (difficulty falling asleep, staying asleep, early morning awakening) occurring at least 3 times a wk	MMSE; Global Deterioration Scale Participants with MMSE <24.0 were evaluated for dementia by expert panel	Insomnia diagnosis was not associated with cognitive impairment	43
Insomnia Interview Schedule and Sleep Impairment Index: onset, maintenance, termination insomnia	Alzheimer disease diagnosis was made according to NINCDS/ADRDA and DSM-IV criteria	Individuals with Alzheimer disease did not differ from the healthy comparison group in terms of the frequency of onset, maintenance, termination of insomnia symptoms	44

Abbreviations: ADRDA, Alzheimer's Disease and Related Disorders Association; BMI, body mass index; BVRT, Benton visual retention test; CASI, cognitive abilities screening instrument; DSM-IV, Diagnostic and Statistical Manual of Mental Disorders, Fourth, Edition; ICD-9, International Classification of Diseases; IST, Isaacs Set Test; MCI, mild cognitive impairment; MMSE, Mini-Mental State Examination; NINCDS, National Institute of Neurological Disorders and Stroke, Ninth, Revision; SPMSQ, short portable mental status questionnaire.

Table 3
Insomnia treatment and cognitive performance

Insomnia Measure	Cognitive Measure	Results	Study
DSM-IV criteria, Pittsburgh Sleep Quality Index, Sleep Disorders Questionnaire. PSG and sleep diaries were also used.	Simple and complex sustained attention assessed via computer. Outcomes: lapses, false-positive responses, and reaction times.	Compared with the waitlist control, insomnia intervention group showed increased reaction time for simple vigilance task and reduced reaction time for complex vigilance task.	31
DSM-IV-TR, ICSD-2 verified by self-report questionnaires and clinical interview. Polysomnography and the Pittsburgh Sleep Quality Index were also used.	Neuropsychological tests assessed 3 cognitive domains: episodic memory, working memory, abstract reasoning.	Insomnia intervention was not associated with greater improved cognitive performance compared with information-only control.	46
DSM-5 criteria, verified by clinical interview. Single night ambulatory monitoring for SDB.	Overall cognitive functioning, attention, processing speed, language, memory, executive functioning.	No significant improvement in overall cognitive functioning or cognitive domains from pretreatment to posttreatment.	47

Abbreviations: DSM-IV-TR, Diagnostic and Statistical Manual of Mental Disorders, Fourth, Edition, text revision; ICSD-2, International Classification of Sleep Disorders, Second Edition.

- Problem solving[65]
- Verbal recall[63,66,67]
- Nonverbal recall[65]
- Episodic memory[62]
- Declarative memory[64]
- Processing speed[64]

Cross and colleagues[64] performed a meta-analysis and review of 13 studies examining neuropsychological performance in older adults with obstructive sleep apnea (OSA). Executive functioning was the most common cognitive domain explored in studies. Overall, OSA had a small but significant impact on executive functioning, processing speed, and declarative memory. The effect of OSA was small and nonsignificant for working memory, global cognition, and motor learning. The meta-analysis did find years of education, mean apnea-hypopnea index (AHI), and proportion of females in study samples to have a significant moderating effect on the association between OSA and neuropsychological performance. The authors suggest differences in study methodology may have contributed to findings, because small case-control studies from

specialized sleep clinics showed significant medium-effect-sized associations between OSA and cognitive functioning, but larger cohort studies from the community obtained null results.[64] Additional meta-analytic data suggest some sex differences in risk of cognitive decline. Women with OSA are more likely to develop mild cognitive impairment than men with OSA.

Although few studies have examined the longitudinal impact of SDB on cognitive performance in older adults, preliminary evidence suggests that SDB can contribute to relevant long-term changes. A systematic review by Bubu and colleagues[68] found three studies that used longitudinal designs. Evidence is mixed with two studies reporting positive findings and one reporting null findings. The first found a modest association between nocturnal hypoxemia and global cognitive decline over 3 years among 2636 cognitively normal older adults.[69] The second study found that higher AHI was associated with a slight decline in attention over 8 years for 559 community-dwelling older adults.[70] The final study containing 966 older adults found no association between OSA severity or nocturnal hypoxemia

Table 4
Cognitive performance in older adults with sleep-disordered breathing

Cognitive Domain	Measures	Outcomes	Representative References
Global functioning	MMSE	EDS is associated with global cognitive decline over 3 y	52,53
		Increased levels of hypoxemia and AHI are associated with lower global cognition functioning	
	Modified Mini-Mental State Exam	Nocturnal hypoxemia associated with global cognitive decline over 3 y	69
Vigilance	Digital Vigilance Test	SDB is associated with decreased vigilance	55,56,60,61
	Psychomotor Vigilance Test	Increased hypoxemia is associated with decreased vigilance	
	Trail-making Test Part A	Increased RDI is associated with decreased attention	
	Digit Symbol Substitution/Coding Subtest	Older adults with SDB have slower reaction times compared with age-matched control subjects and younger adults	
	Vienna Test System		
Executive function	Stroop Color and Word Test	Higher RDI associated with decreased executive function	58,60,62,63
	Trail-making Test Part B	RDI associated with lower cerebral efficiency	
	Similarities Subtest	SDB is associated with a greater decline of executive function over time	
	Raven Progressive Matrices	Severe SDB is associated with poorer executive functioning	
		SDB is associated with poorer problem-solving abilities	
Memory	Hopkins Verbal Learning Test	SDB is associated with lower nonverbal delayed recall	65–67
	Brief Visuospatial Memory Test-Revised	Increased AHI and RDI are associated with decreased verbal delayed recall memory	

(continued on next page)

Cognitive Domain	Measures	Outcomes	Representative References

Table 4
(continued)

Cognitive Domain	Measures	Outcomes	Representative References
	Rey Auditory Verbal Learning Test	Severe SDB is associated with poorer episodic memory over time	
Attention	Trail Making Test Part A Stroop Color-Word Test Part I and II Coding subtest of WAIS-III	AHI was associated with a small decline in attention over 8 y	[70]

Abbreviations: AHI, apnea-hypopnea index; EDS, excessive daytime sleepiness; RDI, respiratory disturbance index.

and cognitive decline over 15 years.[71] The authors note that some discrepancy in the findings may be caused by the methodologic differences, including the use of healthy participants with strict inclusion criteria and differences between excluded participants and those who remained in the study in terms of AHI and indices and hypoxemia, obesity, hypertension.

The long-term impact of SDB may also influence the onset and course of certain neurologic disorders. Individuals with SDB have higher rates of mild cognitive impairment and dementia at an earlier age.[72,73] Evidence also suggests that older adults with neurologic disorders might be more vulnerable to the negative cognitive effects of SDB.[56] For example, SDB can exacerbate cognitive impairments in older adults with dementia.[74] The possible role of SDB in the development of neurologic disorders has led researchers to examine the possible pathways contributing to impairments in cognitive functioning. According to one review, evidence suggests a link between OSA and biomarkers of Alzheimer disease pathology.[68] Although longitudinal evidence is still limited, findings suggest OSA severity is associated with higher amyloid burden over a 2-year period. In an additional longitudinal analysis that included cognitively normal older adults, and those with various dementias, and mild cognitive impairment, self-reported diagnosis of OSA was associated with larger increases in amyloid burden and cerebral spinal fluid concentration over 2.5 years in cognitively normal older adults and older adults with mild cognitive impairment, but not older adults with Alzheimer disease.[68]

Several mechanisms through which SDB contributes to cognitive decline in older adults have been proposed. Evidence suggests that high levels of hypoxemia, an abnormally low level of oxygen in the blood, may play a prominent role. Yaffe and colleagues[73] found that hypoxemia was associated with an increased risk of future mild cognitive impairment and dementia. In addition, increased hypoxemia is associated with greater impairment in global cognitive functioning, and declines in specific cognitive domains.[55,69] However, other studies have found no association between hypoxemia and impaired cognition.[52,67] As a result, sleep fragmentation and excessive daytime sleepiness have been proposed as alternative mechanisms through which SDB may lead to cognitive dysfunction.[75] For example, excessive daytime sleepiness caused by SDB was associated with a decline in global cognitive functioning.[52] Despite these findings, the relative contributions of sleep fragmentation and excessive daytime sleepiness to cognitive impairment remain poorly understood. SDB may manifest differently in men and women, with men displaying more episodic hypoxia and women having more sleep fragmentation. These sex-specific presentations of SDB may be associated with unique cognitive sequela.

Although strong evidence supports an association between SDB and cognitive decline in older adults, not all findings support this association. One study found that although SDB and aging are independently associated with cognitive deficits, age did not interact with SDB to make those cognitive deficits worse.[76] Other studies report similar findings. Boland and colleagues[77] found no evidence for an association between either mild or moderate forms of SDB and cognitive functioning in verbal learning and short-term recall, psychomotor efficiency, or verbal fluency. Similarly, other research found no association between SDB and performance on broad standardized cognitive tests.[78,79] Studies that report no association between SDB and cognitive impairment in older adults contain several methodologic differences. First, they generally lacked comprehensive measures of cognitive functioning or relied on single measures of global functioning.[77] Cognitive impairments in older adults with SDB may be subtle and may not be readily identified by general/global cognitive measures. Second, several of the studies that report no association between SDB and cognition used home-based PSG,[79] which has been shown to differ from laboratory PSG, particularly for adults with severe SDB.[80] In addition, several studies reporting no associations between SDB and cognitive performance only included participants with mild to moderate SDB,[77,78] potentially suggestive of a dose–response association between SDB severity and cognitive performance.

Although the findings are inconsistent, overall, current research suggests that SDB adversely affects cognitive performance in older adults. Cognitive impairments are particularly pronounced in the domains of attention, executive function, and memory; however, these impairments may be sex-specific. These findings are largely consistent with research examining the influence of SDB in young and middle-aged adults.[81,82]

Sleep-Disordered Breathing Severity and Cognitive Performance

Research has explored whether the severity of SDB (as indexed by the AHI or respiratory disturbance index) is related to the level of cognitive impairment in older adults. Studies have found that greater AHI and respiratory disturbance index were associated with poorer global cognitive functioning,[53] and adverse outcomes on specific cognitive domains, such as

- Vigilance[56,59,83]
- Executive functioning[63]
- Language functioning[84]
- Attention[58,60]
- Executive function[58,60]
- Memory[66]

However, one study examining older adults with mostly mild to moderate SDB found no association between SDB severity and cognitive functioning,[77] suggesting that there may be a threshold at which SDB exerts an increasingly negative impact on cognition. Further research investigating SDB severity and cognitive impairment is warranted.

Sleep-Disordered Breathing Treatment and Cognitive Performance

Given the nature of cognitive dysfunction in older adults with SDB, and the association between SDB and neurologic disorders, the influence of SDB treatment on cognitive functioning in older adults has been the subject of recent interest. The most common treatment of SDB is positive airway pressure (PAP) therapy. Although PAP has been shown to decrease some of the primary sequelae of SDB, such as sleep fragmentation and nocturnal oxygen saturation, several studies suggest possible additional benefits of PAP treatment on cognitive performance.

Four studies report improvements in many areas of cognitive functioning following 3 months of PAP treatment.[66,85–87] Improvements were shown in the following domains:

- Episodic learning and memory
- Short-term memory
- Executive functioning
- Working memory
- Attention
- Psychomotor speed
- Nonverbal delayed recall

Despite optimism about the potential benefits of PAP on cognition, some studies have shown more limited and uneven benefits of PAP treatment. For example, Kang and colleagues[88] found that short-term PAP treatment was associated with gains in executive functioning but no other cognitive domains. Moreover, small single-center trials have shown improvement in attention, psychomotor speed, memory, and executive function, whereas larger, multicenter clinical cohorts show significant improvement in only working memory or no significant changes.[68] Low adherence and short-term PAP usage were suspected to have weakened the impact of the intervention. Additionally, authors considered a ceiling effect because of high baseline cognitive scores among participants.

Preliminary evidence suggests that cognitive gains observed with short-term PAP treatment might be maintained over time. PAP treatment over the course of 10 years is associated with better memory, attention, and executive functioning.[62] The long-term benefits of PAP treatment may also extend to older adults with neurologic disorders. Preliminary examination of long-term PAP use among individuals with Alzheimer disease found that treatment can slow cognitive deterioration.[89] Another recent study reported that PAP treatment may delay the age of onset of mild cognitive impairment.[72]

Although the influence of PAP treatment on cognitive outcomes seems promising, noncompliance with the treatment remains prevalent in the general population, and among older adults.[90] Limited compliance may severely limit the benefits of PAP treatment on cognitive abilities. Older

Table 5
Theories on the link between sleep and cognition

Name	Description	Reference
Controlled attention	Monotonous tasks are most affected by sleep loss because of the amount of top-down control needed to sustain attention, whereas more complex/difficult tasks are intrinsically motivating (ie, bottom-up control)	94
Neuropsychological	Sleep loss results in focal impairment in functions subserved by the prefrontal cortex (ie, executive functions), beyond any impairment in attention or vigilance	21,25,95
Vigilance/arousal	Attention, which is needed for the performance of many other cognitive tasks, is mediated by arousal; a common correlated feature of disturbed sleep	96,97
Wake-state instability	Cognitive deficits observed as a result of sleep loss occur because of the interaction of the drive to maintain alertness and the homeostatic drive to initiate sleep	98–100

adults who complied with treatment (average use of 8.5 hours per night) showed greater cognitive abilities compared with individuals who were non-compliant (3.9 hours per night).[66] One hypothesis about PAP compliance is that older adults who notice cognitive gains in readily observable domains, such as attention and memory, may be more likely to comply with PAP treatment.[66]

Although preliminary evidence shows improved cognitive outcomes for older adults treated with PAP, further research is needed to confirm these findings and better understand which cognitive domains are affected. In addition, future research should examine whether other forms of SDB treatment, such as weight loss, oral appliance therapy, positional therapy, and surgical treatments, might lead to similar cognitive gains.

Hypoglossal nerve stimulation (HNS) is a novel, promising treatment of SDB. The treatment uses a surgically implanted device to produce electrical stimulation of the hypoglossal nerve to move the tongue and relieve upper airway obstruction. Two systematic reviews have shown that HNS treatment significantly improves sleep apnea severity and excessive sleepiness in adult populations at 1- and 5-year follow-up.[91,92] Additional evidence is needed to determine the impact of HNS treatment on cognitive functioning among older adults. This is particularly important given recent evidence suggesting that middle-aged and older adults are among those interested in obtaining HNS treatment.[93]

Please note that these theories are not mutually exclusive but attempt to explain similar phenomena in different ways.

UNIFYING THEORIES AND MECHANISMS

There are several informative hypotheses concerning the association between sleep and cognitive functioning. These hypotheses include the controlled attention hypothesis,[94] neuropsychological hypothesis,[21,25,95] vigilance/arousal hypothesis,[96,97] and wake-state instability hypothesis.[98–100] These various theories about the role of sleep processes in regulating and maintaining cognitive functioning may not be mutually exclusive.[21] The controlled attention and

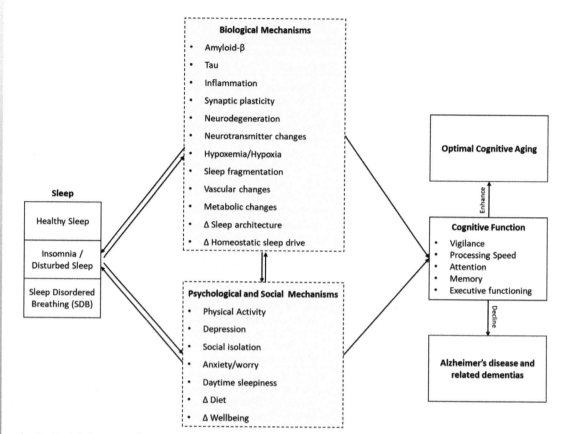

Fig. 2. Model depicting the relationships among healthy sleep, insomnia/disturbed sleep, and sleep-disordered breathing and cognitive functioning, optimal cognitive aging, and Alzheimer disease and related dementias in older adults. Factors listed in *dashed boxes* represent potential biopsychosocial mechanisms through which sleep may impact cognitive functioning.

vigilance/arousal hypotheses are essentially parallel descriptions of the same phenomena. Many higher order cognitive functions may rely on the appropriate levels of attention and arousal. It has been suggested that impairment of the prefrontal cortex may cause decrements in attention and vigilance.[101] Sleep seems to impede arousal/vigilance/attention and prefrontal functioning, potentially through instability of the neurobiologic systems responsible for attentional and sleep drives. **Table 5** provides a description of each sleep-cognition theory. In addition to the sleep-cognition hypotheses discussed previously, there are many suspected mechanisms involved in the sleep-cognition relationship in late life. These mechanisms are graphically depicted in **Fig. 2**.

SUMMARY AND FUTURE DIRECTIONS

Sleep and cognitive functioning are linked in late-life; however, the exact nature of this relationship has yet to be discerned. Future studies should continue to investigate the gamut of sleep-

cognition relationships. Important questions remain concerning (1) the role of normal sleep changes in normal cognitive aging; (2) the role of pathologic sleep changes in the development of dementias; (3) the utility of treating sleep disorders for improving cognitive functioning, warding off unwanted cognitive decline, and slowing the course of neurodegenerative diseases; and (4) sex differences in the association between sleep (healthy and disordered) and cognitive functioning. An intriguing prospect for future study is to examine the additive impact of treating sleep disorders in conjunction with focused cognitive interventions, and treating sleep disorders in older adults with comorbid conditions, such as diabetes, known to be associated with cognitive functioning. Perhaps the combination of interventions that focus on different pathways of change may have a synergistic effect and result in more pronounced cognitive improvements. Increasing knowledge of the ways in which sleep may affect late-life cognitive functioning could have far-reaching benefits.

CLINICS CARE POINTS

- Sleep should be considered and evaluated when working with older adults with cognitive concerns/complaints.
- Treating late-life insomnia and sleep apnea has potential to slow late-life cognitive decline.

DISCLOSURE

Dr J.M. Dzierzewski was supported by a grant from the National Institute on Aging (K23AG049955). Dr N. Dautovich serves as a sleep consultant for the National Sleep Foundation and Merck Sharp & Dohme Corp. Dr. Dzierzewski served on an advisory panel for Eisai Pharmaceuticals. E. Perez and S.G. Ravyts report no commercial or financial conflicts of interest.

REFERENCES

1. Li S-C, Huxhold O, Schmiedek F. Aging and attenuated processing robustness. Gerontology 2003; 50(1):28–34.
2. Nesselroade JR. The warp and the woof of the developmental fabric. Visions Aesthetics, Environ Dev Legacy Joachim F Wohlwill 1991;213–40.
3. Park DC, Smith AD, Lautenschlager G, et al. Mediators of long-term memory performance across the life span. Psychol Aging 1996;11(4):621.
4. Schaie KW, Willis SL, Caskie GI. The Seattle Longitudinal Study: relationship between personality and cognition. Neuropsychol Dev Cogn B Aging Neuropsychol Cogn 2004;11(2–3):304–24.
5. Salthouse TA. What and when of cognitive aging. Curr Dir Psychol Sci 2004;13(4):140–4.
6. Morgan K. Sleep and aging. In: Lichstein K, Morin C, editors. Treatment of late-life insomnia. Sage Publications; 2000.
7. Foley DJ, Monjan AA, Brown SL, et al. Sleep complaints among elderly persons: an epidemiological study of 3 communities. Sleep 1995;18:425–32.
8. Newman AB, Enright PL, Manolio TA, et al. Sleep disturbance, psychosocial correlates, and cardiovascular disease in 5201 older adults: the Cardiovascular Health Study. J Am Geriatr Soc 1997; 45(1):1–7.
9. Young T, Peppard PE, Gottlieb DJ. Epidemiology of obstructive sleep apnea: a population health perspective. Am J Respir Crit Care Med 2002; 165(9):1217–39.
10. Faubel R, López-García E, Guallar-castillÓn P, et al. Usual sleep duration and cognitive function in older adults in Spain. J Sleep Res 2009;18(4): 427–35.
11. Kronholm E, Sallinen M, Suutama T, et al. Self-reported sleep duration and cognitive functioning in the general population. J Sleep Res 2009;18(4): 436–46.
12. Tworoger SS, Lee S, Schernhammer ES, et al. The association of self-reported sleep duration, difficulty sleeping, and snoring with cognitive function in older women. Alzheimer Dis Assoc Disord 2006;20(1):41–8.
13. Bastien CH, Fortier-Brochu É, Rioux I, et al. Cognitive performance and sleep quality in the elderly suffering from chronic insomnia: relationship between objective and subjective measures. J Psychosom Res 2003;54(1):39–49.
14. Devore EE, Grodstein F, Schernhammer ES. Sleep duration in relation to cognitive function among older adults: a systematic review of observational studies. Neuroepidemiology 2016;46(1):57–78.
15. Cox SR, Ritchie SJ, Allerhand M, et al. Sleep and cognitive aging in the eighth decade of life. Sleep 2019;42(4):zsz019.
16. Crenshaw MC, Edinger JD. Slow-wave sleep and waking cognitive performance among older adults with and without insomnia complaints. Physiol Behav 1999;66(3):485–92.
17. Djonlagic I, Mariani S, Fitzpatrick AL, et al. Macro and micro sleep architecture and cognitive performance in older adults. Nat Hum Behav 2021;5(1): 123–45.
18. Blackwell T, Yaffe K, Ancoli-Israel S, et al. Poor sleep is associated with impaired cognitive function in older women: the study of osteoporotic fractures. J Gerontol A Biol Sci Med Sci 2006;61(4): 405–10.
19. McSorley VE, Bin YS, Lauderdale DS. Associations of sleep characteristics with cognitive function and decline among older adults. Am J Epidemiol 2019; 188(6):1066–75.
20. Oosterman JM, van Someren EJ, Vogels RL, et al. Fragmentation of the rest-activity rhythm correlates with age-related cognitive deficits. J Sleep Res 2009;18(1):129–35.
21. Lim J, Dinges DF. A meta-analysis of the impact of short-term sleep deprivation on cognitive variables. Psychol Bull 2010;136(3):375.
22. Webb WB, Levy CM. Age, sleep deprivation, and performance. Psychophysiology 1982;19(3): 272–6.
23. Webb WB. A further analysis of age and sleep deprivation effects. Psychophysiology 1985;22(2): 156–61.
24. Pasula EY, Brown GG, McKenna BS, et al. Effects of sleep deprivation on component processes of

working memory in younger and older adults. Sleep 2018;41(3). https://doi.org/10.1093/sleep/zsx213.

25. Jones K, Harrison Y. Frontal lobe function, sleep loss and fragmented sleep. Sleep Med Rev 2001; 5(6):463–75.

26. Bliese PD, Wesensten NJ, Balkin TJ. Age and individual variability in performance during sleep restriction. J Sleep Res 2006;15(4):376–85.

27. Lowe CJ, Safati A, Hall PA. The neurocognitive consequences of sleep restriction: a meta-analytic review. Neurosci Biobehav Rev 2017;80:586–604.

28. Banks S, Dinges DF. Behavioral and physiological consequences of sleep restriction. J Clin Sleep Med 2007;3(5):519–28.

29. Tucker M, McKinley S, Stickgold R. Sleep optimizes motor skill in older adults. J Am Geriatr Soc 2011;59(4):603–9.

30. Fortier-Brochu E, Beaulieu-Bonneau S, Ivers H, et al. Insomnia and daytime cognitive performance: a meta-analysis. Sleep Med Rev 2012; 16(1):83–94.

31. Altena E, Van Der Werf YD, Strijers RLM, et al. Sleep loss affects vigilance: effects of chronic insomnia and sleep therapy. J Sleep Res 2008; 17(3):335–43.

32. Haimov I, Hanuka E, Horowitz Y. Chronic insomnia and cognitive functioning among older adults. Behav Sleep Med 2008;6(1):32–54.

33. Ling A, Lim ML, Gwee X, et al. Insomnia and daytime neuropsychological test performance in older adults. Sleep Med 2016;17:7–12.

34. Nofzinger EA, Buysse DJ, Germain A, et al. Functional neuroimaging evidence for hyperarousal in insomnia. Am J Psychiatry 2004;161(11):2126–8.

35. Chen P-L, Lee W-J, Sun W-Z, et al. Risk of dementia in patients with insomnia and long-term use of hypnotics: a population-based retrospective cohort study. In: Forloni G, editor. PLoS One 2012;7(11): e49113.

36. Cricco M, Simonsick EM, Foley DJ. The impact of insomnia on cognitive functioning in older adults. J Am Geriatr Soc 2001;49(9):1185–9.

37. Resciniti NV, Yelverton V, Kase BE, et al. Time-varying insomnia symptoms and incidence of cognitive impairment and dementia among older US adults. Int J Environ Res Public Health 2021;18(1):E351.

38. de Almondes KM, Costa MV, Malloy-Diniz LF, et al. Insomnia and risk of dementia in older adults: systematic review and meta-analysis. J Psychiatr Res 2016;77:109–15.

39. Jaussent I, Bouyer J, Ancelin M-L, et al. Excessive sleepiness is predictive of cognitive decline in the elderly. Sleep 2012. https://doi.org/10.5665/sleep.2070.

40. Rao V, Spiro J, Samus QM, et al. Insomnia and daytime sleepiness in people with dementia residing in assisted living: findings from the Maryland assisted living study. Int J Geriatr Psychiatry 2008;23(2): 199–206.

41. Foley D, Monjan A, Masaki K, et al. Daytime sleepiness is associated with 3-year incident dementia and cognitive decline in older Japanese-American men. J Am Geriatr Soc 2001;49(12): 1628–32.

42. Keage HAD, Banks S, Yang KL, et al. What sleep characteristics predict cognitive decline in the elderly? Sleep Med 2012;13(7):886–92.

43. Merlino G, Piani A, Gigli GL, et al. Daytime sleepiness is associated with dementia and cognitive decline in older Italian adults: a population-based study. Sleep Med 2010;11(4):372–7.

44. Ohadinia S, Noroozian M, Shahsavand S, et al. Evaluation of insomnia and daytime napping in Iranian Alzheimer disease patients: relationship with severity of dementia and comparison with normal adults. Am J Geriatr Psychiatry 2004; 12(5):517–22.

45. Xu W, Tan C-C, Zou J-J, et al, Alzheimer's Disease Neuroimaging Initiative. Insomnia moderates the relationship between amyloid-β and cognitive decline in late-life adults without dementia. J Alzheimers Dis 2021;81(4):1701–10.

46. Wilckens KA, Hall MH, Nebes RD, et al. Changes in cognitive performance are associated with changes in sleep in older adults with insomnia. Behav Sleep Med 2016;14(3):295–310.

47. McCrae CS, Curtis AF, Williams JM, et al. Efficacy of brief behavioral treatment for insomnia in older adults: examination of sleep, mood, and cognitive outcomes. Sleep Med 2018. https://doi.org/10.1016/j.sleep.2018.05.018.

48. McCrae CS, Curtis AF, Williams JM, et al. Effects of brief behavioral treatment for insomnia on daily associations between self-reported sleep and objective cognitive performance in older adults. Behav Sleep Med 2020;18(5):577–88.

49. Peppard PE, Young T, Barnet JH, et al. Increased prevalence of sleep-disordered breathing in adults. Am J Epidemiol 2013;177(9):1006–14.

50. Hedden T, Gabrieli JD. Insights into the ageing mind: a view from cognitive neuroscience. Nat Rev Neurosci 2004;5(2):87–96.

51. Ayalon L, Ancoli-Israel S, Drummond SP. Obstructive sleep apnea and age: a double insult to brain function? Am J Respir Crit Care Med 2010;182(3): 413–9.

52. Cohen-Zion M, Stepnowsky C, Marler ST, et al. Changes in cognitive function associated with sleep disordered breathing in older people. J Am Geriatr Soc 2001;49(12):1622–7.

53. Spira AP, Blackwell T, Stone KL, et al. Sleep-disordered breathing and cognition in older women. J Am Geriatr Soc 2008;56(1):45–50.

54. Zimmerman ME, Aloia MS. Sleep-disordered breathing and cognition in older adults. Curr Neurol Neurosci Rep 2012;12(5):537–46.

55. Blackwell T, Yaffe K, Ancoli-Israel S, et al. Associations between sleep architecture and sleep-disordered breathing and cognition in older community-dwelling men: the osteoporotic fractures in men sleep study. J Am Geriatr Soc 2011; 59(12):2217–25.

56. Kim H, Dinges DF, Young T. Sleep-disordered breathing and psychomotor vigilance in a community-based sample. Sleep 2007;30(10): 1309–16.

57. Dealberto MJ, Pajot N, Courbon D, et al. Breathing disorders during sleep and cognitive performance in an older community sample: the EVA Study. J Am Geriatr Soc 1996;44(11):1287–94.

58. Hayward L, Mant A, Eyland A, et al. Sleep disordered breathing and cognitive function in a retirement village population. Age Ageing 1992;21(2):121–8.

59. Saint Martin M, Sforza E, Roche F, et al. Sleep breathing disorders and cognitive function in the elderly: an 8-year follow-up study. The Proof-Synapse Cohort. Sleep 2015;38(2):179–87.

60. Yesavage J, Bliwise D, Guilleminault C, et al. Preliminary communication: intellectual deficit and sleep-related respiratory disturbance in the elderly. Sleep 1985;8(1):30–3.

61. Alchanatis M, Zias N, Deligiorgis N, et al. Comparison of cognitive performance among different age groups in patients with obstructive sleep apnea. Sleep Breath 2008;12(1):17–24.

62. Crawford-Achour E, Dauphinot V, Saint Martin M, et al. Protective effect of long-term CPAP therapy on cognitive performance in elderly patients with severe OSA: the PROOF study. J Clin Sleep Med 2015;11(5):519–24.

63. Ju G, Yoon I-Y, Lee SD, et al. Effects of sleep apnea syndrome on delayed memory and executive function in elderly adults. J Am Geriatr Soc 2012;60(6): 1099–103.

64. Cross N, Lampit A, Pye J, et al. Is obstructive sleep apnoea related to neuropsychological function in healthy older adults? A systematic review and meta-analysis. Neuropsychol Rev 2017;27(4): 389–402.

65. Berry DT, Phillips BA, Cook YR, et al. Geriatric sleep apnea syndrome: a preliminary description. J Gerontol 1990;45(5):M169–74.

66. Aloia MS, Ilniczky N, Di Dio P, et al. Neuropsychological changes and treatment compliance in older adults with sleep apnea. J Psychosomatic Res 2003;54(1):71–6.

67. O'Hara R, Schröder CM, Kraemer HC, et al. Nocturnal sleep apnea/hypopnea is associated with lower memory performance in APOE ε4 carriers. Neurology 2005;65(4):642–4.

68. Bubu OM, Andrade AG, Umasabor-Bubu OQ, et al. Obstructive sleep apnea, cognition and Alzheimer's disease: a systematic review integrating three decades of multidisciplinary research. Sleep Med Rev 2020;50:101250.

69. Blackwell T, Yaffe K, Laffan A, et al. Associations between sleep-disordered breathing, nocturnal hypoxemia, and subsequent cognitive decline in older community-dwelling men: the Osteoporotic Fractures in Men sleep study. J Am Geriatr Soc 2015;63(3):453–61.

70. Martin MS, Sforza E, Roche F, et al, PROOF study group. Sleep breathing disorders and cognitive function in the elderly: an 8-year follow-up study. the proof-synapse cohort. Sleep 2015;38(2):179–87.

71. Lutsey PL, Bengtson LGS, Punjabi NM, et al. Obstructive sleep apnea and 15-year cognitive decline: the Atherosclerosis Risk in communities (ARIC) study. Sleep 2016;39(2):309–16.

72. Osorio RS, Gumb T, Pirraglia E, et al. Sleep-disordered breathing advances cognitive decline in the elderly. Neurology 2015;84(19):1964–71.

73. Yaffe K, Laffan AM, Harrison SL, et al. Sleep-disordered breathing, hypoxia, and risk of mild cognitive impairment and dementia in older women. JAMA 2011;306(6):613–9.

74. Ancoli-Israel S, Ayalon L, Salzman C. Sleep in the elderly: normal variations and common sleep disorders. Harv Rev Psychiatry 2008;16(5):279–86.

75. Yaffe K, Falvey CM, Hoang T. Connections between sleep and cognition in older adults. Lancet Neurol 2014;13(10):1017–28.

76. Mathieu A, Mazza S, Décary A, et al. Effects of obstructive sleep apnea on cognitive function: a comparison between younger and older OSAS patients. Sleep Med 2008;9(2):112–20.

77. Boland LL, Shahar E, Iber C, et al. Measures of cognitive function in persons with varying degrees of sleep-disordered breathing: the Sleep Heart Health Study. J Sleep Res 2002;11(3): 265–72.

78. Sforza E, Roche F, Thomas-Anterion C, et al. Cognitive function and sleep related breathing disorders in a healthy elderly population: the SYN-APSE study. Sleep 2010;33(4):515–21.

79. Foley DJ, Masaki K, White L, et al. Sleep-disordered breathing and cognitive impairment in elderly Japanese-American men. Sleep 2003; 26(5):596–9.

80. Portier F, Portmann A, Czernichow P, et al. Evaluation of home versus laboratory polysomnography in the diagnosis of sleep apnea syndrome. Am J Respir Crit Care Med 2000;162(3):814–8.

81. Beebe DW, Groesz L, Wells C, et al. The neuropsychological effects of obstructive sleep apnea: a meta-analysis of norm-referenced and case-controlled data. Sleep 2003;26(3):298–307.

82. Bucks RS, Olaithe M, Eastwood P. Neurocognitive function in obstructive sleep apnoea: a meta-review. Respirology 2013;18(1):61–70.

83. Ingram F, Henke KG, Levin HS, et al. Sleep apnea and vigilance performance in a community-dwelling older sample. Sleep 1994;17(3):248–52.

84. Kim SJ, Lee JH, Lee DY, et al. Neurocognitive dysfunction associated with sleep quality and sleep apnea in patients with mild cognitive impairment. Am J Geriatr Psychiatry 2011;19(4):374–81.

85. Dalmases M, Solé-Padullés C, Torres M, et al. Effect of CPAP on cognition, brain function, and structure among elderly patients with OSA: a randomized pilot study. Chest 2015;148(5):1214–23.

86. Martínez-García MÁ, Chiner E, Hernández L, et al. Obstructive sleep apnoea in the elderly: role of continuous positive airway pressure treatment. Eur Respir J 2015;46(1):142–51.

87. Richards KC, Gooneratne N, Dicicco B, et al. CPAP adherence may slow 1-year cognitive decline in older adults with mild cognitive impairment and apnea. J Am Geriatr Soc 2019;67(3):558–64.

88. Kang S-H, Yoon I-Y, Lee SD, et al. Effects of continuous positive airway pressure treatment on cognitive functions in the Korean elderly with obstructive sleep apnea. Sleep Med Res 2016; 7(1):10–5.

89. Cooke JR, Ancoli-Israel S, Liu L, et al. Continuous positive airway pressure deepens sleep in patients with Alzheimer's disease and obstructive sleep apnea. Sleep Med 2009;10(10):1101–6.

90. Russo-Magno P, O'Brien A, Panciera T, et al. Compliance with CPAP therapy in older men with obstructive sleep apnea. J Am Geriatr Soc 2001; 49(9):1205–11.

91. Certal VF, Zaghi S, Riaz M, et al. Hypoglossal nerve stimulation in the treatment of obstructive sleep apnea: a systematic review and meta-analysis. Laryngoscope 2015;125(5):1254–64.

92. Costantino A, Rinaldi V, Moffa A, et al. Hypoglossal nerve stimulation long-term clinical outcomes: a systematic review and meta-analysis. Sleep Breath 2020;24(2):399–411.

93. Dzierzewski JM, Soto P, Vahidi N, et al. Clinical characteristics of older adults seeking hypoglossal nerve stimulation for the treatment of obstructive sleep apnea. Ear Nose Throat J 2021;31. https://doi.org/10.1177/01455613211042126.

94. Pilcher JJ, Band D, Odle-Dusseau HN, et al. Human performance under sustained operations and acute sleep deprivation conditions: toward a model of controlled attention. Aviat Space Environ Med 2007;78(Supplement 1):B15–24.

95. Harrison Y, Horne JA. The impact of sleep deprivation on decision making: a review. J Exp Psychol Appl 2000;6(3):236.

96. Bonnet MH, Arand DL. 24-hour metabolic-rate in insomniacs and matched normal sleepers. Sleep 1995;18:581–8.

97. Richardson GS. Human physiological models of insomnia. Sleep Med 2007;8(Supplement 4): S9–14.

98. Dinges DF, Pack F, Williams K, et al. Cumulative sleepiness, mood disturbance and psychomotor vigilance performance decrements during a week of sleep restricted to 4-5 hours per night. Sleep 1997. Available at: http://psycnet.apa.org/psycinfo/1997-06077-003. Accessed September 27, 2016.

99. Durmer JS, Dinges DF. Neurocognitive consequences of sleep deprivation. In: Seminars in neurology, vol. 25. New York: Thieme Medical Publishers, Inc.; 2005. p. 117–29. Available at: https://www.thieme-connect.com/products/ejournals/html/10.1055/s-2005-867080. Accessed September 27, 2016.

100. Goel N, Rao H, Durmer JS, et al. Neurocognitive consequences of sleep deprivation. In: Seminars in neurology, 29. copyright Thieme Medical Publishers; 2009. p. 320–39. Available at: https://www.thieme-connect.com/products/ejournals/html/10.1055/s-0029-1237117. Accessed October 3, 2016.

101. Boonstra TW, Stins JF, Daffertshofer A, et al. Effects of sleep deprivation on neural functioning: an integrative review. Cell Mol Life Sci 2007;64(7–8): 934–46.

Sleep in Hospitalized Older Adults

Nancy H. Stewart, DO, MS[a], Vineet M. Arora, MD, MAPP[b],*

KEYWORDS

• Sleep • Hospitalized adults • Geriatrics • Older adults • Patients • Hospitals

KEY POINTS

- Despite the need for rest and recovery during acute illness, hospitalization is a period of acute sleep deprivation for older adults owing to environmental, medical, and patient factors.
- Sleep loss in the hospital for older adults is associated with worse health outcomes, including cardiometabolic derangements and an increased risk of delirium.
- Both pharmacologic and nonpharmacologic interventions have shown promise in improving sleep loss for hospitalized older adults.

INTRODUCTION

Nearly 70 million Americans suffer from a chronic disorder of sleep that adversely affects their health.[1] The National Academy of Medicine estimates that hundreds of billions of dollars per year are spent caring for patients with sleep disorders. For example, 1 in 5 of all injuries owing to serious car crashes are owing to drowsy driving.[1] Despite this, most people with underlying sleep disorders remain undiagnosed. Awareness of diagnoses and treatment of sleep disorders among health care professionals and the public remains very low.

Sadly, the patients most at risk for poor, nonrestorative sleep are often acutely ill and hospitalized, when they arguably need sleep to recover from their acute illness. Acute sleep loss in the hospital has been associated with poor patient outcomes, including cardiometabolic effects such as high blood pressure and hyperglycemia, as well as delirium.[2] For instance, Krumholz[3] coined the term "posthospital syndrome" to highlight the increased risk of readmission for the nearly 3 million hospitalized seniors for diseases unrelated to the index admission. Although studies of long-term consequences of acute sleep loss of hospitalization are lacking, in-hospital sleep loss has been implicated as a potential mediator of posthospital syndrome.

Prior research has demonstrated that sleep loss is associated with worse cardiometabolic outcomes in the hospital,[4] that hospitalization is a period of acute sleep loss that does not recover in the week after discharge,[5] and that 40% of medical patients without a known sleep disorder are actually at high risk for sleep-disordered breathing.[6] Therefore, the hospital setting is a missed opportunity to optimize the sleep environment for better sleep in the hospital and after discharge, but also to improve diagnosis and treatment of previously unrecognized sleep disorders and potentially reduce unnecessary hospital readmissions.[7]

SLEEP LOSS IN OLDER ADULTS

Changes in sleep among healthy older adults are highly relevant when considering disturbed sleep among older adults in the hospital setting. Sleep in older adults is characterized by decreased slow wave (deep) sleep (stage N3 sleep),

Sleep Med Clin 13 (2018) 127-135 https://doi.org/10.1016/j.jsmc.2017.09.012 1556-407X/18/© 2017 Elsevier Inc. All rights reserved.

[a] Department of Medicine, University of Kansas Medical Center, 400 Cambridge Street, Mailstop 3007, Kansas City, KS 66160, USA; [b] Department of Medicine, University of Chicago, 5841 South Maryland Avenue, MC 2007 AMB W216, Chicago, IL 60637, USA
* Corresponding author.
E-mail address: varora@uchicago.edu

Sleep Med Clin 17 (2022) 223–232
https://doi.org/10.1016/j.jsmc.2022.02.002
1556-407X/22/© 2022 Elsevier Inc. All rights reserved.

increased amounts of lighter sleep, more frequent awakenings, less rapid eye movement (REM) sleep, and less total sleep time.[8] In addition, complaints of insomnia are more frequent in older adults. Older patients are also more easily aroused from sleep by environmental stimuli such as noise or light exposure (which is common in the hospital setting). As a result, sleep becomes increasingly fragmented and sleep efficiency decreases. The circadian sleep-wake cycle also frequently advances with age, resulting in a tendency to fall asleep and awaken earlier, and circadian rhythms are more sensitive to disruption in older adults. These changes occur in nearly all older adults, independent of any medical or psychiatric pathology.[9] Anxiety, depression, loss of social support, pain, and acute illness can all further contribute to sleep disturbances in older patients.

Given the increasing recognition that sleep disturbance in older patients can be considered as part of a geriatric syndrome,[10] it is important to optimize sleep in older patients, especially during times of care transitions, such as admission and discharge from the hospital. Unfortunately, obtaining a good night's sleep in the hospital is often difficult.

HEALTH EFFECTS OF SLEEP LOSS FOR HOSPITALIZED OLDER ADULTS

Although there is a paucity of literature regarding the effects of sleep loss in hospitalized patients, a model of 2 possible pathways by which sleep loss may impair recovery and function in hospitalized older patients can be proposed (**Fig. 1**). First, laboratory and epidemiologic studies provide evidence to suggest that sleep deprivation itself can lead to a variety of intrinsic negative health consequences (eg, development of delirium, metabolic derangements in blood sugar or blood pressure).[11–14] Interestingly, these health consequences that are linked to sleep deprivation and fragmentation (eg, delirium, hypertension, and hyperglycemia) are also known complications of hospitalization in older patients.[15–17] In addition, these conditions often are associated with the administration of additional medications or higher dosages of existing medications for older people (eg, antipsychotics for delirium, insulin for hyperglycemia, or antihypertensives for elevated blood pressure). Furthermore, a significant portion of these medications may be continued after discharge and subsequently result in patient harm.[18] Another possible pathway by which sleep loss can impair recovery in hospitalized older patients is due to fatigue and excessive daytime sleepiness, which may hinder patients'

participation in recovery activities (eg, physical therapy), or could diminish patients' desire and ability to be an active participant in their care (ie, ask informed questions, understand medication changes, follow-up tests).[19,20] Understanding this pathway is especially important because diminished daytime physical activity is a known contributor to functional decline, a well-known negative consequence of hospitalization in older adults. In addition, hospitalized older patients who are less empowered and informed regarding their hospital care are more likely to experience readmission.[21]

In addition to these factors, sleep loss has been associated with a variety of important outcomes of relevance for hospitalized older adults as they recover from acute illness. In addition to delirium discussed, sleep loss has been implicated in other geriatric syndromes, such as falls, that are also prevalent in hospitalized older patients. For example, in 1 study women with shorter sleep duration or lower sleep efficiency were more likely to suffer from falls in the subsequent year compared with women with normal sleep duration (>7 hours) and sleep efficiency (>70%).[22] In addition, sleep loss has also been associated with impaired immune function in animals and healthy humans, which may have implications for hospitalized older adults.[23] For example, scientists have shown that more sleep after infection yields better survival in fruit flies.[24]

BARRIERS TO PROPER SLEEP FOR HOSPITALIZED OLDER ADULTS

Obtaining a good night's sleep in the hospital is far from easy. Among the factors that are likely to disrupt sleep are environmental factors (eg, noise, light disruptions), medical care-related factors (eg, early morning vital signs, phlebotomy), and patient factors (eg, pain). Patients in a variety of acute care settings report difficulty falling and staying asleep, not feeling rested, increased daytime napping, and a reduction in sleep quality.[25]

Medical Care Interruptions

Frequent awakenings by care providers represent a significant barrier to sleep in the hospital. Patients who are awakened often may be unable to complete an entire sleep cycle, leading to further deprivation of N3 and REM sleep. Routine nighttime awakenings by care providers are often used to complete tasks needed for clinicians during the day, such as vital signs or blood draws. Interruptions in observational studies of wards and intensive care units (ICUs) are so prevalent that patients rarely received 2 to 3 hours of uninterrupted sleep.[26,27]

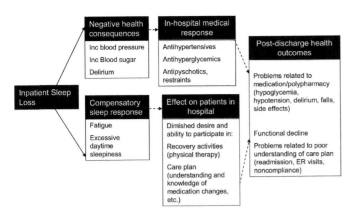

Fig. 1. Potential mechanisms for effects of inpatient sleep loss on older patients. ER, emergency room; Inc, increased.

Patient Factors

Issues such as poor health, anxiety, and depression that are often associated with acute and chronic illnesses contribute to sleep disturbances among older inpatients.[28] Studies show that poor self-rated health and the presence of chronic conditions (eg, cardiovascular disease, chronic obstructive pulmonary disease, gastroesophageal reflux, and arthritis) are associated with complaints of poor sleep.[29] Pain is also frequently reported by inpatients as a major cause of poor sleep and nighttime awakenings.[30]

Environmental Disruptions

Hospital noise is more than just an annoyance.[31] The auditory environment should exemplify high and compassionate standards of patient care. Failure to provide patients with quiet rooms affects clinical outcomes through several mechanisms, including increased physiologic arousal and stress responses,[32] medical errors, sleep disruption, and interference with speech privacy.[33] Although the United States Environmental Protection Agency recommends a maximum noise level of 45 dB (dB) throughout the day and 35 dB at night, most hospitals today have noise levels from 50 to 70 dB during the day and an average of 67 dB at night.[34] Medicare has made patient-reported noise a publicly reported quality measure as part of its Hospital Compare program.[35] Unfortunately, these data demonstrate that only 58% of hospitalized Americans report their room as quiet at night, which is the worst performing patient experience measure in the entire Hospital Consumer Assessment of Healthcare Providers and Systems (HCAHPS) Survey. Further, a study in the ICU setting found that 51% of noise was modifiable, with patients reporting staff conversation and television noise as the most irritating disturbances, and interfered with sleep in electroencephalogram

recordings.[36] In addition, patients in the loudest rooms get significantly less sleep.[37] In addition, the absence or reduced amplitude of diurnal light–dark cycles in hospital environments can result in the disruption of the circadian regulation of sleep.[38] This is especially problematic in ICU settings, whereby circadian rhythms in patients are particularly abnormal.[39]

PREVALENCE OF SLEEP DISORDERS AMONG HOSPITALIZED OLDER ADULTS

Hospitalization also represents a missed opportunity to screen patients for sleep disorders. The high prevalence of untreated sleep disorders may often complicate or worsen patients' existing conditions. For example, as many as 80% of patients are apparently at risk for obstructive sleep apnea (OSA) according to a recent small single-institution study that screened patients using the STOP-BANG questionnaire.[40] Despite this high prevalence, very few had been evaluated with a sleep study, diagnosed with OSA, or were receiving treatment with continuous positive airway pressure (CPAP) therapy, which is known to improve quality of life and reduce complications.[41,42] The prevalence of insomnia is also high; a recent study suggested that nearly 2 of every 5 patients screened positive for insomnia.[43,44] In another study of hospitalized patients, although one-half of inpatients reported chronic sleep complaints with nearly one-third screening positive for insomnia, there was no mention of a sleep complaint in the admission record.[45] To make matters worse, even if sleep disorders are recognized in hospitalized patients, therapy is often suboptimal. For example, in a nationally representative sample of nearly 300,000 discharges of patients with OSA from nonfederal acute care hospitals in the United States, only 5.8% of patients were identified as receiving

CPAP therapy.[46] Given that sleep disorders may exacerbate cardiopulmonary health conditions that actually result in hospitalization, such as congestive heart failure or chronic obstructive pulmonary disease, it is critical to recognize that sleep disorders complicate patient's underlying medical conditions.[47] For example, patients with OSA who undergo surgery are at greater risk of having postoperative hypoxemia, ICU transfers, and longer durations of hospital stay.[48–50] Certain inpatient medical diagnoses, such as acute stroke or heart failure, are associated with a higher prevalence of sleep-disordered breathing.[51–56] In addition, hospitalized medical ward patients with COPD have higher risk of OSA and insomnia and worse in-hospital sleep quality and quantity compared with hospitalized medical patients without COPD.[57] Moreover, treatment of OSA with CPAP in patients with postacute stroke or systolic heart failure improves outcomes.[42,58,59] The presence of a highly treatable and very prevalent disorder such as sleep-disordered breathing in such patients warrants a process for better and earlier recognition and treatment.[60]

Perhaps most concerning is that acute sleep loss in the hospital may be associated with the development of chronic insomnia after discharge, especially among those with preexisting poor sleep hygiene.[61] This factor is especially problematic given the association between chronic insomnia and poor long-term health outcomes, highlighting the need for early recognition of insomnia.[62] Moreover, among older patients discharged from the hospital, nighttime sleep duration and efficiency and daytime sleep duration were similar in-hospital to postdischarge; however, physical activity was greater postdischarge and increased more rapidly in-hospital than postdischarge.[63] Last, poor self-reported sleep quality predicts 1-year mortality among older adults who received inpatient rehabilitation.[64] A similar study demonstrated that sleep disturbance as determined by hourly observations of patients in a geriatric hospital were associated with higher mortality at 2 years.[65]

INTERVENTIONS TO IMPROVE SLEEP IN HOSPITALIZED ADULTS

In general, interventions to improve sleep in hospitalized older adults can be classified as pharmacologic or nonpharmacologic interventions. Although some patients do request pharmacologic sleep aids, it is generally recommended that nonpharmacologic interventions be the first line of therapy.[66] In the event a pharmacologic sleep aid is needed, the choice of drug should be customized based on the patient profile to minimize any side effects, especially given the degree of polypharmacy common in hospitalized older adults.

Pharmacologic Interventions

Melatonin
If a pharmacologic sleep aid is deemed necessary, melatonin is well-tolerated and considered by some as the first choice to consider in older adults owing to its minimal side effect profile, low likelihood of drug–drug interactions, and the possibility to improve circadian rhythms.[67,68] Small, randomized studies conducted with ICU patients, hospitalized patients, and in simulated sleep environments showed improvements in sleep duration (as measured by polysomnography) and sleep quality (as measured by actigraphy) when initiating 1 to 5 mg of melatonin at night.[69–71] Although dosing has not yet been standardized, the typical dose is 1 to 3 mg dispensed between 9 PM and 10 PM, depending on the sleeping habits of the patient, and should be given 30 minutes before the desired bedtime.

Sleep aids
Sleep aid medications are commonly prescribed in the hospital setting, although they are generally not recommended owing to concerns about side effects. A retrospective single-center study from 2014 found that, over a 2-month period, 26.2% of patients received a sleep aid, with trazodone being the most commonly prescribed (30.4% of the time).[72] A meta-analysis by Glass and colleagues[73] in 2005 evaluated the risks and benefits of sedative-hypnotics in people over the age of 60, and found a statistically significant improvement in sleep quality and sleep duration with sedative use compared with placebo, although the magnitude of the effect was small, and the risks (including falls and cognitive impairment) were great. Although 3 classes of medications for insomnia have been approved by the US Food and Drug Administration (benzodiazepines, nonbenzodiazepines, and melatonin-receptor agonists), 2 of these classes are on the Beers Criteria list from the American Geriatrics Society to avoid in older adults (benzodiazepines and nonbenzodiazepines).[74,75] Assessing Care of Vulnerable Elders 3 (ACOVE 3) quality measures regarding sleep disorders suggests avoidance of anticholinergic medications owing to their side effect profile. In 2015, the American Geriatrics Society released the updated Beers Criteria for identifying medications to avoid in the older adult population. Medications used for upper respiratory infections such as anticholinergics (including antihistamines) should be avoided.[75] Medications for insomnia such as

antihistamines, oral decongestants (eg, pseudoephedrine and ephedrine), and stimulants (eg, amphetamine and methylphenidate) make insomnia worse in the older population, are associated with anticholinergic side effects, and should be avoided.[75,76] Use of other agents as sleep aids, such as tricyclic antidepressants, antipsychotics, atypical antipsychotics, and anticholinergics, should also be avoided owing to their adverse side effect profile.[75]

Pain treatment
The treatment of pain is recommended in the hospital setting, because pain can interfere with the ability to fall asleep, and is a potentially reversible cause of sleep disturbance. Pharmacologic and nonpharmacologic management options should be evaluated for the treatment of pain in the older patient population.[76]

Nonpharmacologic Interventions

Because nonpharmacologic therapies are the mainstay of treatment of sleep disturbances among older adults in the hospital, there is great interest in evidence-based interventions that demonstrate improvement in sleep or related outcomes among hospitalized patients. To this end, 2 relevant systematic reviews have summarized the evidence. First, a Cochrane review on improving sleep in the ICU setting resulted in the review of interventions including ventilator type, eye masks in collaboration with ear plugs, relaxation therapy, sleep-inducing music, massage, foot baths, aromatherapy, acupressure, and visiting time of family members, although the quality of the evidence was low.[77] Another systematic review published found only 13 intervention studies, 4 of which were randomized, controlled trials.[78] Although the evidence was poor, some evidence existed for improving sleep quality, interventions to improve sleep hygiene or reduce interruptions, and daytime bright light exposure. Each of these nonpharmacologic interventions is discussed in further detail.

Relaxation techniques
Several methods of relaxation techniques have been proposed, although the data are limited and the quality of evidence is low. A systematic review of nonpharmacologic interventions by Tamrat and colleagues[78] reviewed 4 randomized control trials on relaxation techniques and found a 0% to 28% improvement of overall sleep quality. A study by Soden and colleagues[79] evaluated the use of aromatherapy, aromatherapy plus massage, or usual care, and no overall differences were found between the groups. When guided imagery for 20 minutes daily was compared with a solitary activity of choice, no difference between groups was found.[80] Last, a study that randomized patients who under coronary artery bypass grafting to 30 minutes of rest, a soothing music video, or 30 minutes of music through headphones demonstrated a 28% improvement in self-reported sleep quality in the group that watched a soothing music video compared with the control group.[81]

Sleep hygiene program
A randomized control trial by Lareau and colleagues[82] evaluated a nighttime intervention of decreasing light and noise, clustering nursing care, and minimizing unnecessary patient contact, compared with usual care. The intervention was associated with an improvement of sleep quality by 7% and a decrease in the use of sleep aid medications. Edinger and colleagues[83] evaluated an inpatient sleep hygiene program to usual care for hospitalized psychiatric patients. The intervention included the standardization of sleep and wake times, including removal of daytime napping. The intervention was associated with an increase of 18 minutes (5%) of total sleep time, although neither sleep quality nor significance testing was reported.

Bright light therapy
Three small studies evaluated bright light therapy (3000–5000 lux) use during daytime hours. Mishima and colleagues[84] exposed patients with dementia in a psychiatric hospital to bright light therapy between 9 and 11 AM for 4 weeks and found an improvement in average total sleep time among intervention patients. Wakamura and colleagues[85] exposed 7 hospitalized patients to 5 hours of bright light therapy during daytime hours and noted a 7% increase in total sleep time in the intervention arm. Twenty-seven patients with Alzheimer's disease were exposed to bright light therapy by Yamadera and colleagues,[86] and were noted to have an increase in total nighttime sleep. Although these studies all reported an increase in total sleep time after exposure to bright light therapy, the effects are modest and the strength of the evidence is low based on potential bias, along with measurement and reporting inconsistencies.[78]

Noise reduction
Several studies assessing modalities for noise reduction in the ICU have been performed. These approaches include the use of ear plugs in conjunction with eye masks,[87] use of "white noise" (otherwise known as sound masking),[88,89] and the installation of sound-proof materials.[90] The overall quality of evidence with these approaches is also

low, and the outcomes used have primarily been subjective sleep measures.[91]

Reducing nighttime interruptions

Two reported studies evaluated the reduction of nighttime nursing interruptions, by altering workflow and reducing patient interactions during typical sleeping hours. These studies suggest that, by reducing nighttime interruptions, there is a reduction in sedatives requested by patients, although sleep duration and quality did not improve.[92,93] One study implemented an electronic health record (EHR) order set aimed to decrease nocturnal phlebotomy. This study demonstrated over 25% fewer routine nocturnal lab draws while improving sleep-friendly orders in hospitalized patients.[94] Further studies are needed in this area to best determine how to reduce nighttime patient interactions so as to improve sleep quality and duration.

Sleep education and empowerment

In a recent randomized trial, non-ICU patients who received sleep-enhancing tools (eye mask, ear plugs, and a white noise machine) plus education reported less fatigue and sleep impairment than those who just received the sleep-enhancing tools alone.[95] A study aimed at decreasing nocturnal awakenings and medications evaluated nursing coaching, empowerment, and "nudges" showed a unit-based nursing empowerment approach was associated with fewer nighttime room entries and improved patient experience via increased HCAPS scores.[96] A pilot study evaluating the feasibility and acceptability of a multi-component intervention (I-SLEEP) that educates and empowers inpatients to advocate for fewer nighttime disruptions to improve sleep showed the intervention was well received and enabled hospitalized patients to advocate for reducing nighttime sleep disruptions.[97] Another patient empowerment study evaluated a "sleep menu" for patients to request certain options of an intervention which demonstrated a decrease in nighttime noise and interruptions and an increase in HCAHPS quiet-at-night scores.[98]

Multifaceted Protocols

An example of a multifaceted protocol is the "Somerville" approach, whereby several components were implemented such as an 8-h quiet time, fewer disruptions for routine vitals and medications, and noise control. The investigators noted that fewer patients reported sleep disruption from hospital staff and also fewer patients received as-needed sedatives.[99]

Assessment and Treatment of Underlying Sleep Disorders

Several studies suggest that early recognition and treatment of underlying sleep disorders in hospitalized patients is associated with improved outcomes after discharge. For example, in a very small study, Konikkara and associates[100] showed that, compared with patients not compliant with CPAP therapy, patients with chronic obstructive pulmonary disease who were compliant with CPAP therapy had fewer emergency room and readmission visits 6 months after discharge. In a larger study of hospitalized patients with congestive heart failure, patients compliant with CPAP for a minimum of 4 hours 70% of the time in the first month after discharge had fewer readmissions compared with those not compliant with CPAP therapy after discharge.[101] Likewise, a study of early diagnosis of sleep-disordered breathing in hospitalized cardiac patients using in-hospital portal sleep studies demonstrated that patients who were adherent to CPAP had fewer 30-day readmissions.[102]

CLINICS CARE POINTS

- Older adults are at greater risk for sleep disruptions in hospital.
- Non-pharmacologic sleep interventions are recommended as first line treatments in hospital.
- Address and treat patient pain appropriately, as it can inpact patient sleep.

SUMMARY

Sleep disturbance is common in hospitalized older adults owing to a variety of factors, including environmental, medical, and patient issues. Sleep loss in the hospital is associated with worse health outcomes, including cardiometabolic derangements and increased risk of delirium. In addition, the hospital setting may represent an important opportunity to identify previously unrecognized sleep disorders, such as OSA, that can impact important patient outcomes. Finally, a growing body of evidence suggests that nonpharmacologic interventions should be the first choice to improve sleep in hospitalized older adults.

DISCLOSURE

The authors have no relevant disclosures related to this article.

REFERENCES

1. Colten HR, Altevogt BM, editors. Sleep disorders and sleep deprivation. An unmet public health problem. Institute of Medicine (US) Committee on Sleep Medicine and Research. Washington, DC: National Academies Press (US); 2006.
2. Pilkington S. Causes and consequences of sleep deprivation in hospitalised patients. Nurs Stand 2013;27(49):35–42.
3. Krumholz HM. Post-hospital syndrome-an acquired, transient condition of generalized risk. N Engl J Med 2013;368(2):100–2.
4. Arora VM, Chang KL, Fazal AZ, et al. Objective sleep duration and quality in hospitalized older adults: associations with blood pressure and mood. J Am Geriatr Soc 2011;59(11):2185–6.
5. Shah MS, Spampinato LM, Beveridge C, et al. Quan tifying post hospital syndrome: sleeping longer and physically stronger? [abstract]. J Hosp Med 2016;11(Suppl 1). Available at: http://www.shmabstracts.   com/abstract/ quantifying-post-hospital-syndrome-   sleeping- longer-and-physically-stronger/. Accessed March 24, 2016.
6. Shear TC, Balachandran JS, Mokhlesi B, et al. Risk of sleep apnea in hospitalized older patients. J Clin Sleep Med 2014;10(10):1061–6.
7. Sharma S. Hospital sleep medicine: the elephant in the room? J Clin Sleep Med 2014;10:1067–8.
8. Wolkove N, Elkholy O, Baltzan M, et al. Sleep and aging: 1. Sleep disorders commonly found in older people. CMAJ 2007;176(9):1299–304.
9. Bliwise DL. Sleep in normal aging and dementia. Sleep 1993;16(1):40–81.
10. Vaz Fragoso CA, Gill TM. Sleep complaints in community-living older persons: a multifactorial geri atric syndrome. J Am Geriatr Soc 2007; 55(11):1853–66.
11. Knutson KL, Spiegel K, Penev P, et al. The metabolic consequences of sleep deprivation. Sleep Med Rev 2007;11(3):163–78.
12. Spiegel K, Leproult R, Van Cauter E. Impact of sleep debt on metabolic and endocrine function. Lancet 1999;354:1435–9.
13. Meisinger C, Heier M, Loewel H. Sleep disturbance as a predictor of type 2 diabetes mellitus in men and women from the general population. Diabetologia 2005;48(2):235–41.
14. Yaggi HK, Araujo AB, McKinlay JB. Sleep duration as a risk factor for the development of type 2 dia betes. Diabetes Care 2006;29(3):657–61.
15. Inzucchi SE. Management of hyperglycemia in the hospital setting. N Engl J Med 2006;355(18): 1903–11.
16. Inouye SK. Prevention of delirium in hospitalized older patients: risk factors and targeted intervention strategies. Ann Med 2000;32(4):257–63.
17. Jaiswal SJ, Kang DY, Wineinger NE, et al. Objectively measured sleep fragmentation is associated with incident delirium in older hospitalized patients: analysis of data collected from an randomized controlled trial. J Sleep Res 2021;30(3): e13205.
18. Bell CM, Fischer HD, Gill SS, et al. Initiation of benzodiazepines in the elderly after hospitalization. J Gen Intern Med 2007;22(7):1024–9.
19. Ancoli-Israel S, Cooke JR. Prevalence and comorbidity of insomnia and effect on functioning in elderly populations. J Am Geriatr Soc 2005;53(7 Suppl):S264–71.
20. Gooneratne NS, Weaver TE, Cater JR, et al. Func tional outcomes of excessive daytime sleepiness in older adults. J Am Geriatr Soc 2003;51(5):642–9.
21. Coleman EA, Parry C, Chalmers S, et al. The care transitions intervention: results of a randomized controlled trial. Arch Intern Med 2006;166(17): 1822–8.
22. Stone KL, Ancoli-Israel S, Blackwell T, et al. Acti gra-phy-measured sleep characteristics and risk of falls in older women. Arch Intern Med 2008; 168(16):1768–75.
23. Spiegel K, Sheridan JF, Van Cauter E. Effect of sleep deprivation on response to immunization. JAMA 2002;288(12):1471–2.
24. Kuo TH, Williams JA. Increased sleep promotes survival during a bacterial infection in Drosophila. Sleep 2014;37(6):1077–86, 1086A-1086D.
25. Redeker NS. Sleep in acute care settings: an inte grative review. J Nurs Scholarsh 2000;32(1):31–8.
26. Tamburri LM, DiBrienza R, Zozula R, et al. Nocturnal care interactions with patients in critical care units. Am J Crit Care 2004;13(2):102–12.
27. Friese RS, Diaz-Arrastia R, McBride D, et al. Quan tity and quality of sleep in the surgical intensive care unit: are our patients sleeping? J Trauma 2007;63(6):1210–4.
28. Beck-Little R, Weinrich SP. Assessment and management of sleep disorders in the elderly. J Gerontol Nurs 1998;24(4):21–9.
29. Blazer DG, Hays JC, Foley DJ. Sleep complaints in older adults: a racial comparison. J Gerontol A Biol Sci Med Sci 1995;50(5):M280–4.
30. Ersser S, Wiles A, Taylor H, et al. The sleep of older people in hospital and nursing homes. J Clin Nurs 1999;8(4):360–8.
31. Grumet GW. Pandemonium in the modern hospital. N Engl J Med 1993;328(6):433–7.
32. Buxton OM, Ellenbogen JM, Wang W, et al. Sleep disruption due to hospital noises: a prospective evaluation. Ann Intern Med 2012;157(3):170–9.

33. Mazer S. Speech privacy: beyond architectural solu-tions. Available at: http://www.healinghealth.com/images/uploads/files/Mazer_SpeechPrivacy.pdf. Accessed June 1, 2016.

34. Tullmann DF, Dracup K. Creating a healing environ ment for elders. AACN Clin Issues 2000;11(1):34–50.

35. U.S. Department of health & human services. Hospital Compare. Available at: http://www.hospital-compare.hhs.gov/. Accessed June 1, 2016.

36. Kahn DM, Cook TE, Carlisle CC, et al. Identification and modification of environmental noise in an ICU setting. Chest 1998;114(2):535–40.

37. Yoder JC, Staisiunas PG, Meltzer DO, et al. Noise and sleep among adult medical inpatients: far from a quiet night. Arch Intern Med 2012;172(1):68–70.

38. Monk TH, Buysse DJ, Billy BD, et al. The effects on human sleep and circadian rhythms of 17 days of continuous bedrest in the absence of daylight. Sleep 1997;20(10):858–64.

39. Shilo L, Dagan Y, Smorjik Y, et al. Patients in the intensive care unit suffer from severe lack of sleep associated with loss of normal melatonin secretion pattern. Am J Med Sci 1999;317(5):278–81.

40. Kumar S, McElligott D, Goyal A, et al. Risk of obstructive sleep apnea (OSA) in hospitalized pa tients. Chest 2010;138(4 supp):779. Available at: http://journal.publications.chestnet.org/article.aspx? articleID = 1087266. Accessed June 1, 2016.

41. Javaheri S, Caref EB, Chen E, et al. Sleep apnea testing and outcomes in a large cohort of Medi-care beneficiaries with newly diagnosed heart fail- ure. Am J Respir Crit Care Med 2011;183(4):539–46.

42. Kaneko Y, Floras JS, Usui K, et al. Cardiovascular ef-fects of continuous positive airway pressure in patients with heart failure and obstructive sleep ap nea. N Engl J Med 2003;348(13):1233–41.

43. Kokras N, Kouzoupis AV, Paparrigopoulos T, et al. Predicting insomnia in medical wards: the effect of anxiety, depression and admission diagnosis. Gen Hosp Psychiatry 2011;33(1):78–81.

44. Isaia G, Corsinovi L, Bo M, et al. Insomnia among hospitalized elderly patients: prevalence, clinical characteristics and risk factors. Arch Gerontol Geriatr 2011;52(2):133–7.

45. Meissner HH, Riemer A, Santiago SM, et al. Failure of physician documentation of sleep complaints in hospitalized patients. West J Med 1998;169(3):146–9.

46. Spurr KF, Graven MA, Gilbert RW. Prevalence of un specified sleep apnea and the use of continuous positive airway pressure in hospitalized patients: 2004 national hospital discharge survey. Sleep Breath 2008;12(3):229–34.

47. Gay PC. Sleep and sleep-disordered breathing in the hospitalized patient. Respir Care 2010;55(9):1240–54.

48. Kaw R, Pasupuleti V, Walker E, et al. Postoperative complications in patients with obstructive sleep ap nea. Chest 2012;141(2):436–41.

49. Liao P, Yegneswaran B, Vairavanathan S, et al. Post operative complications in patients with obstructive sleep apnea: a retrospective matched cohort study. Can J Anaesth 2009;56(11):819–28.

50. Hwang D, Shakir N, Limann B, et al. Association of sleep-disordered breathing with postoperative com plications. Chest 2008;133(5):1128–34.

51. Mohsenin V, Valor R. Sleep apnea in patients with hemispheric stroke. Arch Phys Med Rehabil 1995;76:71–6.

52. Harbison J, Ford G, James O, et al. Sleep-disor-dered breathing following acute stroke. QJM 2002;95:741–7.

53. Bassetti C, Aldrich M. Sleep apnea in acute cere-bro vascular diseases: final report on 128 patients. Sleep 1999;22:217–23.

54. Good D, Henkle J, Gelber D, et al. Sleep-disor-dered breathing and poor functional outcome after stroke. Stroke 1996;27:252–9.

55. Sahlin C, Sandberg O, Gustafson Y, et al. Obstruc-tive sleep apnea is a risk factor for death in patients with stroke: a 10-year follow-up. Arch Intern Med 2008;168:297–301.

56. Oldenburg O, Lamp B, Faber L, et al. Sleep-disor-dered breathing in patients with symptomatic heart failure: a contemporary study of prevalence in and characteristics of 700 patients. Eur J Heart Fail 2007;9:251–7.

57. Stewart NH, Walters RW, Mokhlesi B, et al. Sleep in hospitalized patients with chronic obstructive pul-monary disease: an observational study. J Clin Sleep Med 2020;16(10):1693–9.

58. Bravata DM, Concato J, Fried T, et al. Continuous Positive airway pressure: evaluation of a novel ther- apy for patients with acute ischemic stroke. Sleep 2011;34:1271–7.

59. Mansfield DR, Gollogly NC, Kaye DM, et al. Controlled trial of continuous positive airway pres sure in obstructive sleep apnea and heart failure. Am J Respir Crit Care Med 2004;169:361–6.

60. White J, Cates C, Wright J. Continuous positive air-ways pressure for obstructive sleep apnoea. Cochrane Database Syst Rev 2002;(2):CD001106.

61. Griffiths MF, Peerson A. Risk factors for chronic insomnia following hospitalization. J Adv Nurs 2005;49(3):245–53.

62. Morin CM, Benca R. Chronic insomnia. Lancet 2012;379(9821):1129–41.

63. Kessler R, Knutson KL, Mokhlesi B, et al. Sleep and activity patterns in older patients discharged from the hospital. Sleep 2019;42(11):zsz153.

64. Martin JL, Fiorentino L, Jouldjian S, et al. Poor self-reported sleep quality predicts mortality within one year of inpatient post-acute rehabilitation among older adults. Sleep 2011;34(12):1715–21.

65. Manabe K, Matsui T, Yamaya M, et al. Sleep patterns and mortality among elderly patients in a geriatric hospital. Gerontology 2000;46(6):318–22.

66. Lenhart SE, Buysse DJ. Treatment of insomnia in hospitalized patients. Ann Pharmacother 2001; 35(11):1449–57.

67. Brzezinski A, Vangel MG, Wurtman RJ, et al. Effects of exogenous melatonin on sleep: a meta-analysis. Sleep Med Rev 2005;9(1):41–50.

68. Zhdanova IV, Wurtman RJ, Regan MM, et al. Melatonin treatment for age-related insomnia. J Clin En Docrinol Metab 2001;86(10):4727–30.

69. Andrade C, Srihari BS, Chandramma L. Melatonin in medically ill patients with insomnia: a double-blind, placebo-controlled study. J Clin Psychiatry 2001;62(1):41–5.

70. Shilo L, Dagan Y, Smorjik Y, et al. Effect of melatonin on sleep quality of COPD intensive care patients: a pilot study. Chronobiol Int 2000;17(1): 71–6.

71. Huang HW, Zheng BL, Jiang L, et al. Effect of oral melatonin and wearing earplugs and eye masks on nocturnal sleep in healthy subjects in a simulated intensive care unit environment: which might be a more promising strategy for ICU sleep deprivation? Crit Care 2015;19(1):1.

72. Gillis CM, Poyant JO, Degrado JR, et al. Inpatient pharmacological sleep aid utilization is common at a tertiary medical center. J Hosp Med 2014; 9(10):652–7.

73. Glass J, Lanctot KL, Herrmann N, et al. Sedative hypnotics in older people with insomnia: meta-analysis of risks and benefits. BMJ 2005; 331(7526):1169.

74. Young JS, Bourgeois JA, Hilty DM, et al. Sleep in hospitalized medical patients, part 2: behavioral and pharmacological management of sleep disturbances. J Hosp Med 2009;4(1):50–9.

75. Radcliff S, Yue J, Rocco G, et al. American Geriatrics Society 2015 updated beers criteria for potentially inappropriate medication use in older adults. J Am Geriatr Soc 2015;63(11):2227–46.

76. Martin JL, Fung CH. Quality indicators for the care of sleep disorders in vulnerable elders. J Am Geriatr Soc 2007;55(Suppl 2):S424–30.

77. Hu R, Jiang X, Chen J, et al. Non-pharmacological interventions for sleep promotion in the intensive care unit. Cochrane Database Syst Rev 2015;(10):CD008808.

78. Tamrat R, Huynh-Le MP, Goyal M. Non-pharmacologic interventions to improve the sleep of hospitalized patients: a systematic review. J Gen Intern Med 2014;29(5):788–95.

79. Soden K, Vincent K, Craske S, et al. A randomized controlled trial of aromatherapy massage in a hospice setting. Palliat Med 2004;18(2):87–92.

80. Toth M, Wolsko PM, Foreman J, et al. A pilot study for a randomized, controlled trial on the effect of guided imagery in hospitalized medical patients. J Altern Complement Med 2007;13(2):194–7.

81. Zimmerman L, Nieveen J, Barnason S, et al. The effects of music interventions on postoperative pain and sleep in coronary artery bypass graft (CABG) patients. Sch Inq Nurs Pract 1996;10(2):153–70.

82. Lareau R, Benson L, Watcharotone K, et al. Examining the feasibility of implementing specific nursing interventions to promote sleep in hospitalized elderly patients. Geriatr Nurs 2008;29(3): 197–206.

83. Edinger JD, Lipper S, Wheeler B. Hospital ward policy and patients' sleep patterns: a multiple baseline study. Rehabil Psychol 1989;34(1):43.

84. Mishima K, Okawa M, Hishikawa Y, et al. Morning bright light therapy for sleep and behavior disorders in elderly patients with dementia. Acta Psychiatr Scand 1994;89(1):1–7.

85. Wakamura T, Tokura H. Influence of bright light during daytime on sleep parameters in hospitalized elderly patients. J Physiol Anthropol Appl Human Sci 2001;20(6):345–51.

86. Yamadera H, Ito T, Suzuki H, et al. Effects of bright light on cognitive and sleep-wake (circadian) rhythm disturbances in Alzheimer-type dementia. Psychiatry Clin Neurosci 2000;54(3):352–3.

87. Richardson A, Allsop M, Coghill E, et al. Earplugs and eye masks: do they improve critical care patients' sleep? Nurs Crit Care 2007;12(6):278–86.

88. Gragert MD. The use of a masking signal to enhance the sleep of men and women 65 years of age and older in the critical care environment. In: INTER- NOISE and NOISE-CON Congress and Conference Proceedings, vol. 1. Inst Noise Control Eng 1990;315–20.

89. Stanchina ML, Abu-Hijleh M, Chaudhry BK, et al. The influence of white noise on sleep in subjects exposed to ICU noise. Sleep Med 2005;6(5):423–8.

90. Blomkvist V, Eriksen CA, Theorell T, et al. Acoustics and psychosocial environment in intensive coronary care. Occup Environ Med 2005;62(3):e1.

91. Xie H, Kang J, Mills GH. Clinical review: the impact of noise on patients' sleep and the effectiveness of noise reduction strategies in intensive care units. Crit Care 2009;13(2):1.

92. Yoder JC, Yuen TC, Churpek MM, et al. A prospective study of nighttime vital sign monitoring frequency and risk of clinical deterioration. JAMA Intern Med 2013;173(16):1554–5.

93. Le A, Friese RS, Hsu CH, et al. Sleep disruptions and nocturnal nursing interactions in the intensive care unit. J Surg Res 2012;177(2):310–4.

94. Tapaskar N, Kilaru M, Puri TS, et al. Evaluation of the order SMARTT: an initiative to reduce phlebotomy and improve sleep-friendly labs on general medicine services. J Hosp Med 2020;15(8): 479–82.

95. Farrehi PM, Clore KR, Scott JR, et al. Efficacy of sleep tool education during hospitalization: a randomized controlled trial. Am J Med 2016;129(12). 1329.e9–1329.e17.

96. Arora VM, Machado N, Anderson SL, et al. Effectiveness of SIESTA on objective and subjective metrics of nighttime hospital sleep disruptors. J Hosp Med 2019;14(1):38–41.

97. Mason NR, Orlov NM, Anderson S, et al. Piloting I-SLEEP: a patient-centered education and empowerment intervention to improve patients' in-hospital sleep. Pilot Feasibility Stud 2021;7(1):161.

98. Antonio CK. Improving quiet at night on a telemetry unit: introducing a holistic sleep menu intervention. Am J Nurs 2020;120(10):58–64.

99. Bartick MC, Thai X, Schmidt T, et al. Decrease in as-needed sedative use by limiting nighttime sleep disruptions from hospital staff. J Hosp Med 2010;5(3):E20–4.

100. Konikkara J, Tavella R, Willes L, et al. Early recognition of obstructive sleep apnea in patients hospitalized with COPD exacerbation is associated with reduced readmission. Hosp Pract (1995) 2016;44(1):41–7.

101. Sharma S, Mather P, Gupta A, et al. Effect of early intervention with positive airway pressure therapy for sleep disordered breathing on six-month readmission rates in hospitalized patients with heart failure. Am J Cardiol 2016;117(6):940–5.

102. Kauta SR, Keenan BT, Goldberg L, et al. Diagnosis and treatment of sleep disordered breathing in hospitalized cardiac patients: a reduction in 30-day hospital readmission rates. J Clin Sleep Med 2014;10(10):1051–9.

Insomnia in the Older Adult

Glenna S. Brewster, PhD, RN, FNP-BC[a,b],*, Barbara Riegel, PhD, RN[a,1],
Philip R. Gehrman, PhD, CBSM[b,c]

KEYWORDS

- Sleep onset latency • Sleep efficiency • Benzodiazepines • Sleep diary • Pharmacotherapy
- Cognitive behavioral therapy for insomnia (CBTi) • Wake after sleep onset

KEY POINTS

- The incidence of insomnia increases with aging. Insomnia can include difficulty falling asleep at the start of the sleep period, waking up during the night and having difficulty falling back asleep, and waking up early and being unable to get back to sleep. Difficulty staying asleep and early morning insomnia are common in older adults with insomnia disorder.
- When diagnosing insomnia, health care providers need to collect a thorough health history and include questions about the older adult's sleep, medical, and psychiatric history.
- Cognitive behavioral therapy for insomnia, which consists of stimulus control, sleep restriction, sleep hygiene, and cognitive therapy, is the recommended first-line therapy for treatment of insomnia in older adults.
- Because of higher risk for adverse effects in older patients, medications should be used sparingly and, when possible, discontinued.
- Cognitive behavioral therapy for insomnia has been shown to be more efficacious than medications for the long-term management of insomnia in older adults.

INTRODUCTION
Prevalence and Diagnosis of Insomnia

Sleep changes with aging. Specifically, babies sleep between 10 and 14 hours per day, whereas the recommended sleep duration for older adults is between 7 and 8 hours daily.[1] Many older adults experience dissatisfaction with the quantity and quality of sleep even with adequate opportunity to sleep; when this is accompanied by daytime impairment over a period of time, they may meet criteria for insomnia disorder (**Table 1**). Compared with younger adults, the prevalence of insomnia is higher in middle and older adults[2,3] and increases with age. Up to 50% of older adults report insomnia symptoms; however, this does not mean that insomnia is a normal part of aging.[4]

Sleep onset or initial insomnia is manifested by difficulty falling asleep that occurs at the start of the sleep period.[5–7] Sleep maintenance or middle insomnia involves multiple and prolonged awakenings during the night.[5–7] Late insomnia or early morning awakenings is waking up early on

Publisher's Disclaimer: This is a PDF file of an unedited article that has been accepted for publication. As a service to our customers we are providing this early version of the article. The article will undergo copyediting, typesetting, and review of the resulting proof before it is published in its final citable form. Please note that during the production process errors may be discovered that could affect the content and all legal disclaimers that apply to the journal pertain.

This article previously appeared in *Sleep Med Clin.* 2018 March ; 13(1): 13–19.

[a] Nell Hodgson Woodruff School of Nursing, 1520 Clifton Road, Atlanta, GA 30322, USA; [b] Center for Sleep and Circadian Neurobiology, Perelman School of Medicine of the University of Pennsylvania, Philadelphia, PA, USA; [c] Department of Psychiatry, Perelman School of Medicine of the University of Pennsylvania, 3535 Market Street, Suite 670, Philadelphia, PA 19104, USA

[1] Present address: Room 418 Curie Boulevard, 335 Fagin Hall, Philadelphia, PA 19104.

* Corresponding author. 3624 Market Street, Suite 205, Philadelphia, PA 19104. .

E-mail address: glenna.brewster@emory.edu

Sleep Med Clin 17 (2022) 233–239
https://doi.org/10.1016/j.jsmc.2022.03.004
1556-407X/22/© 2022 Elsevier Inc. All rights reserved.

Table 1
Diagnostic criteria for insomnia

Diagnostic Criteria for Chronic Insomnia (ICSD-3)[44]	Diagnostic Criteria for Chronic Insomnia (DSM-5)[5]

Criteria A–F must be met
A. The patient reports, or the patient's parent or caregiver observes, one or more of the following:
  1. Difficulty initiating sleep
  2. Difficulty maintaining sleep
  3. Waking up earlier than desired
  4. Resistance to going to bed on appropriate schedule
  5. Difficulty sleeping without parent or caregiver intervention
B. The patient reports, or the patient's parent or caregiver observes, one or more of the following related to the night time sleep difficulty:
  1. Fatigue/malaise
  2. Attention, concentration, or memory impairment
  3. Impaired social, family, occupational, or academic performance
  4. Mood disturbance/irritability
  5. Daytime sleepiness
  6. Behavioral problems (eg, hyperactivity, impulsivity, aggression)
  7. Reduced motivation/energy/initiative
  8. Proneness for errors/accidents
  9. Concerns about or dissatisfaction with sleep
C. The reported sleep/wake complaints cannot be explained purely by inadequate opportunity (ie, enough time is allotted for sleep) or inadequate circumstances (ie, the environment is safe, dark, quiet, and comfortable) for sleep.
D. The sleep disturbance and associated daytime symptoms occur at least 3 times per week
E. The sleep disturbance and associated daytime symptoms have been present for at least 3 mo
F. The sleep/wake difficulty is not explained more clearly by another sleep disorder
	307.42 (F51.01)
	1. A predominant complaint of dissatisfaction with sleep quantity or quality, associated with one (or more) of the following symptoms:
	  1. Difficulty initiating sleep. (In children, this may manifest as difficulty initiating sleep without caregiver intervention.)
	  2. Difficulty maintaining sleep, characterized by frequent awakenings or problems returning to sleep after awakenings. (In children, this may manifest as difficulty returning to sleep without caregiver intervention.)
	  3. Early morning awakening with inability to return to sleep.
	2. The sleep disturbance causes clinically significant distress or impairment in social, occupational, educational, academic, behavioral, or other important areas of functioning.
	3. The sleep difficulty occurs at least 3 nights per week.
	4. The sleep difficulty is present for at least 3 mo.
	5. The sleep difficulty occurs despite adequate opportunity for sleep.
	6. The insomnia is not better explained by and does not occur exclusively during the course of another sleep-wake disorder (eg, narcolepsy, a breathing-related sleep disorder, a circadian rhythm sleep-wake disorder, a parasomnia).
	7. The insomnia is not attributable to the physiologic effects of a substance (eg, a drug of abuse, a medication).
	8. Coexisting mental disorders and medical conditions do not adequately explain the predominant complaint of insomnia.
	Specify if:
	• *Episodic:* symptoms last at least 1 mo but <3 mo.
	• *Persistent:* symptoms last 3 mo or longer.
	• *Recurrent:* two (or more) episodes within the space of 1 y.

mornings and being unable to return to sleep.[5–7] Older adults tend to have more challenges with sleep maintenance compared with younger adults,[3,4,8] which results in reductions in total sleep time and sleep efficiency.[8] Insomnia can also be situational, persistent, or recurrent.[5] Situational insomnia is usually acute insomnia, which lasts a few days or weeks and is associated with changes in the sleep schedule or the sleep environment.[5,8] Life events such as retirement, hospitalizations, and new-onset illnesses can precipitate situational insomnia. Usually when the

event that triggers the insomnia is resolved, so too does the insomnia. If the insomnia does not resolve, it evolves into chronic insomnia.[5] Recurrent insomnia is episodic and often returns with the occurrence of stressful life events.[5]

Risk Factors of Insomnia

Multiple factors increase the risk for older adults developing insomnia, which include environmental, behavioral, medical, and social factors[8] (**Table 2**). For example, older adults may change

Table 2
Risk factors for insomnia in older adults[2,5,8,9,34]

Environment	Excessive noise, hot or cold temperatures, light during the sleep period, moving to a new home or downsizing to a smaller space or a retirement community or related facility Institutionalization
Behavioral/ Social	Irregular sleep schedules, caffeine use later in the day, alcohol close to bedtime Caregiving, hospitalizations, new medical problems Retirement or lifestyle change Death of a family member or friend Inappropriate use of social drugs, for example, alcohol (Note that alcohol is frequently used to self-medicate for sleep problems. It helps with falling asleep; however, when the effect wears off, sleep becomes light and disrupted.) Napping
Demographics	Female gender
Medical	Medications: Theophylline, thyroid hormone, anticholinergics, stimulants, oral decongestants, antidepressants, corticosteroids, antihypertensives, opioids, nonsteroidal antiinflammatory drugs Sleep disorders: sleep apnea, restless leg syndrome, periodic limb movement disorder, rapid eye movement disorder, age-related circadian rhythm change (phase advance) Psychiatric and cognitive conditions: depression, anxiety, mania, panic attacks, schizophrenia, substance abuse, dementia Other medical conditions: diabetes, fibromyalgia, hypertension, cardiovascular disease, stroke, chronic pain

their usual bed and wake time after they retire. Also, older adults also tend to have more comorbid disorders and are using multiple medications, which further increases their risk for sleep disturbances.[2,3]

Evaluation of Insomnia

Insomnia is diagnosed through a detailed clinical history taken from the patient and their bed partner.[9] In order to diagnose the specific type of insomnia, it is important for clinicians to ask about the history of insomnia, insomnia symptoms, sleep-wake routines and patterns, other sleep-related symptoms, daytime functioning and consequences, and previous treatments.[9,10] Older adults should also be asked about whether they snore or have leg discomfort.[11] Clinicians need to also identify whether there are comorbid medical, substance, and/or psychiatric conditions affecting sleep[10] using screening tests such as the Patient Health Questionnaire-9,[12] the Geriatric Depression Scale,[13] and the General Anxiety Disorder Questionnaire.[14] It is also important to assess daytime activities, as older adults may be less active during the day and consequently spend more time napping or dozing.

Subjective measures that can be used to evaluate sleep include sleep questionnaires, such as the Pittsburgh Sleep Quality Index (PSQI) and the Insomnia Severity Index (ISI), and sleep diaries. The PSQI is a 19-item instrument that assesses sleep quality and disturbances over a 1-month interval.[15] Scores can range between 0 and 21 with a score of 5 or more suggesting poor sleep quality.[15] The ISI is a 7-item questionnaire that assesses the nighttime symptoms and impact of insomnia over the previous month.[16] Scores range from 0 to 28, with values greater than 14 that suggest moderate to severe insomnia.[16]

Sleep diaries allow for the prospective tracking of an individual's sleep/wake patterns. They capture information such as bedtime, time to fall asleep, number and duration of nightly awakenings, wake-up time, out-of-bed time, and times and duration of daytime naps or dozing.[9,17] Sleep diaries may also include questions about sleep quality and types and amounts of medications, caffeine, and alcohol consumed.[9] Sleep diaries completed for approximately 2 weeks allows for the recognition of sleep patterns and variability.[9] Older patients sometime shave difficulties completing sleep diaries due to visual impairments, and large print is sometimes used to make it easier for older patients to complete sleep diaries.

Objective assessments of sleep such as actigraphy and polysomnography are not necessary for routine diagnosis and assessment of insomnia, but they may be helpful to rule out other comorbid sleep disorders such as sleep-disordered breathing or circadian rhythm sleep wake disorders.[18–20]

Treatments for Insomnia

The goal of insomnia treatment is the improvement of sleep quality and/or quantity and reduction in insomnia-related daytime impairments.[9] The patient should be involved in the development of the treatment plan and decisions about which treatment goals to pursue, as buy-in from the patient is critical for success.[21] The choice of treatment depends on the severity and duration of the insomnia symptoms, coexisting disorders, willingness of the patient to engage in behavioral therapies, and vulnerability of the patient to the adverse effects of medications.[9] It is important to emphasize to patients that it is normal to have occasional nights of poor sleep during and after the completion of treatment so that they will have realistic expectations about treatment and cope better during treatment.[21]

Sleep diaries and questionnaires can be used to evaluate how the treatment is progressing and to determine when there has been sufficient improvement to warrant discontinuation of treatment.[9] After treatment is discontinued, it is important to conduct periodic follow-ups to identify potential recurrence and precipitating events due to changes in health or lifestyle.

Nonpharmacologic Treatment Options

Cognitive behavioral therapy for insomnia (CBTi) is a multicomponent intervention involving cognitive and behavioral techniques such as stimulus control therapy, sleep restriction therapy, relaxation training, cognitive restructuring, and sleep hygiene education.[22] The goal of CBTi is to replace maladaptive thoughts and sleep habits and to reduce arousal associated with sleep.[22] CBTi has produced both short-term and long-term improvement in sleep.[23] Although CBTi is effective for insomnia, many health care providers are neither aware of the existence of CBTi nor know how to refer patients for treatment.[24]

- Stimulus control aims to strengthen the association between the bed/bedroom and sleep and to produce a consistent sleep-wake schedule. Instructions for stimulus control include the following: minimize napping; go to bed only when sleepy; get out of bed if unable to sleep; use the bed/bedroom only for sleep and sex; and wake up at the same time each day.[22]
- Sleep restriction is used to increase homeostatic drive for sleep in order to improve sleep quality. The time spent in bed is reduced to the actual sleep duration based on sleep diaries, which creates some mild sleep deprivation. The time in bed is then gradually increased until the individual achieves an optimal sleep duration.[22] There is strong support for sleep restriction in older adults with insomnia.[25] Sleep compression is an alternative technique to sleep restriction where time in bed is gradually reduced until the older adult achieves an optimal sleep duration.[26]
- Relaxation training is done to reduce tension and intrusive thoughts that interfere with the ability to sleep. Relaxation techniques used include deep breathing exercises, progressive muscle relaxation, biofeedback, and guided imagery.[22]
- Cognitive restructuring aims to reduce worry and change misconceptions associated with sleep and insomnia using Socratic questioning.[22] Challenging inaccurate patterns of thinking can change in how older adults perceive the effect of sleep on their lives.
- Sleep hygiene education provides some guidelines about factors that may help or interfere with sleep. They include not eating a heavy meal or drinking alcohol within 2 hours of bedtime; limiting caffeine intake after lunchtime; exercising regularly but not within 2 hours of bedtime; and keeping the bedroom quiet, dark, and at a cool, comfortable temperature.[22]

Mindfulness-based stress reduction techniques aim to change reactions to stress by teaching purposeful awareness and acceptance of the present state[27] and includes techniques such as breathing, body scan, and walking meditations and Hatha Yoga.[28] These techniques have been effective in reducing insomnia in older adults.[28]

Bright light therapy helps to strengthen circadian rhythms and establish a healthy sleep-wake cycle.[29,30] Results have been mixed on its efficacy for treatment of insomnia in older adults[29,30] but in general, may have a favorable effect when used with older adults.[29] Health care practitioners provide white light sources with a bluish tint that provide at least 1000 lux at the eye during daytime hours, at a time that is most convenient for the patient, on mornings after awakening if the circadian timing of the patient is unknown, or during the time interval the patient tends to be more tired.[29]

Acupuncture is a traditional Chinese technique in which specific points on the body are stimulated usually by inserting thin needles through the skin.[31] It has been shown to be effective in improving insomnia symptoms in older adults.[31]

Pharmacologic Treatment Options

Benzodiazepines, such as Lorazepam, Temazepam, and Clonazepam, decrease sleep latency and decrease nocturnal awakenings, but they also reduce rapid eye movement sleep.[32] In older adults, they increase the risk for memory impairment, falls, fractures, and motor vehicle accidents, and avoidable emergency department visits and hospital admissions; therefore, their use should be avoided in older adults.[33,34] Between 5.3% and 10.8% of adults 50 years and older use benzodiazepines.[35] Long-term use of benzodiazepines can promote psychological dependence, and there is an increased risk of addiction and abuse.[36] Tolerance can also develop over time, thus requiring larger doses to sustain efficacy.[36] It is necessary to educate older adults about the effects of benzodiazepine use and encourage discontinuation through tapering.[33,37] Although there is no current standard for tapering benzodiazepines, some providers recommend establishing a longer tapering schedule over 4 to 5 months for older patients and tapering the dose by 25% every 2 weeks.[33,37,38] While tapering health care providers could provide cognitive behavioral therapy for insomnia.[37,38]

Nonbenzodiazepine hypnotics reduce sleep latency.[32] These medications, which include eszopiclone, zolpidem, and zaleplon, should be avoided in older adults without consideration of the duration of use (no more than 90 days) because they can cause confusion and they increase the risk of falls and fractures; this should be avoided in older adults with dementia and cognitive impairment.[34]

Melatonin receptor agonists reduce sleep latency and increase sleep duration. An example is ramelteon. *Potential* adverse effects include mild gastrointestinal disturbances and nervous system effects such as dizziness, headache, somnolence, and fatigue with no evidence of significant rebound insomnia or withdrawal effects.[39] Ramelteon has been shown to decrease sleep latency in older adults.[39]

Many *antidepressants* have sedating effects and are sometimes used to treat insomnia, often at lower doses than used for depression. Antidepressants often have overall REM-suppressing effects, can decrease slow-wave sleep latency, and duration of slow wave sleep.[32] In the absence of an underlying depressive disorder, antidepressants should also be avoided in older adults because they are highly anticholinergic, sedating, increase the risk of falls, and cause orthostatic hypotension.[34]

Antihistamines decrease sleep latency[32]; however, these over-the-counter sleep medications such as diphenhydramine produce rapid tolerance and are highly anticholinergic.[34] Anticholinergic effects include blurred vision, dizziness, difficulty urinating, dry mouth, and constipation. Anticholinergic medications can also increase the risk for cognitive impairment and decline; therefore, drugs with a high anticholinergic profile such as antihistamines and antidepressants should be avoided in older adults.[34]

Melatonin and Valerian Root are classified as complementary and alternative medications. They are supplements and are not regulated by the Food and Drug Administration. The doses and the preparations available to consumers usually vary significantly. Melatonin is an endogenous hormone secreted by the pineal gland but is also used as an exogenous supplement.[40,41] Melatonin decreases subjective sleep latency in some studies, although it may cause headaches and drowsiness.[40,41] Valerian root has been shown to improve subjective sleep parameters but the research is less consistent with objective sleep parameters. Rare side effects reported for valerian root include gastrointestinal upset, contact allergies, headache, and restless sleep.[40] Individuals using complementary and alternative medications should always inform their health care provider and consider the interactions between herbal remedies and prescription medications.[40]

Pharmacologic treatments should only be used for short-term management of insomnia. When pharmacotherapy is used, health care providers should consider the insomnia symptoms, whether other treatments are available, how the patient responded to previous treatments, the side-effect profile of the medication, and medication interactions.[36] Older adults have better response rates with lower dosages because decreased lean body mass, increased body fat, and reduction in plasma proteins may increase blood concentration of unbound drugs and drug half-life.[36] Therefore, when prescribing medications for insomnia for older adults, start with the lowest dose and titrate upward.[36] Given the side effects and concerns about long-term safety, it is recommended that pharmacotherapy for insomnia be avoided or be used only for short periods of time.[34,42]

COMPARATIVE EFFECTIVENESS OF COGNITIVE BEHAVIORAL THERAPY FOR INSOMNIA AND MEDICATIONS

A comparative effectiveness study of CBTi compared with sleep medications (zopiclone, zolpidem, temazepam, or triazolam) found that CBTi is as effective for short-term treatment of insomnia as medications.[24,43] The effects of CBTi may also be more long-lasting than medications.[22,24] Although medications produce more rapid improvements compared with CBTi, over the long-term, CBTi has more durable and sustained effects on sleep quality and outcomes. The therapeutic effects of medications are usually not maintained after the medication is discontinued.[24]

SUMMARY

Aging is associated with several changes in sleep continuity and architecture parameters. Many older adults experience difficulties with falling asleep, staying asleep, or waking up too early, which leads to daytime impairment and warrant a diagnosis of insomnia. Factors such as the sleep environment, medications, and medical and psychiatric disorders can increase the risk for insomnia. Therefore, health care providers should obtain a comprehensive health and sleep history from older adults in order to correctly diagnose insomnia and identify the potential correlates of the disorder. After diagnosing insomnia, first-line treatment is CBTi. Medications such as benzodiazepines and nonbenzodiazepines should be avoided in older adults, given their potential for significant adverse consequences and clinical guidelines recommending against their use.

ACKNOWLEDGMENTS

Glenna Brewster is a Ruth L. Kirschstein NRSA Postdoctoral Research Fellow (T32HL07713; PI: Pack, A.) Funded by the National Institute on Aging (K23AG070378, PI: Brewster).

DISCLOSURE

The authors have no financial or commercial disclosures.

REFERENCES

1. Hirshkowitz M, Whiton K, Albert SM, et al. National Sleep Foundation's sleep time duration recommendations: methodology and results summary. Sleep Health 2015;1(1):40–3 [PubMed: 29073412].
2. Blay SL, Andreoli SB, Gastal FL. Prevalence of self-reported sleep disturbance among older adults and the association of disturbed sleep with service demand and medical conditions. Int Psychogeriatr 2008;20(3):582–95 [PubMed: 18053289].
3. Leblanc M-F, Desjardins S, Desgagné A. Sleep problems in anxious and depressive older adults. Psychol Res Behav Manag 2015;8:161–9 [PubMed: 26089709].
4. Ohayon MM. Epidemiology of insomnia: what we know and what we still need to learn. Sleep Med Rev 2002;6(2):97–111 [PubMed: 12531146].
5. American Psychiatric Association. Sleep-Wake Disorders. In Diagnostic and Statistical Manual of Mental Disorders (5th ed.). 2013. Available at: https://doi.org/10.1176/appi.books.9780890425596.dsm12.
6. Lichstein KL, Durrence HH, Taylor DJ, et al. Quantitative criteria for insomnia. Behav Res Ther 2003;41(4):427–45 [PubMed: 12643966].
7. Lineberger MD, Carney CE, Edinger JD, et al. Defining insomnia: quantitative criteria for insomnia severity and frequency. Sleep 2006;29(4):479–85 [PubMed: 16676781].
8. Vitiello MV. Sleep in normal aging. Sleep Med Clin. 2006;7(3):539–544.
9. Schutte-Rodin S, Broch L, Buysse D, et al. Clinical guideline for the evaluation and management of chronic insomnia in adults. J Clin Sleep Med 2008;4(5):487–504 [PubMed: 18853708].
10. Mai E, Buysse DJ. Insomnia: prevalence, impact, pathogenesis, differential diagnosis, and evaluation. Sleep Med Clin 2008;3(2):167–74 [PubMed: 19122760].
11. McCall WV. Sleep in the elderly: burden, diagnosis, and treatment. Prim Care Companion J Clin Psychiatry 2004;6(1):9–20.
12. Kroenke K, Spitzer RL, Williams JBW. The PHQ-9: validity of a brief depression severity measure. J Gen Intern Med 2001;16(9):606–13 [PubMed: 11556941].
13. Yesavage JA, Brink TL, Rose TL, et al. Development and validation of a geriatric depression screening scale: a preliminary report. J Psychiatr Res 1982;17(1):37–49 [PubMed: 7183759].
14. Wild B, Eckl A, Herzog W, et al. Assessing generalized anxiety disorder in elderly people using the GAD-7 and GAD-2 scales: results of a validation study. Am J Geriatr Psychiatry 2014;22(10):1029–38 [PubMed: 23768681].
15. Buysse DJ, Reynolds CF 3rd, Monk TH, et al. The Pittsburgh Sleep Quality Index: a new instrument for psychiatric practice and research. Psychiatry Res 1989;28(2):193–213 [PubMed: 2748771].
16. Bastien CH, Vallieres A, Morin CM. Validation of the Insomnia Severity Index as an outcome measure for insomnia research. Sleep Med 2001;2(4):297–307 [PubMed: 11438246].
17. Carney CE, Buysse DJ, Ancoli-Israel S, et al. The consensus sleep diary: standardizing prospective

sleep self-monitoring. Sleep 2012;35(2):287–302 [PubMed: 22294820].

18. Littner M, Hirshkowitz M, Kramer M, et al. Practice parameters for using polysomnography to evaluate insomnia: an update. Sleep 2003;26(6):754–60 [PubMed: 14572131].

19. Ancoli-Israel S, Cole R, Alessi C, et al. The role of actigraphy in the study of sleep and circadian rhythms. Sleep 2003;26(3):342–92 [PubMed: 12749557].

20. Roehrs T. Sleep physiology and pathophysiology. Clin Cornerstone 2000;2(5):1–15.

21. Gooneratne NS, Vitiello MV. Sleep in older adults: normative changes, sleep disorders, and treatment options. Clin Geriatr Med 2014;30(3):591–627 [PubMed: 25037297].

22. Morin CM, Bootzin RR, Buysse DJ, et al. Psychological and behavioral treatment of insomnia:update of the recent evidence (1998–2004). Sleep 2006; 29(11):1398–414 [PubMed: 17162986].

23. Alessi C, Martin JL, Fiorentino L, et al. Cognitive behavioral therapy for insomnia in older veterans using nonclinician sleep coaches: randomized controlled trial. J Am Geriatr Soc 2016;64(9):1830–8 [PubMed: 27550552].

24. Mitchell MD, Gehrman P, Perlis M, et al. Comparative effectiveness of cognitive behavioral therapy for insomnia: a systematic review. BMC Fam Pract 2012;13:40 [PubMed: 22631616].

25. McCurry SM, Logsdon RG, Teri L, et al. Evidence-based psychological treatments for insomnia in older adults. Psychol Aging 2007;22(1):18–27 [PubMed: 17385979].

26. Lichstein KL, Riedel BW, Wilson NM, et al. Relaxation and sleep compression for late-life insomnia: a placebo-controlled trial. J Consult Clin Psychol 2001;69(2):227–39 [PubMed: 11393600].

27. Ong JC, Manber R, Segal Z, et al. A randomized controlled trial of mindfulness meditation for chronic insomnia. Sleep 2014;37(9):1553–63 [PubMed: 25142566].

28. Zhang JX, Liu XH, Xie XH, et al. Mindfulness-based stress reduction for chronic insomnia in adults older than 75 years: a randomized, controlled, single-blind clinical trial. Explore (NY) 2015;11(3):180–5.

29. Sloane PD, Figueiro M, Cohen L. Light as therapy for sleep disorders and depression in older adults. Clin Geriatr 2008;16(3):25–31 [PubMed: 24285919].

30. Gammack JK. Light therapy for insomnia in older adults. Clin Geriatr Med 2008;24(1):139–49. viii. [PubMed: 18035237].

31. Kwok T, Leung PC, Wing YK, et al. The effectiveness of acupuncture on the sleep quality of elderly with dementia: a within-subjects trial. Clin Interventions Aging 2013;8:923–9 [PubMed: 23940415].

32. Pagel JF, Parnes BL. Medications for the treatment of sleep disorders: an overview. Prim Care Companion J Clin Psychiatry 2001;3(3):118–25.

33. Tannenbaum C. Inappropriate benzodiazepine use in elderly patients and its reduction. J Psychiatry Neurosci 2015;40(3):E27–8 [PubMed: 25903036].

34. By the american geriatrics society beers criteria update expert P. American geriatrics society 2015 updated beers criteria for potentially inappropriate medication Use in older adults. J Am Geriatr Soc 2015;63(11):2227–46 [PubMed: 26446832].

35. Olfson M, King M, Schoenbaum M. Benzodiazepine use in the United States. JAMA Psychiatry 2015; 72(2):136–42 [PubMed: 25517224].

36. Kamel NS, Gammack JK. Insomnia in the elderly: cause, approach, and treatment. Am J Med 2006; 119(6):463–9 [PubMed: 16750956].

37. Bélanger L, Belleville G, Morin C. Management of hypnotic discontinuation in chronic insomnia. Sleep Med Clin 2009;4(4):583–92 [PubMed: 20607118].

38. Paquin AM, Zimmerman K, Rudolph JL. Risk versus risk: a review of benzodiazepine reduction in older adults. Expert Opin Drug Saf 2014;13(7):919–34 [PubMed: 24905348].

39. Roth T, Seiden D, Sainati S, et al. Effects of ramelteon on patient- reported sleep latency in older adults with chronic insomnia. Sleep Med 2003;7(4):312–8.

40. Gooneratne NS. Complimentary and alternative medicine for sleep disturbances in older adults. Clin Geriatr Med 2008;24(1):121. viii. [PubMed: 18035236].

41. Buscemi N, Vandermeer B, Hooton N, et al. The efficacy and safety of exogenous melatonin for primary sleep disorders: a meta-analysis. J Gen Intern Med 2005;20(12):1151–8 [PubMed: 16423108].

42. Perlis M, Gehrman P, Riemann D. Intermittent and long-term use of sedative hypnotics. Curr Pharm Des 2008;14(32):3456–65 [PubMed: 19075721].

43. Sivertsen B, Omvik S, Pallesen S, et al. Cognitive behavioral therapy vs zopiclone for treatment of chronic primary insomnia in older adults: a randomized controlled trial. JAMA 2006;295(24):2851–8 [PubMed: 16804151].

44. American Academy of Sleep Medicine. International classification of sleep disorders. 3. Darien. IL: American Academy of Sleep Medicine; 2014.

Circadian Rhythm Sleep–Wake Disorders in Older Adults

Jee Hyun Kim, MD, PhD[a], Alexandria R. Elkhadem[b],
Jeanne F. Duffy, MBA, PhD[c],*

KEYWORDS

- Circadian rhythm sleep disorders • Advanced sleep phase • Delayed sleep phase • Melatonin
- Circadian rhythm disruption • Alzheimer's disease • Light therapy

KEY POINTS

- The circadian timing system regulates the timing, structure, and consolidation of sleep, in conjunction with a sleep–wake homeostatic process.
- There are age-related changes in the circadian regulation of sleep, in sleep homeostatic regulation of sleep, and in the interaction between these 2 processes.
- Circadian rhythm sleep–wake disorders result from a mismatch between the desired timing of sleep and the ability to fall asleep or remain asleep.
- Advanced sleep–wake phase disorder and irregular sleep–wake rhythm disorder are more common in older adults than in young adults.
- Jet lag disorder and shift-work disorder are more commonly experienced by travelers and workers as they age.

INTRODUCTION

The timing, duration, and consolidation of human sleep result largely from the interaction of 2 sleep regulatory systems: the sleep–wake homeostat and the circadian timing system. When these 2 processes are aligned and functioning optimally, they allow adults to achieve a long, consolidated bout of wakefulness throughout the day and a long and consolidated sleep episode at night. Changes to either process, or a change in how the 2 processes interact, can result in an inability to fall asleep at the desired time, difficulty remaining asleep, or difficulty remaining awake throughout the desired wake episode. This mismatch between the desired timing of sleep (and wakefulness) and the ability to fall asleep and remain asleep is a hallmark of a distinct class of sleep disorders called the circadian rhythm sleep–wake disorders (CRSWDs). This article discusses the circadian timing system, the role played by the circadian system in sleep–wake regulation, typical changes in the circadian regulation of sleep with aging, the CRSWDs and how age influences their diagnosis and treatment, and how neurologic diseases in older patients affect circadian rhythms and sleep.

Circadian Rhythm Sleep–wake Disorders

Although surveys[1] suggest that less than 3% of the adult population have a CRSWD, the CRSWDs are often confused with insomnia, resulting in underestimates of the true prevalence. Some

Published: November 23, 2017 DOI: https://doi.org/10.1016/j.jsmc.2017.09.004.
^a Department of Neurology, Ewha Womans University Seoul Hospital, Ewha Womans University College of Medicine, Gonghangdae-ro 260, Gangseo-gu, Seoul, Republic of Korea; ^b Division of Sleep and Circadian Disorders, Department of Medicine, Brigham and Women's Hospital, 221 Longwood Avenue BLI438, Boston, MA 02115, USA; ^c Division of Sleep Medicine, Harvard Medical School, Boston, MA, USA
* Corresponding author: Division of Sleep and Circadian Disorders, Department of Medicine, Brigham and Women's Hospital, 221 Longwood Avenue BLI438, Boston, MA 02115.
E-mail address: jduffy@research.bwh.harvard.edu

estimates are that up to 10% of adult patients with sleep disorders may have a CRSWD.[2] Although some CRSWDs (such as jet lag) can be self-limiting, others, when untreated, can lead to adverse medical, psychological, and social consequences for affected patients. The International Classification of Sleep Disorders classifies CRSWDs as disorders related to the timing of sleep and wakefulness, with 6 subtypes[3]: delayed sleep–wake phase disorder, advanced sleep–wake phase disorder, irregular sleep–wake rhythm disorder, non–24-h sleep–wake rhythm disorder, jet lag disorder, and shift-work disorder (**Table 1**). The primary clinical characteristic of all CRSWDs is an inability to fall asleep, remain asleep, and/or wake at the desired time. CRSWDs are thought to arise from a problem with the internal biological clock (circadian timing system) and/or misalignment between the circadian timing system and the external 24-h environment. This misalignment can be the result of biological and/or behavioral factors,[4] and the rates of different CRSWDs vary across age groups.

The Circadian Timing System in Humans

The circadian timing system refers to near-24-h rhythmicity in many aspects of physiology and behavior, including not only sleep and waking, but hormone secretion, body temperature, and urine production.[5–7] These rhythms are features of individual cells[8] and arise through transcription–translation feedback loops.[9] Coordination of the rhythms among cells within an organ, and between the organ systems of the body, is achieved through signals from a central pacemaker in the hypothalamus, the suprachiasmatic nucleus (SCN).[10] The SCN not only coordinates the rhythmic activity of the cells and organs within the body but also synchronizes the near-24-h rhythmic activity of the body with the 24-h cycle of the external environment, a process called entrainment. A functional circadian timing system allows the organism to predict regular changes that occur in the environment (eg, sunlight, food availability, presence of predators) and to prepare for those changes, thus providing an adaptive advantage.[11]

Because the underlying rhythmicity is close to, but not exactly, 24 hours in cycle length, it must be synchronized or *entrained* to the external 24-h day on a regular basis. Entrainment of the near-24-h circadian system to the 24-h day occurs typically through exposure to signals from the environment, and in the case of humans (as in most other mammals) this is largely conducted via regular exposure to light during the day and darkness at night. Studies in healthy sighted adults have shown that the period (cycle length) of the circadian system averages around 24.2 hours across age groups.[12] This finding implies that the average adult's circadian system needs to be reset about 10 minutes earlier each day to remain synchronized to external clock time, and, if it is not, then the circadian system may drift out of synchrony with external clock time. One example of this desynchronization is what happens to many blind individuals. They complain of cyclic sleep–wake problems, alternating periods when they can sleep well at night and are alert during the day with times when their nighttime sleep is very disturbed and they struggle to remain awake throughout the day.[13]

Although on average human circadian period is 24.2 hours, the range between individuals is about an hour, from approximately 23.5 to 24.5 hours.[12] This means that individuals with the shortest and longest periods need to reset by half an hour each day to remain entrained, and, without that regular resetting, they are even more likely than the average person to drift out of synchronization. Individuals with the shortest and longest periods are, therefore, most susceptible to non–24-h sleep–wake rhythm disorder. On average, the circadian period in women is shorter than in men, and significantly more women than men have a period that is less than 24 hours.[12] This difference predisposes women to advanced sleep–wake phase disorder.

Circadian Regulation of Sleep and Wakefulness

- The circadian timing system coregulates the timing, structure, and consolidation of sleep
- The circadian timing system interacts with the sleep–wake homeostat to allow consolidated wakefulness during the day and consolidated sleep at night

The circadian system is a major determinant of the timing of sleep and internal sleep structure in humans.[14] Specialized experimental techniques have been used to separate the circadian and sleep–wake homeostatic influences on sleep to understand how each independently influences sleep and wakefulness. Those studies have revealed that although most aspects of sleep are influenced by the biological time at which sleep occurs, the circadian system has its strongest impact on rapid eye movement (REM) sleep, sleep latency, and sleep consolidation.[15] The rhythm in circadian sleep–wake propensity is such that the strongest drive for wakefulness occurs in the evening, close to the end of the usual wake episode

Table 1
Characteristics of circadian rhythm sleep–wake disorders with special considerations for older patients

Circadian Rhythm Sleep–Wake Disorder	Basic Characteristics	Age-Related Considerations
Delayed sleep–wake phase disorder	Sleep timing occurs later than desired or required	Less common in older adults
Advanced sleep–wake phase disorder	Sleep timing occurs earlier than desired or required	More common in older adults
Irregular sleep–wake rhythm disorder	Irregularity in sleep–wake timing, often including multiple irregular short sleep bouts within a day	More common in older adults, particularly in the context of dementia and institutionalization
Non–24-h sleep–wake rhythm disorder	Sleep timing moves progressively later each night (or rarely, moves earlier each night)	More common in older adults, particularly in the context of vision loss
Jet lag disorder	Inability to sleep at night and/ or remain awake throughout the day after traveling across several time zones. This condition is caused by the abrupt mismatch between internal biological time and external time resulting from rapid travel across time zones and is typically self-limiting.	Older adults more affected due to decreased ability to sleep at adverse circadian time
Shift-work disorder	Inability to obtain sufficient sleep during the day and difficulty remaining awake at night to perform night work. Shift work disorder can also impact day workers whose early morning shifts require very early rise times	Older adults may be more susceptible due to decreased ability to sleep during the day

All circadian rhythm sleep–wake disorders are characterized by an inability to fall asleep, remain asleep, and/or awaken at the desired or required time

(creating the wake maintenance zone or forbidden zone for sleep). Similarly, the strongest drive for sleep occurs in the late night/early morning hours, close to the time of the end of the usual sleep episode. When this rhythm in sleep–wake propensity interacts with the sleep–wake homeostatic process, it results in an ability to remain awake across a long episode each day and to remain asleep for a long and consolidated time each night. Laboratory studies have shown that the ability to have a long consolidated sleep episode is critically dependent on the proper alignment of the timing of sleep with respect to the underlying circadian rhythm of sleep–wake propensity.[15,16] Misalignment, as occurs when night-shift workers attempt to sleep during the day, typically produces an inability to sleep for more than a few hours,[17] and can result in shift-work disorder.

Age-related Changes in Circadian Rhythms

- There are age-related changes in the phase (timing) of circadian rhythms
- There are age-related changes in the amplitude of circadian rhythms
- There are age-related changes in how the circadian and sleep homeostatic systems interact
- With advancing age, the ability to sleep at adverse circadian phases is compromised, even in healthy individuals

The timing of the circadian rhythms of body temperature, melatonin, and cortisol have been shown to move earlier, or advance, in older adults when compared with young adults.[18] In addition, there are numerous reports that the amplitude of circadian rhythms, including those of body temperature, melatonin, and other hormones, are reduced in older adults.[18] Studies in animals suggest that these age-related changes in rhythms may be caused by changes in the SCN.[19] In addition to changes in the timing of physiologic rhythms controlled by the circadian timing system, there are also reports that the relative timing of rhythms with respect to sleep–wake timing change with age.[20] This latter finding means that older adults are not only sleeping at a different clock time than young adults, they are also sleeping at a different biological time.

Laboratory studies have shown that the sleep of older adults is much more sensitive to the circadian time at which it occurs than is the sleep of young adults,[16] thus making older adults more vulnerable to the CRSWDs jet lag disorder and shift work disorder (discussed later). Studies for which the circadian time of sleep is systematically manipulated have revealed that there may be an age-related reduction in the amplitude of the circadian rhythm of sleep–wake propensity that not only makes it more difficult to sleep at an adverse circadian time but makes the consolidation of an extended nighttime sleep episode more difficult.[16,21]

Diagnosis of Circadian Rhythm Sleep–wake Disorders

As described earlier, CRSWDs are assumed to result from a mismatch between the timing of sleep (and wakefulness) and the underlying circadian rhythm of sleep–wake propensity. Despite this, current standards[3,22] for diagnosis of a CRSWD do not require the assessment of circadian rhythmicity but instead focus on the timing of sleep alone. This lack of circadian rhythm assessment may contribute to the poor treatment outcomes of some patients with CRSWDs.[4,23]

Diagnosis of all CRSWDs requires that 3 main criteria are met:

- The complaint is chronic
- The affected patient has problems with sleep (difficulty falling asleep, difficulty remaining asleep, or waking too early), difficulty remaining awake (excessive daytime sleepiness), or both
- The sleep–wake problem causes clinically significant distress or impairment of one or more areas of functioning

Depending on the CRSWD, there are additional and/or specific criteria used to make a diagnosis. These are outlined in **Box 1**.

Prevalence of Circadian Rhythm Sleep–wake Disorders in Older Adults

- Although CRSWD diagnoses are not common, older adults are much more likely than young adults to be diagnosed with advanced sleep–wake phase disorder and irregular sleep–wake rhythm disorder
- Older individuals are more prone to jet lag disorder and shift-work disorder than their younger counterparts (and even more prone than when they were younger) because of a reduced ability to sleep at adverse circadian phases

Early morning awakening (EMA) is common among older adults.[24] Although some surveys of older adults indicate that 20% to 30% of them report EMA, when individuals with comorbidities such as depression, pain, physical limitations, and respiratory symptoms are excluded, less than 4% of those remaining have EMA.[25] It is impossible to determine from these subjective complaints whether circadian changes underlie the EMA, although in some cases the EMA meets the criteria for advanced sleep–wake phase disorder. Data from the Münich Chronotype Questionnaire[26] show that about 2% of the overall population have a mid-sleep time on free days earlier than 2 AM

Advanced sleep–wake phase disorder is found more frequently in older adults than in young adults.[1,27,28] As outlined in **Box 1**, delayed sleep–wake phase disorder is found rarely in older adults.[27,29] Non–24-h sleep–wake rhythm disorder, although rare in sighted older adults, may develop secondary to loss of vision.[30] Irregular sleep–wake rhythm disorder is also rare and is found most frequently in patients with dementias and in institutionalized individuals,[31] likely in part because of the lack of strong daily environmental and behavioral influences that typically synchronize circadian rhythms.[32] Jet lag disorder and shift-work disorder may affect individuals to a greater extent as they age,[33,34] because of typical age-related changes in sleep. This is because the sleep of older adults, even those who are in good health and without sleep disorders, is more vulnerable to misalignment with the circadian rhythm of sleep–wake propensity.[16,20,21] As a consequence, older shift workers report more sleep problems[35] and have higher rates of hypnotic use than younger shift workers.[36] In addition, irregular sleep–wake patterns are more prevalent in older adults with current or remitted depression,[37] and older adults with a lifetime of major depression

Box 1
Diagnostic criteria for circadian rhythm sleep–wake disorders most common in older adults

- Main criteria for all CRSWDs:

  o The sleep–wake complaint is chronic

  o The patient has a problem with sleep (difficulty falling asleep, remaining asleep, or waking too early), difficulty remaining awake (excessive daytime sleepiness), or both

  o The sleep–wake problem causes clinically significant distress or impairment of one or more areas of daytime functioning

- Advanced sleep–wake phase disorder, additional criteria:

  o An advance in the timing of sleep relative to the desired or required timing, both by history and as evidenced using actigraphy and/or a daily sleep log for at least 1 week

  o Symptoms/complaints present for at least 3 months

  o When allowed to sleep without timing constraints, the patient is able to achieve a sleep episode of good quality and sufficient duration, although the timing is advanced

  o The sleep problem is not explained by any other sleep, medical, neurologic, or psychological disorder, by medication, or by substance use/abuse

- Irregular sleep–wake rhythm disorder, additional criteria:

  o Irregular sleep and wake episodes throughout the 24-h day, both by history and as evidenced using actigraphy and/or a daily sleep log for at least 1 week; 3 or more sleep episodes per 24 hours, difficulty sleeping/remaining asleep at night, difficulty remaining awake during the day

  o Symptoms/complaints present for at least 3 months

  o The sleep problem is not explained by any other sleep, medical, neurologic, or psychological disorder, by medication, or by substance use/abuse

- Shift-work disorder, additional criteria:

  o When working a particular shift (night shift or day shift with early morning start time), difficulty sleeping and/or excessive sleepiness, with overall reduced sleep duration by history and as evidenced using actigraphy and/or a daily sleep log for at least 1 week

  o Symptoms/complaints present for at least 3 months when on the work schedule

  o The sleep problem is not explained by any other sleep, medical, neurologic, or psychological disorder, by medication, by substance use/abuse, or by the patient forgoing daytime sleep to work a second job or perform childcare or other activities

- Jet lag disorder, additional criteria:

  o Difficulty sleeping and/or excessive sleepiness, with overall reduced sleep duration following rapid travel across 2 or more time zones

  o Impairment of function that appears within a few days of the travel

  o The sleep problem is not explained by any other sleep, medical, neurologic, or psychological disorder, by medication, or by substance use/abuse

Note that the assessment of endogenous circadian rhythmicity (eg, timing of evening melatonin secretion onset) is not required for diagnosis.[4]

have been reported to show different timings of melatonin onset than healthy individuals.[38]

Neurologic Implications of Circadian Rhythm Changes in Older Adults

- Patients with neurodegenerative diseases show changes in rest-activity patterns and sleep disruptions, and these may be caused by circadian disruption
- Changes in sleep may be an early sign of future neurodegenerative changes
- Changes in sleep often precede cognitive decline, and more severe sleep changes are associated with faster/greater cognitive decline
- Postoperative delirium, with associated sleep pattern changes, may be a warning sign for later cognitive decline.

As described earlier, it is typical for older adults to experience circadian rhythm changes, and most often these changes go unrecognized unless they are accompanied by significant sleep disturbances or daytime dysfunction. However, there is growing evidence from numerous epidemiologic studies that sleep problems in older adults, including modest circadian rhythm changes, might represent an early sign of cognitive decline, potential development of a neurodegenerative disease, and might also be associated with increased mortality.[39–46] A bidirectional relationship between sleep and neurodegeneration has been suggested based on evidence from studies in animals.[47–49] These findings may relate to the discovery of the brain glymphatic system, hypothesized to be responsible for eliminating metabolic waste, including amyloid-β and tau proteins, from the brain during sleep.[49,50]

How circadian rhythm changes are associated with the sleep-cognitive decline relationship are not well understood, because few studies have attempted to measure circadian rhythms.[40,42,43] Although actigraphy cannot assess the function of the underlying endogenous circadian pacemaker, rest-activity monitoring by actigraphy is the most commonly reported measure used to monitor the sleep–wake rhythm in older adults. There is evidence from the general population that rest-activity patterns show certain systematic changes with aging, including reduced amplitude and advanced acrophase.[51] Many studies have extracted variables from activity that are associated with cognitive changes in older adults, including interdaily stability (IS, a measure of rest-activity rhythm synchronization to 24-h clock time), intradaily variability (IV, a measure of rhythm fragmentation), amplitude, as well as acrophase or nadir of activity.[42,43,52–54] Recently, researchers have attempted to use features of rest-activity patterns measured by actigraphy to predict the development of cognitive decline or dementia in patients with preclinical Alzheimer's disease (AD) or mild cognitive impairment, although those methods remain experimental. One study presented increased rest-activity rhythm fragmentation without phase change or amplitude was associated with the presence of preclinical amyloid plaque pathology proved by positive amyloid PET finding.[55,56] Whether those rest-activity changes relate to changes in the circadian timing system remains to be determined. However, 2 studies of patients with probable AD found that the acrophase (ie, timing of the rhythm peak) of the core body temperature rhythms of patients with AD was delayed compared with controls,[57,58] suggesting that there may be circadian changes that underlie the sleep–wake changes.

Another hint that changes in sleep–wake behavior are associated with subsequent cognitive decline occurs in patients experiencing delirium during hospitalization or after major surgery. The sleep–wake behavior in patients experiencing delirium shares similar features with sundown syndrome/day–night reversal. One study followed the cognitive status in previously high-functioning patients who experienced postoperative delirium during a hospital stay and found they showed an approximately 3-fold greater rate of decline of cognition in the 36 months after surgery.[59] Difficulty falling asleep in community-dwelling older adults is also associated with memory problems,[25] and thus these 2 lines of evidence hint that a phase delay or circadian disruption, manifested through altered sleep timing, is associated with cognitive decline. Whether the altered sleep timing (and presumed circadian alteration) is a cause or a symptom of the cognitive decline remains to be determined.

In summary, although it is not always clear that a change in rest-activity patterns represents a change in circadian rhythms, a delay of the rest-activity pattern seems to precede a later cognitive decline in the older population. For otherwise healthy older patients who present features of a CRSWD, especially a phase delay, careful assessment and monitoring of their cognitive status may be warranted, because the sleep–wake timing change may be an early indicator of neurodegenerative changes. Longitudinal studies with careful clinical observations that include robust sleep and circadian rhythm measures (such as melatonin secretion) will provide greater insights into how circadian and sleep changes may be associated with neurodegeneration.

Circadian Rhythm Disruption in Older Patients with Neurodegenerative Disease

Patients with neurodegenerative disease commonly present with sleep–wake disturbances and/or sleep disorders (including insomnia, excessive daytime sleepiness, sudden sleep attacks, and REM behavior disorder) at an early stage. These disorders may result from structural changes in the SCN and/or in the way SCN cells communicate,[19] because the SCN in patients with AD shows more severe changes compared with age-matched adults without AD.[60,61] Recent studies suggest that changes in the melanopsin-containing retinal ganglion cells may also occur in patients with neurodegenerative diseases,[62,63] thereby contributing to circadian disruption.

As described earlier, studies that have assessed the rhythm of core body temperature have found a significant delay of the rhythm in patients with probable[58] or actual[64] AD. Some studies have reported that the disruption of rhythms in AD may be caused by pathologic changes to structures in the light input pathway from the eye to the SCN.[65–67]

Sleep disturbance is the most common nonmotor manifestation of Parkinson's disease (PD), with an incidence of 60% to 80%.[68,69] A recent prospective study found that lower overall activity and a reduction in the day–night difference in actigraphy was associated with a significantly increased risk of developing PD.[46] Insomnia, dream-enacting behaviors, excessive daytime sleepiness, snoring/apnea, restless legs syndrome, and sudden sleep attacks are common sleep complaints in PD. REM behavior disorder is now recognized as an important early nonmotor phenomenon associated with the later development of PD and Parkinson-Plus syndrome. However, few studies have been conducted to evaluate circadian markers in patients with PD. Changes in phase and amplitude of the melatonin rhythm in patients with PD have been reported,[70,71] suggesting that circadian dysfunction may be a feature of PD, although further studies are needed to understand whether the observed changes are not only prodromal nonmotor features of PD but may also be therapeutic targets. There are also reports of circadian alterations in other neurodegenerative disorders such as progressive supranuclear palsy[72] and Huntington disease.[73–75]

In summary, patients with certain neurodegenerative diseases show sleep–wake changes, and there is some evidence that there may also be circadian changes. However, additional studies measuring circadian markers in connection with clinical features are needed to understand what role the circadian system plays in the sleep–wake changes associated with those neurodegenerative diseases.

Treatment of Circadian Sleep–wake Disorders in Older Adults

- Treatments focus on resetting and/or synchronizing circadian rhythms
- Light therapy and/or melatonin are common strategies
- Much more research is needed to develop clinical guidelines and protocols for the use of light therapy and other treatments for CRSWDs in older adults

As outlined in **Table 2**, the most common treatments used for CRSWDs are designed to reset or synchronize the circadian timing system. A basic strategy used in all CRSWDs is to have the patient select a sleep time and attempt to strictly adhere to it. In addition, therapies that shift rhythm timing are often used, including bright light therapy and melatonin administration. In some cases, hypnotics to promote sleep and/or stimulants to promote wakefulness are also used. However, much more research is needed to identify new ways to diagnose and choose the best treatment of CRSWDs in patients of all ages.[4]

Light Therapy

The timing of light exposure is crucial when using light therapy for the treatment of CRSWDs.[76–80]

Table 2
Common treatments for circadian rhythm sleep–wake disorders

CRSWD	Common Recommendations and Treatments
Advanced sleep–wake phase disorder	• Adhere to a fixed sleep schedule • Evening bright light
Irregular sleep–wake rhythm disorder	• Adhere to a fixed sleep schedule • Daytime bright light • Evening melatonin
Non–24-h sleep–wake rhythm disorder	• Adhere to a fixed sleep schedule • Chronotherapy • Evening melatonin • Morning bright light exposure
Jet lag disorder	• Adhere to a fixed sleep schedule • Appropriately timed melatonin • Hypnotics • Timed light exposure (including minimizing exposure to bright light at certain times) • Caffeine and other stimulants
Shift-work disorder	• Timed light exposure (including minimizing exposure to bright light on the commute home in the morning) • Appropriately timed melatonin • Modafinil • Strategic napping • Caffeine

According to the phase response curves to light, evening/early night light delays the circadian phase, whereas late night/early morning light advances the circadian phase.[81] In young adults, duration-dependent responses to light have been reported,[82,83] with the maximal responses occurring in the initial minutes of light exposure. In fact, Najjar and Zeitzer[84] reported that intermittent flashes of light can produce significant circadian effects. Although additional studies in clinical populations need to be performed, such findings suggest that patients might not need to remain fixed in front of a light box to achieve phase shifts, improving practicality and compliance. In terms of the optimal intensity for light therapy, there are some reports that older adults may be less sensitive to light than young adults,[77,85,86] although not all studies have identified an age difference.[77,79] There is evidence that light transmission is affected by typical age-related changes in the lens of the eye, which may contribute to differential impacts of light therapy between young and older adults.[87]

Despite findings from laboratory studies, there are few randomized trials in clinical populations that show the benefit of light therapy for older adults with advanced sleep–wake phase disorder,[88] and some studies show little to no impact.[89,90] Clinical treatment guidelines suggest that there is only weak evidence for evening light therapy in advanced sleep–wake phase disorder,[91] and there are no detailed guidelines for the intensity, duration or timing for light therapy.[4]

However, rather than use timed light exposures to shift rhythms, one use of light therapy may be to enhance the overall robustness of circadian rhythmicity in older adults, especially those who are institutionalized, as described later in discussion.

Treatment of Irregular Sleep–wake Disorder in Older Adults

Irregular sleep–wake disorder in older adults is most common in patients with neurodegenerative disease, including AD and other dementias, especially as the disease advances. The disruptive impact of the irregular sleep pattern is one of the main reasons for institutionalization.[92,93] Several studies have been performed to test whether light interventions improve sleep in such patients, and there is some evidence that bright light exposure can reduce sleep disturbances and improve rest-activity patterns.[94–97] Combined light and melatonin interventions have also been tested, with some finding improvements in sleep and/or behavior.[98–100] Related interventions that include limits on daytime time in bed, increased light exposure during the day and decreased disruptions at night (eg, noise, caregiver interventions) have been reported to improve sleep–wake function.[101]

Treatment of Shift Work Sleep Disorder in Older Adults

Older adults are reported to be less tolerant to shift work,[34,102] and this is typically attributed to the decreased ability of older individuals to sleep at an adverse circadian phase.[16]

Nonpharmacologic interventions to treat shift work disorder include bright light exposure in the nighttime work environment and avoiding light on the morning commute home, strategic napping, as well as the use of caffeine and other stimulants.[103–105] Although few of those studies have focused on older shift workers exclusively, one study found that a combined intervention of enhanced lighting and scheduled afternoon–evening sleep was effective in improving night-shift alertness and performance in older individuals.[106] When they tested the impact of moving sleep to afternoon–evening hours alone, all participants showed longer actigraphically recorded sleep, with those instructed to remain in bed for 8 hours showing the longest sleep and best night shift performance.[107,108] Additional studies testing interventions in older shift workers are needed.[109]

SUMMARY

The circadian timing system has a strong impact on the timing, structure, and consolidation of sleep, and interacts with a sleep–wake homeostatic process to allow extended sleep and wake episodes. With age, there are changes to both of these sleep regulatory processes, as well as a change in the way they interact. Those age-related changes in sleep make it more likely that older adults will experience certain CRSWDs, particularly advanced sleep–wake phase disorder, jet lag disorder, and shift-work disorder. In addition, other medical changes that occur with aging can contribute to a greater likelihood of the CRSWD irregular sleep–wake rhythm disorder. Although sleep hygiene, bright light therapy, melatonin administration, and other therapies are used to treat the CRSWDs, few systematic studies have been performed to determine the optimal strategy for treating CRSWDs, and few studies have specifically tested the therapies in older adults.[4] These deficiencies are compounded by current standards not requiring the assessment of circadian rhythmicity in the diagnosis of CRSWDs, mainly because of the time and expense of doing so.[4] Thus, there remain significant knowledge gaps in the diagnosis and treatment of CRSWDs, especially in older patients.[110]

DISCLOSURE

The authors have nothing to disclose.

ACKNOWLEDGMENTS

The authors wish to thank Mr. J. Wise for assistance with the references. Supported in part by US NIH grants R01 AG044416, R01 HL148704, and P01 AG09975.

REFERENCES

1. Schrader H, Bovim G, Sand T. The prevalence of delayed and advanced sleep phase syndromes. J Sleep Res 1993;2:51–5.
2. Barion A, Zee PC. A clinical approach to circadian rhythm sleep disorders. Sleep Med 2007;8(6):566–77.
3. American Academy of Sleep Medicine. International classification of sleep disorders. Darien, IL: American Academy of Sleep Medicine; 2014.
4. Duffy JF, Abbott SM, Burgess HJ, et al. Workshop report. Circadian rhythm sleep-wake disorders: gaps and opportunities. Sleep 2021;44(5).
5. Czeisler CA, Klerman EB. Circadian and sleep-dependent regulation of hormone release in humans. Recent Prog Horm Res 1999;54:97–132.
6. Czeisler CA, Gooley JJ. Sleep and circadian rhythms in humans. Cold Spring Harb Symp Quant Biol 2007;72:579–97.
7. Czeisler CA, Buxton OM. Human circadian timing system and sleep-wake regulation. In: Kryger MH, Roth T, Dement WC, editors. Principles and practice of sleep medicine. 6th ed. Philadelphia: W.B. Saunders Company; 2017. p. 362–76.
8. Ko CH, Takahashi JS. Molecular components of the mammalian circadian clock. Hum Mol Genet 2006;15(Spec No 2):R271–7.
9. Dibner C, Schibler U, Albrecht U. The mammalian circadian timing system: organization and coordination of central and peripheral clocks. Annu Rev Physiol 2010;72:517–49.
10. Menaker M, Takahashi JS, Eskin A. The physiology of circadian pacemakers. Annu Rev Physiol 1978;40:501–26.
11. DeCoursey PJ. Survival value of suprachiasmatic nuclei (SCN) in four wild sciurid rodents. Behav Neurosci 2014;128(3):240–9.
12. Duffy JF, Cain SW, Chang AM, et al. Sex difference in the near-24-hour intrinsic period of the human circadian timing system. Proc Natl Acad Sci U S A 2011;108(suppl. 3):15602–8.
13. Lockley SW, Arendt J, Skene DJ. Visual impairment and circadian rhythm disorders. Dialogues Clin Neurosci 2007;9(3):301–14.
14. Czeisler CA, Dijk DJ. Human circadian physiology and sleep-wake regulation. In: Takahashi JS, Turek FW, Moore RY, editors. Handbook of behavioral neurobiology: circadian clocks. New York: Plenum Publishing Co.; 2001. p. 531–69.
15. Dijk DJ, Czeisler CA. Contribution of the circadian pacemaker and the sleep homeostat to sleep propensity, sleep structure, electroencephalographic slow waves, and sleep spindle activity in humans. J Neurosci 1995;15(5):3526–38.
16. Dijk DJ, Duffy JF, Riel E, et al. Ageing and the circadian and homeostatic regulation of human sleep during forced desynchrony of rest, melatonin and temperature rhythms. J Physiol 1999;516(2):611–27.
17. Luckhaupt SE. Short sleep duration among workers – United States, 2010. MMWR. Morb Mortal Wkly Rep 2012;61(16):281–5.
18. Duffy JF, Zitting KM, Chinoy ED. Aging and circadian rhythms. Sleep Med Clin 2015;10(4):423–34.
19. Engelberth RCGJ, Bezerra de Pontes AL, Porto Fiuza F, et al. Changes in the suprachiasmatic nucleus during aging: implications for biological rhythms. Psychol Neurosci 2013;6(3):287–97.
20. Duffy JF, Dijk DJ, Klerman EB, et al. Later endogenous circadian temperature nadir relative to an earlier wake time in older people. Am J Physiol 1998;275:R1478–87.
21. Dijk DJ, Duffy JF, Czeisler CA. Age-related increase in awakenings: impaired consolidation of nonREM sleep at all circadian phases. Sleep 2001;24(5):565–77.
22. Morgenthaler TI, Lee-Chiong T, Alessi C, et al. Practice parameters for the clinical evaluation and treatment of circadian rhythm sleep disorders. Sleep. 2007;30(11):1445–59.
23. Rahman SA, Kayumov L, Tchmoutina EA, et al. Clinical efficacy of dim light melatonin onset testing in diagnosing delayed sleep phase syndrome. Sleep Med 2009;10(5):549–55.
24. Foley DJ, Monjan AA, Brown SL, et al. Sleep complaints among elderly persons: an epidemiologic study of three communities. Sleep 1995;18(6):425–32.
25. Foley D, Ancoli-Israel S, Britz P, et al. Sleep disturbances and chronic disease in older adults: results of the 2003 national sleep foundation sleep in America survey. J Psychosom Res 2004;56(5):497–502.
26. Roenneberg T, Kuehnle T, Pramstaller PP, et al. A marker for the end of adolescence. Curr Biol 2004;14(24):R1038–9.
27. Sack RL, Auckley D, Auger RR, et al. Circadian rhythm sleep disorders: part II, advanced sleep phase disorder, delayed sleep phase disorder, free-running disorder, and irregular sleep-wake rhythm. an American academy of sleep medicine review. Sleep 2007;30(11):1484–501.
28. Curtis BJ, Ashbrook LH, Young T, et al. Extreme morning chronotypes are often familial and not exceedingly rare: the estimated prevalence of advanced sleep phase, familial advanced sleep phase, and advanced sleep-wake phase disorder in a sleep clinic population. Sleep 2019;42(10).
29. Monk TH, Buysse DJ. Chronotype, bed timing and total sleep time in seniors. Chronobiol Int 2014;31(5):655–9.
30. Uchiyama M, Lockley SW. Non-24-hour sleep-wake rhythm disorder in sighted and blind patients. Sleep Med Clin 2015;10(4):495–516.

31. Zee PC, Vitiello MV. Circadian rhythm sleep disorder: irregular sleep wake rhythm type. Sleep Med Clin 2009;4(2):213–8.

32. Ancoli-Israel S, Klauber MR, Jones DW, et al. Variations in circadian rhythms of activity, sleep, and light exposure related to dementia in nursing-home patients. Sleep 1997;20(1):18–23.

33. Sack RL, Auckley D, Auger RR, et al. Circadian rhythm sleep disorders: part I, basic principles, shift work and jet lag disorders. an American academy of sleep medicine review. Sleep 2007;30(11):1460–83.

34. Duffy JF. Shift work and aging: roles of sleep and circadian rhythms. Clin Occup Environ Med 2003;3:311–32.

35. Schuster M, Oberlinner C, Claus M. Shift-specific associations between age, chronotype and sleep duration. Chronobiol Int 2019;36(6):784–95.

36. Härmä M, Tenkanen L, Sjöblom T, et al. Combined effects of shift work and life-style on the prevalence of insomnia, sleep deprivation and daytime sleepiness. Scand J Work Environ Health 1998;24:300–7.

37. Pye J, Phillips AJ, Cain SW, et al. Irregular sleep-wake patterns in older adults with current or remitted depression. J Affect Disord 2021;281:431–7.

38. Hoyos CM, Gordon C, Terpening Z, et al. Circadian rhythm and sleep alterations in older people with lifetime depression: a case-control study. BMC Psychiatry 2020;20(1):192.

39. Blackwell T, Yaffe K, Ancoli-Israel S, et al. Poor sleep is associated with impaired cognitive function in older women: the study of osteoporotic fractures. J Gerontol A Biol Sci Med Sci 2006;61(4):405–10.

40. Yaffe K, Blackwell T, Barnes DE, et al. Preclinical cognitive decline and subsequent sleep disturbance in older women. Neurology 2007;69(3):237–42.

41. Tranah GJ, Blackwell T, Ancoli-Israel S, et al. Circadian activity rhythms and mortality: the study of osteoporotic fractures. J Am Geriatr Soc 2010;58(2):282–91.

42. Tranah GJ, Blackwell T, Stone KL, et al. Circadian activity rhythms and risk of incident dementia and mild cognitive impairment in older women. Ann Neurol 2011;70(5):722–32.

43. Lim AS, Yu L, Costa MD, et al. Increased fragmentation of rest-activity patterns is associated with a characteristic pattern of cognitive impairment in older individuals. Sleep 2012;35(5):633–640B.

44. Blackwell T, Yaffe K, Laffan A, et al. Associations of objectively and subjectively measured sleep quality with subsequent cognitive decline in older community-dwelling men: the MrOS sleep study. Sleep 2014;37(4):655–63.

45. Diem SJ, Blackwell TL, Stone KL, et al. Measures of sleep-wake patterns and risk of mild cognitive impairment or dementia in older women. Am J Geriatr Psychiatry 2016;24(3):248–58.

46. Leng Y, Blackwell T, Cawthon PM, et al. Association of circadian abnormalities in older adults with an increased risk of developing Parkinson disease. JAMA Neurol 2020;77(10):1270–8.

47. Kang JE, Lim MM, Bateman RJ, et al. Amyloid-beta dynamics are regulated by orexin and the sleep-wake cycle. Science 2009;326(5955):1005–7.

48. Roh JH, Huang Y, Bero AW, et al. Disruption of the sleep-wake cycle and diurnal fluctuation of beta-amyloid in mice with Alzheimer's Disease pathology. Sci Transl Med 2013;4(150):1–10.

49. Holth JK, Fritschi SK, Wang C, et al. The sleep-wake cycle regulates brain interstitial fluid tau in mice and CSF tau in humans. Science 2019;363(6429):880–4.

50. Xie L, Kang H, Xu Q, et al. Sleep drives metabolite clearance from the adult brain. Science 2013;342(6156):373–7.

51. Li J, Somers VK, Lopez-Jimenez F, et al. Demographic characteristics associated with circadian rest-activity rhythm patterns: a cross-sectional study. Int J Behav Nutr Phys Act 2021;18(1):107.

52. Van Someren EJ. Actigraphic monitoring of sleep and circadian rhythms. Handb Clin Neurol 2011;98:55–63.

53. Oosterman JM, van Someren EJ, Vogels RL, et al. Fragmentation of the rest-activity rhythm correlates with age-related cognitive deficits. J Sleep Res 2009;18(1):129–35.

54. Wang JL, Lim AS, Chiang WY, et al. Suprachiasmatic neuron numbers and rest-activity circadian rhythms in older humans. Ann Neurol 2015;78(2):317–22.

55. Musiek ES, Bhimasani M, Zangrilli MA, et al. Circadian rest-activity pattern changes in aging and pre-clinical Alzheimer disease. JAMA Neurol 2018;75(5):582–90.

56. Li P, Gao L, Gaba A, et al. Circadian disturbances in Alzheimer's disease progression: a prospective observational cohort study of community-based older adults. Lancet Healthy Longev 2020;1(3):e96–105.

57. Satlin A, Volicer L, Stopa EG, et al. Circadian locomotor activity and core-body temperature rhythms in Alzheimer's disease. Neurobiol Aging 1995;16(5):765–71.

58. Harper DG, Volicer L, Stopa EG, et al. Disturbance of endogenous circadian rhythm in aging and Alzheimer disease. Am J Geriatr Psychiatry 2005;13(5):359–68.

59. Inouye SK, Marcantonio ER, Kosar CM, et al. The short-term and long-term relationship between delirium and cognitive trajectory in older

surgical patients. Alzheimers Dement 2016; 12(7):766–75.

60. Swaab DF, Fliers E, Partiman TS. The suprachiasmatic nucleus of the human brain in relation to sex, age and senile dementia. Brain Res 1985; 342:37–44.

61. Baloyannis SJ, Mavroudis I, Mitilineos D, et al. The hypothalamus in Alzheimer's disease: a golgi and electron microscope study. Am J Alzheimers Dis Other Demen 2015;30(5):478–87.

62. Joyce DS, Feigl B, Kerr G, et al. Melanopsin-mediated pupil function is impaired in Parkinson's disease. Sci Rep 2018;8(1):7796.

63. La Morgia C, Ross-Cisneros FN, Sadun AA, et al. Retinal ganglion cells and circadian rhythms in Alzheimer's disease, Parkinson's disease, and beyond. Front Neurol 2017;8:162.

64. Harper DG, Stopa EG, McKee AC, et al. Differential circadian rhythm disturbances in men with Alzheimer disease and frontotemporal degeneration. Arch Gen Psychiatry 2001;58(4):353–60.

65. Gao L, Liu Y, Li X, et al. Abnormal retinal nerve fiber layer thickness and macula lutea in patients with mild cognitive impairment and Alzheimer's disease. Arch Gerontol Geriatr 2015;60(1):162–7.

66. Coppola G, Di Renzo A, Ziccardi L, et al. Optical coherence tomography in Alzheimer's disease: a meta-analysis. PLoS one 2015;10(8):e0134750.

67. La Morgia C, Ross-Cisneros FN, Koronyo Y, et al. Melanopsin retinal ganglion cell loss in Alzheimer disease. Ann Neurol 2016;79(1):90–109.

68. Chahine LM, Amara AW, Videnovic A. A systematic review of the literature on disorders of sleep and wakefulness in Parkinson's disease from 2005 to 2015. Sleep Med Rev 2016;35:33–50. epub ahead of print.

69. Gros P, Videnovic A. Overview of sleep and circadian rhythm disorders in Parkinson disease. Clin Geriatr Med 2020;36(1):119–30.

70. Videnovic A, Noble C, Reid KJ, et al. Circadian melatonin rhythm and excessive daytime sleepiness in Parkinson disease. JAMA Neurol 2014; 71(4):463–9.

71. Bordet R, Devos D, Brique S, et al. Study of circadian melatonin secretion pattern at different stages of Parkinson's disease. Clin Neuropharmacol 2003; 26(2):65–72.

72. Walsh CM, Ruoff L, Varbel J, et al. Rest-activity rhythm disruption in progressive supranuclear palsy. Sleep Med 2016;22:50–6.

73. Aziz NA, Pijl H, Frolich M, et al. Delayed onset of the diurnal melatonin rise in patients with Huntington's disease. J Neurol 2009;256(12):1961–5.

74. Morton AJ, Rudiger SR, Wood NI, et al. Early and progressive circadian abnormalities in Huntington's disease sheep are unmasked by social environment. Hum Mol Genet 2014;23(13):3375–83.

75. van Wamelen DJ, Aziz NA, Anink JJ, et al. Suprachiasmatic nucleus neuropeptide expression in patients with Huntington's Disease. Sleep 2013;36(1): 117–25.

76. Czeisler CA, Allan JS, Strogatz SH, et al. Bright light resets the human circadian pacemaker independent of the timing of the sleep-wake cycle. Science 1986;233:667–71.

77. Duffy JF, Zeitzer JM, Czeisler CA. Decreased sensitivity to phase-delaying effects of moderate intensity light in older subjects. Neurobiol Aging 2007;28:799–807.

78. Kim SJ, Benloucif S, Reid KJ, et al. Phase-shifting response to light in older adults. J Physiol 2014; 592(Pt 1):189–202.

79. Benloucif S, Green K, L'Hermite-Baleriaux M, et al. Responsiveness of the aging circadian clock to light. Neurobiol Aging 2006;27(12):1870–9.

80. Klerman EB, Duffy JF, Dijk DJ, et al. Circadian phase resetting in older people by ocular bright light exposure. J Investig Med 2001;49:30–40.

81. Khalsa SBS, Jewett ME, Cajochen C, et al. A phase response curve to single bright light pulses in human subjects. J Physiol 2003;549(Pt 3):945–52.

82. Chang AM, Santhi N, St Hilaire M, et al. Human responses to bright light of different durations. J Physiol 2012;590(Pt 13):3103–12.

83. Dewan K, Benloucif S, Reid K, et al. Light-induced changes of the circadian clock of humans: increasing duration is more effective than increasing light intensity. Sleep 2011;34(5):593–9.

84. Najjar RP, Zeitzer JM. Temporal integration of light flashes by the human circadian system. J Clin Invest 2016;126(3):938–47.

85. Herljevic M, Middleton B, Thapan K, et al. Light-induced melatonin suppression: age-related reduction in response to short wavelength light. Exp Gerontol 2005;40(3):237–42.

86. Sletten TL, Revell VL, Middleton B, et al. Age-related changes in acute and phase-advancing responses to monochromatic light. J Biol Rhythms 2009;24(1):73–84.

87. Kessel L, Siganos G, Jorgensen T, et al. Sleep disturbances are related to decreased transmission of blue light to the retina caused by lens yellowing. Sleep 2011;34(9):1215–9.

88. Campbell SS, Dawson D, Anderson MW. Alleviation of sleep maintenance insomnia with timed exposure to bright light. J Am Geriatr Soc 1993;41: 829–36.

89. Suhner AG, Murphy PJ, Campbell SS. Failure of timed bright light exposure to alleviate age-related sleep maintenance insomnia. J Am Geriatr Soc 2002;50:617–23.

90. Pallesen S, Nordhus IH, Skelton SH, et al. Bright light treatment has limited effect in subjects over

55 years with mild early morning awakening. Percept Mot Skills 2005;101(3):759–70.

91. Auger RR, Burgess HJ, Emens JS, et al. Clinical practice guideline for the treatment of intrinsic circadian rhythm sleep-wake disorders: advanced sleep-wake phase disorder (ASWPD), delayed sleep-wake phase disorder (DSWPD), non-24-hour sleep-wake rhythm disorder (N24SWD), and irregular sleep-wake rhythm disorder (ISWRD). An update for 2015: an American Academy of sleep medicine clinical practice guideline. J Clin Sleep Med 2015;11(10):1199–236.

92. Pollak CP, Perlick D. Sleep problems and institutionalization of the elderly. J Geriatr Psychiatry Neurol 1991;4:204–10.

93. Pollak CP, Perlick D, Linsner JP, et al. Sleep problems in the community elderly as predictors of death and nursing home placement. J Community Health 1990;15(2):123–35.

94. Mishima K, Okawa M, Hishikaa Y, et al. Morning bright light therapy for sleep and behaviour disorders in elderly patients with dementia. Acta Psychiatr Scand 1994;89:1–7.

95. Satlin A, Volicer L, Ross V, et al. Bright light treatment of behavioral and sleep disturbances in patients with Alzheimer's disease. Am J Psychiatry 1992;149:1028–32.

96. Figueiro MG, Plitnick B, Roohan C, et al. Effects of a tailored lighting intervention on sleep quality, rest-activity, mood, and behavior in older adults with Alzheimer disease and related dementias: a randomized clinical trial. J Clin Sleep Med 2019;15(12):1757–67.

97. Endo T, Matsumura R, Tokuda IT, et al. Bright light improves sleep in patients with Parkinson's disease: possible role of circadian restoration. Sci Rep 2020;10(1):7982.

98. Dowling GA, Burr RL, Van Someren EJ, et al. Melatonin and bright-light treatment for rest-activity disruption in institutionalized patients with Alzheimer's disease. J Am Geriatr Soc 2008;56(2):239–46.

99. Riemersma-van der Lek RF, Swaab DF, Twisk J, et al. Effect of bright light and melatonin on cognitive and noncognitive function in elderly residents of group care facilities: a randomized controlled trial. JAMA 2008;299(22):2642–55.

100. Figueiro MG, Plitnick BA, Lok A, et al. Tailored lighting intervention improves measures of sleep, depression, and agitation in persons with Alzheimer's disease and related dementia living in long-term care facilities. Clin Interv Aging 2014;9:1527–37.

101. Alessi CA, Martin JL, Webber AP, et al. Randomized, controlled trial of a nonpharmacological intervention to improve abnormal sleep/wake patterns in nursing home residents. J Am Geriatr Soc 2005;53(5):803–10.

102. Clendon J, Walker L. Nurses aged over 50 years and their experiences of shift work. J Nurs Manag 2013;21(7):903–13.

103. Richter K, Acker J, Adam S, et al. Prevention of fatigue and insomnia in shift workers-a review of nonpharmacological measures. EPMA J 2016;7:16.

104. Crowley SJ, Lee C, Tseng CY, et al. Combinations of bright light, scheduled dark, sunglasses, and melatonin to facilitate circadian entrainment to night shift work. J Biol Rhythms 2003;18(6):513–23.

105. Walsh JK, Muehlbach MJ, Schweitzer PK. Hypnotics and caffeine as countermeasures for shiftwork-related sleepiness and sleep disturbance. J Sleep Res 1995;4(Suppl. 2):80–3.

106. Chinoy ED, Harris MP, Kim MJ, et al. Scheduled evening sleep and enhanced lighting improve adaptation to night shift work in older adults. Occup Environ Med 2016;73(12):869–76.

107. Isherwood CM, Chinoy ED, Murphy AS, et al. Scheduled afternoon-evening sleep leads to better night shift performance in older adults. Occup Environ Med 2020;77(3):179–84.

108. St Hilaire MA, Lammers-van der Holst HM, Chinoy ED, et al. Prediction of individual differences in circadian adaptation to night work among older adults: application of a mathematical model using individual sleep-wake and light exposure data. Chronobiol Int 2020;37(9–10):1404–11.

109. Karoly L, Panis C. Shifting demographic patterns shaping the future workforce. The 21st century at work: forces shaping the future workforce and workplace in the United States. Santa Monica (CA): RAND Corporation; 2004.

110. Fung CH, Vitiello MV, Alessi CA, et al. Report and research agenda of the American geriatrics society and national institute on aging bedside-to-bench conference on sleep, circadian rhythms, and aging: new avenues for improving brain health, physical health, and functioning. J Am Geriatr Soc 2016;64(12):e238–47.

Sleep Deprivation and Circadian Disruption Stress, Allostasis, and Allostatic Load

Bruce S. McEwen, PhD[a], Ilia N. Karatsoreos, PhD[b],*

KEYWORDS

- Sleep deprivation • Hippocampus • Allostasis • Allostatic load • Glycogen • Oxidative stress
- Proinflammatory cytokines • Circadian disruption

KEY POINTS

- Allostatic load/overload refers to the cumulative wear and tear on body systems caused by too much stress and/or inefficient management of the systems that promote adaptation through allostasis.
- Circadian disruption is a broad problem that alters allostasis and elevates allostatic load, affecting brain and body systems. Sleep deprivation is an all-too-common example of a process that includes circadian disruption.
- Even a few days of sleep deprivation or circadian misalignment in young healthy volunteers have been reported to increase appetite and calorie intake, increase levels of proinflammatory cytokines, decrease parasympathetic and increase sympathetic tone, increase blood pressure, increase evening cortisol levels, as well as elevate insulin and blood glucose levels.
- Chronic circadian disruption and reduced sleep time are associated with elevated cortisol levels, increased obesity, and reduced volume of the temporal lobe.
- Mood disorders involve disrupted circadian rhythmicity and altered sleep-wake patterns; yet, acute sleep deprivation can have rapid antidepressant effects and manipulating the timing of the secretion or exogenous administration of melatonin can be beneficial in mood disorders.
- Repeated stress in animal models causes brain regions involved in memory and emotions, such as hippocampus, amygdala, and prefrontal cortex, to undergo structural remodeling with the result that memory is impaired and anxiety and aggression are increased. Structural and functional MRI studies in depression and Cushing disease, as well as anxiety disorders and in air crews with jet lag, provide evidence that the human brain may be similarly affected.
- Brain regions such as the hippocampus are sensitive to glucose and insulin, and both type I and type II diabetes are associated with cognitive impairment and (for type II diabetes) an increased risk for Alzheimer disease. Insofar as poor sleep and circadian disruption also exacerbate metabolic dysregulation and contribute to other aspects of physiologic dysregulation, they must be considered contributors to risk for dementia.
- Animal models of chronic sleep deprivation indicate that memory is impaired along with depletion of glycogen stores and increases in oxidative stress and free radical production.

This article previously appeared in *Sleep Med Clin* 10 (2015) 1–10.
[a] Harold and Margaret Milliken Hatch Laboratory of Neuroendocrinology, The Rockefeller University, 1230 York Avenue, New York, NY 10065, USA; [b] Department of Psychological and Brain Sciences, Neuroscience and Behavior Program, University of Massachusetts Amherst, Tobin Hall, 135 Hicks Way, Amherst, MA 01003, USA
* Corresponding author.
E-mail address: ikaratsoreos@umass.edu

Sleep Med Clin 17 (2022) 253–262
https://doi.org/10.1016/j.jsmc.2022.03.005

INTRODUCTION

Anecdotally, there can be little doubt that sleep plays a role in maintaining a good mood and cognitive acuity. Sleep deprivation one night followed by "getting a good night's sleep" on the next clearly impacts neurobehavioral function as well as promotes physiologic balance and resilience. These subjective impressions are supported by numerous laboratory studies of endocrine function and metabolism as well as by investigations of sleep deprivation effects on cognitive and neural function, including research on the brain that shows a variety of substantial changes resulting from sleep restriction, with reversal after recovery sleep. Similarly, being "out of phase" with local time, be it from a week of night shift work following a week of day shift work or transmeridian air travel across multiple time zones, demonstrates that there are both neural and physiologic effects of internal circadian (daily) time being misaligned with external environmental time. This article reviews selected aspects of the current state of knowledge in these areas and then evaluates what is known using the model of allostasis and allostatic load that emphasizes the "wear and tear" on the brain and body from coping with stress.

ALLOSTASIS AND ALLOSTATIC OVERLOAD

The maintenance of homeostasis, defined as those aspects of physiology that must remain stable to keep us alive (eg, oxygen tension, body temperature, pH), is an active process requiring coordinated action of many different systems, including the autonomic nervous system and neuroendocrine and immune systems. This active process is called "allostasis" or "maintaining stability through change."[1–3] Allostatic mediators work as a nonlinear, sometimes reciprocating, network (Fig. 1), meaning that too much or too little of each mediator can perturb the entire network, leading to harmful consequences. Take for example the relationship between cytokines and the glucocorticoids. Proinflammatory cytokines stimulate the production of cortisol, which then suppresses inflammatory cytokine production.[4,5] Similarly, increased activity of the sympathetic nervous system increases proinflammatory cytokine production, whereas parasympathetic activity has the opposite effect.[6,7] This balance is particularly important, because during an infection, the proinflammatory response that is essential to mounting an immune defense is normally contained by cortisol and also by parasympathetic activity.[4,6] Inadequate containment can lead to

septic shock and death. Treatment with cortisol, or elevation of parasympathetic activity, is a pathway that can reduce the exaggerated inflammatory response.[4] However, at the opposite extreme, too much cortisol can suppress proinflammatory responses, thus compromising immune defenses.[4,8]

Allostatic overload, which is wear and tear produced by imbalances in the mediators of allostasis, is perfectly illustrated by these 2 examples: too much or too little activity of certain mediators of allostasis.[9] Other examples of allostatic overload include conditions such as hypertension, atherosclerosis, diabetes, and the metabolic syndrome as well as stress-induced remodeling in brain regions that support memory, executive function, and anxiety.[3,10] One of the key mediators of allostasis is cortisol (corticosterone in rodent species), and conditions in which corticosteroid balance is affected lead to many such changes in physiologic function and brain structure. Cushing disease and anxiety/depressive disorders are 2 such conditions that affect multiple allostatic mediators, including the corticosteroids.

Cushing disease, broadly defined as hypercortisolemia induced by organic (eg, pituitary or adrenal tumor) or iatrogenic (eg, high doses of corticosteroids to reduce inflammation) factors, is accompanied by several cognitive and emotional symptoms, including depression. Intriguingly, depressive symptoms can be relieved by surgical correction of hypercortisolemia.[11] In major depressive illness as well as in Cushing disease, the duration of the illness and not the age of the subject predicts a progressive reduction in hippocampal volume and is observed by structural MRI.[12] Moreover, there are a variety of other anxiety-related disorders, such as posttraumatic stress disorder (PTSD), in which atrophy of the hippocampus has been reported,[13,14] suggesting that this is a common process reflecting chronic imbalance in the activity of adaptive systems. These chronic imbalances include the hypothalamic-pituitary-adrenal (HPA) axis, and also endogenous neurotransmitters, such as glutamate.[12] Metabolic symptoms are also reported in both Cushing and major depression, because both are associated with chronic elevation of cortisol that results in gradual loss of minerals from the bone, and increases in abdominal obesity.

CIRCADIAN DISRUPTION AND ALLOSTATIC LOAD AND OVERLOAD

When exploring how the brain and body are affected by stress, it is often overlooked that they may be directly regulated by the time of

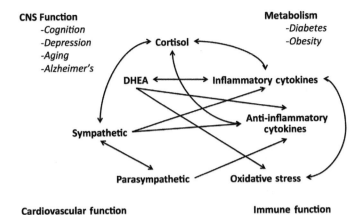

CNS Function
- *Cognition*
- *Depression*
- *Aging*
- *Alzheimer's*

Metabolism
- *Diabetes*
- *Obesity*

Cortisol

DHEA → Inflammatory cytokines

Anti-inflammatory cytokines

Sympathetic

Parasympathetic   Oxidative stress

Cardiovascular function
- *Endothelial cell damage*
- *Atherosclerosis*

Immune function
- *Enhancement*
- *Suppression*

Fig. 1. Nonlinear network of mediators of allostasis involved in the stress response. Arrows indicate that each system regulates the others in a reciprocal manner, creating a nonlinear network. Moreover, there are multiple pathways for regulation (eg, inflammatory cytokine production is negatively regulated via anti-inflammatory cytokines as well as via parasympathetic and glucocorticoid pathways), whereas sympathetic activity increases inflammatory cytokine production. Parasympathetic activity, in turn, contains sympathetic activity. CNS, central nervous system; DHEA, dehydroepiandrosterone. (*Adapted from* Karatsoreos IN, McEwen BS. Psychobiological allostasis: resistance, resilience and vulnerability. Trends Cogn Sci 2011;15:576-84; with permission.)

day. All the systems that are modulators of allostasis show rhythms of activity over the sleep-wake cycle. For instance, cortisol (corticosterone in rodents; CORT) shows a clear circadian pattern, with the peak of CORT occurring just before waking in both nocturnal animals (such as rats and mice) and diurnal animals (such as humans). Circadian rhythms are observed in almost all physiologic measures, including endocrine and immune mediators.[15–17] Many of these factors are also impacted by sleep deprivation, as is discussed later. The circadian system in mammals is centered in the suprachiasmatic nucleus (SCN), with both neural and hormonal projections throughout the brain and body, and impacts many of the systems involved in mediating allostasis; disruption of the circadian system can place the organism into a state of high allostatic load. Indeed, if circadian patterns of CORT are disrupted by adrenalectomy (ADX) and tonic replacement of CORT via a pellet implant providing no diurnal rhythm, a "sluggish" HPA axis response results, with poor shutoff of adrenocorticotropic hormone following termination of a stressor, in contrast to the situation in which the ADX animal drinks CORT in the water in a diurnal pattern.[18] That CORT is also able to reset peripheral oscillators in other body tissues lends credence to an important relationship between disrupted rhythms and allostatic load; this is important because circadian disruption (eg, shift work and jet lag) and sleep deprivation are not uncommon in the modern world and constitute an increasing health concern.[19,20]

The master circadian clock is located in the SCN of the hypothalamus and drives all rhythms in physiology and behavior.[21–23] In addition to the master SCN clock, "peripheral" circadian clocks, in tissues throughout the body, serve to set local time. These peripheral clocks are synchronized to the SCN by a multitude of signals, including glucocorticoids, which are able to "reset" some peripheral clocks in the brain and body (eg, liver), but not others.[24] In the brain, it has been shown that rhythms in glucocorticoids modulate clock protein expression in the oval nucleus of the bed nucleus of the stria terminalis as well as the central amygdala (CEA).[25] It is also known that the basolateral nuclei of the amygdala and the dentate gyrus of the hippocampus express opposite diurnal rhythms of PERIOD2 (a core clock component) when compared with the CEA and that the CEA rhythm is further influenced by ADX.[26] The differential regulation of cellular rhythms in different brain regions is of particular interest when considering that "healthy" regulation of HPA function requires rhythmic glucocorticoids, as discussed earlier.[18] It is posited that if efficient regulation of the HPA axis is a hallmark of a "healthy" response, then disrupted circadian patterns (or, in this case, a lack of a pattern) can result in an unhealthy regulation of the HPA and thus could contribute to allostatic load.[27] Thus, both disruption of the HPA axis and disruption of circadian rhythms could have interacting effects and contribute to shifts in resilience and vulnerability.

Both descriptive and epidemiologic studies show that individuals who suffer from repeated chronic circadian misalignment show negative physiologic, neural, and behavioral effects. In humans, a study of flight crews showed that those who endure more bouts of jet lag (transmeridian, short-recovery crews) show shrunken medial temporal lobes, increased reaction time, and poorer performance in visual-spatial cognitive tasks compared with long recovery crews. In addition to the neurobehavioral effects, short-recovery individuals displayed a significant correlation between salivary cortisol levels and medial temporal cortex volume, whereas this effect was not observed in long-recovery crews. Thus, rapid and repeated shifting of the circadian clock through jet lag is related to reductions in volume of the medial temporal lobe and shifts in behavioral performance on attentional tasks. Moreover, the brain effects are correlated with plasma cortisol levels. What is the significance of these neural and physiologic changes? It is intriguing to speculate that perhaps such shrunken temporal lobes may impart decreased resilience to negative outcomes of stress, as has been observed in PTSD.[28,29] In addition, sleep deprivation seems to increase the amygdalar response to negative emotional stimuli because of an amygdala-prefrontal disconnect.[30] Such effects could also exacerbate cardiovascular reactivity, which may contribute to pathophysiology.[31–33] Sleep deprivation studies have investigated the effects of chronic deprivation on cognitive performance, in both animal and human subjects, but in many cases, the stressful effects of the methods used to induce sleep deprivation confound these studies. Thus, a different approach must be applied to help disentangle these effects.

To directly probe how disruption of the circadian clock affects neurobehavioral function, new models need to be applied and new hypotheses need to be tested. Karatsoreos and coworkers[34] characterized a mouse model of chronic environmental circadian desynchronization (eCD) that has provided several novel insights. This model induces disruption by housing mice in a light-dark cycle of 20 hours (10 hours light, 10 hours dark) compared with laboratory standard 24-hour cycles. After only 5 weeks of this environmental disruption, eCD mice begin showing metabolic signs of allostatic load, including increased weight, adiposity, and leptin levels. A significant effect is also observed in glucose metabolism, because eCD mice also show an imbalance between insulin and plasma glucose, suggesting development of a prediabetic state. Strikingly, the observed metabolic changes are accompanied by changes in prefrontal cortex cellular morphology, mirroring those observed in chronic stress. eCD animals show shrunken and less complex apical dendritic trees of cells in layer II/III of the medial prefrontal cortex,[34] with no apparent effects on basal dendrites. eCD animals further show behavioral abnormalities, with marked cognitive rigidity in a modified Morris water maze. Specifically, eCD mice demonstrate normal performance on the learning phase of the initial task, but are slower to adapt to the hidden platform being moved to a novel location. These changes were mostly due to the mice making more perseverative errors by returning to the original location of the platform.[34] In addition to the cognitive flexibility problems, eCD mice display what may be considered an "impulsive"-like phenotype in the light-dark box, while not showing any overt anxietylike phenotype.[34] Taken in a wider context, these effects of eCD are remarkably similar to those observed in 21 days of chronic restraint stress in rodents, which results in morphologic simplification of prefrontal cortical neurons and impairment in prefrontal-mediated behaviors, such as attentional set-shifting or other working memory tasks.[35–37] When discussing such models of eCD, it is important to note that, just as total hippocampal lesions provided insight into the role of this brain structure in learning and memory, circadian models are purposefully "exotic" (ie, shortened 20-hour days are not expected to become a common occurrence in human society). These models should provide important proof-of-principle concepts that should set the stage for more ecologically relevant and more refined models to be developed.

The specific mechanisms by which disrupted circadian clocks cause changes in brain, behavior, and peripheral physiology remain unknown. One hypothesis is that disrupted light-dark cycles lead to a gradual loss of cohesion between circadian clocks in the brain (eg, the SCN) and those in the body (eg, liver). This loss of cohesion results in central and peripheral oscillators eventually becoming out of phase with each other, creating internal desynchrony. In the brain, this could lead to changes in synchrony between various nodes of a neural circuit (eg, the prefrontal cortex and amygdala drifting out of phase). Over many cycles, such loss of cohesion could lead to changes in neurobehavioral function (as evidenced in Ref.[34]). In addition to long-term, chronic circadian disruption, shorter durations of circadian disruption could lead to changes in these circuits that make them more vulnerable to further insult and could be a more insidious mechanism of circuit level disruption, setting the stage for other stressors (eg, metabolic stress, immune stress) to overwhelm an already compromised network. Extending this model to the periphery, disruption of peripheral body clocks could lead to changes in the way the stress system responds to environmental or psychological stressors. Together, this model illustrates how circadian disruption could lead to neural circuits becoming more vulnerable to insult as well as pathways by which disruption could compromise allostatic responses engaged to help an organism adapt to environmental challenge. In this schema, circadian disruption effects may be similar to the diathesis-stress models, which could explain many of the epidemiologic findings of increased risk for development of psychiatric, cardiovascular, or other physiologic syndromes in populations undergoing chronic circadian disruption , such as shift workers.[20,38–40]

METABOLIC AND HORMONAL RESPONSES TO SLEEP DEPRIVATION AND CIRCADIAN DISRUPTION

Sleep deprivation produces an allostatic overload that can have deleterious consequences. Increases in blood pressure, decreases in parasympathetic tone, and increases in evening cortisol are all observed after only 4 hours of sleep deprivation. Metabolic effects of this short-duration deprivation also include increased insulin levels and increased appetite, possibly through the elevation of ghrelin, a proappetitive hormone, and decreased levels of leptin.[41–43] These short-term effects of sleep deprivation are significant when one considers epidemiologic evidence showing that reduced sleep duration is associated with increased body mass and obesity in the National Health and Nutrition Examination Survey (NHANES) study.[44] However, these relationships are by no means simple. For instance, in adolescents, sleep reduction is associated with measurable changes in insulin sensitivity,[45] whereas durations of sleep longer than average are not associated with such changes. Similarly, a study by St-Onge and colleagues[46] in adults suggests that short-term sleep deprivation is not the cause of altered insulin sensitivity per se, but instead may contribute to overeating, potentially via different mechanisms in men and women. An important study by Vetrivelan and colleagues[47] showed that chronic partial sleep loss in a rat model of spontaneous short sleep did not lead to changes in metabolism, with the investigators suggesting that observed effects on metabolism in sleep deprivation studies may instead be due to other factors, such as circadian disruption , changes in diet, or reduced activity levels. This work is clearly supported by the earlier eCD work of Karatsoreos and McEwen,[27] in which mice that were circadian disrupted, but not explicitly sleep deprived, gained weight and had altered levels of plasma insulin and leptin.

Sleep deprivation also has marked effects on other circulating messengers, in addition to metabolic effects. Specifically, immune mediators are also altered following sleep deprivation. Proinflammatory cytokine levels are increased, along with deterioration in performance as measured by tests of psychomotor vigilance, and this has been reported to result from a modest sleep restriction to 6 hours per night.[48] In humans, poor sleep and

sleep deprivation in aging women have been associated with elevated levels of interleukin (IL)-6.[49] Indeed, recent work has demonstrated that eCD can lead to significant changes in immune challenges while not dramatically altering basal inflammatory tone.[50,51] Thus, clear links exist between sleep deprivation, circadian disruption , and neurobehavioral, metabolic, and immune function.

SLEEP DEPRIVATION AND CIRCADIAN DISRUPTION IN MOOD DISORDERS

There is wide agreement that psychiatric illness, including depression, involves disruption in rhythms of body temperature, mood, and sleep.[52,53] Moreover, acute sleep deprivation is effective in 40% to 60% of depressed subjects in improving mood within 24 to 48 hours, in contrast to antidepressant medications that typically require 2 to 8 weeks to have an effect.[54,55] New research also indicates that sleep deprivation in patients with major depressive disorder can lead to clear plasticity in the cortex.[56] The mechanisms underlying the mood-improving effects of this sudden acute circadian "shock" are as yet unknown, but suggest that directly manipulating the sleep-circadian system may be a pathway to explore. Along these lines, light (photic) therapy is another form of circadian manipulation that is effective in some depressed patients, and there are pharmaceutical agents for mood disorders, such as agomelatine, that interact with the melatonin system[57] as well as the use of melatonin itself for circadian phase shifting in seasonal affective disorder.[52]

Gross circadian disruption, as measured by changes in sleep activity cycles, are not the only rhythms that are perturbed in mood disorders. Psychotic major depression involves elevated evening cortisol levels, whereas the nonpsychotic form does not,[58] and elevated evening cortisol as well as circadian disruption are linked to metabolic syndrome.[59] Moreover, glucocorticoids are able to reset and synchronize the circadian clocks of peripheral tissues, including the liver, although the central pacemaker clock of the SCN does not respond to glucocorticoid.[24] Because almost every cell in the body expresses clock genes and glucocorticoid receptors are ubiquitous, the effects of circadian disruption can be profound: for example, in hamsters living in a light-dark cycle 2 hours different from the period of their normal clock, cardiac hypertrophy and renal failure are observed.[60]

NEURAL RESPONSES TO SLEEP DEPRIVATION

The brain is the master regulator of the neuroendocrine, autonomic, and immune systems. It is important to remember that it is also the master regulator of behaviors that contribute to unhealthy or healthy lifestyles, which, in turn, influence the physiologic processes of allostasis.[3] Therefore, chronic stress can have direct and indirect effects on cumulative allostatic overload. There are many disparate changes driven by allostatic overload resulting from chronic stress. In animal models, chronic stress causes atrophy of neurons in the prefrontal cortex and hippocampus, brain regions involved in executive function, selective attention, and memory. On the other hand, chronic stress leads to hypertrophy of neurons in the amygdala, a region involved in fear, anxiety, and aggression.[61] Thus, chronic stress compromises the ability of an organism to learn, remember, and make decisions, as well as increases the levels of anxiety and aggression.

Although not as much work has been conducted, it is obvious that the results of sleep deprivation, and perhaps to a lesser extent circadian disruption, share certain characteristics with chronic stress. For instance, there is recent evidence not only for cognitive impairment resulting from sleep restriction in animal models but also for altered levels of cytokines, oxidative stress markers, glycogen levels, and structural changes in the form of reduced dentate gyrus neurogenesis. Specifically, increases in brain levels of mRNA of the proinflammatory cytokine IL-1b are reported following sleep deprivation by gentle handling and is reported to be higher in daytime (during the normal sleep period in rodents) than in darkness (during the normal activity time for rodents).[62] Closely related to inflammatory processes, through the actions of NADPH oxidase,[63,64] is oxidative stress involving the generation of free radicals. Seventy-two hours of "flower pot" or platform sleep deprivation has been reported to increase oxidative stress in the mouse hippocampus, as measured by increased lipid peroxidation and increased ratios of oxidized to reduced glutathione.[65] Glycogen, found predominantly in white matter, is also profoundly affected by sleep deprivation and is reported to decrease by as much as 40% in rats deprived of sleep for 24 hours by novelty and gentle handling, an effect reversed by recovery sleep.[66,67] The specific consequences of this effect are not yet elucidated, although it is noteworthy that glycogen in astrocytes is able to sustain axon function during glucose deprivation in central nervous system white matter.[68]

With respect to memory and cognitive performance, there are numerous reports of impairments following sleep deprivation. For example, sleep deprivation by the platform (or flower pot)

method leads to impaired performance of spatial memory in the Morris water maze[69] and reduced CA1 hippocampal long-term potentiation (LTP).[70] Sleep deprivation using these methods also impairs retention of passive avoidance memory, a context-dependent fear-memory task.[65] A different method of sleep deprivation, by gentle stimulation or novelty, following contextual fear conditioning impairs memory consolidation.[71] A 6-hour period of total sleep deprivation by novelty exposure impaired acquisition of a spatial task in the Morris water maze.[72] A 4-hour period of sleep deprivation by gentle stimulation impaired the late-phase LTP in the dentate gyrus 48 hours later but had the opposite effect to enhance late-phase LTP in the prefrontal cortex.[73] Some of these effects might be related to changes in beta-adrenergic activity, at least in the hippocampus.[74] There is also good evidence suggesting that sleep deprivation can affect heterosynaptic metaplasticity in mouse hippocampal slices,[75] although new work also suggests that epigenetic modifications might play a critical role in synaptic plasticity following sleep deprivation.[76] Emotional behaviors are also affected by sleep deprivation. Increases in fighting behavior are observed following rapid eye movement sleep deprivation[77]; there is also a report of increased aggression in the form of phencyclidine-induced muricide after sleep deprivation.[78,79] These findings harken to the results of increased aggression among cage mates in rats subjected to 21 days of 6 hours per day of chronic restraint stress during the resting period when some sleep deprivation may occur.[80] Thus, the effects of sleep deprivation are not simple and are influenced by their type, intensity, and duration and the types of behavioral outcomes measured.

The neural mechanisms of the effects of sleep deprivation on behavior are still not understood. However, sleep deprivation in rats using a treadmill for 96 hours has been reported to decrease proliferation of cells in the dentate gyrus of the hippocampal formation by as much as 50%.[81] In addition, there are significant changes in other measures of synaptic plasticity in these models, including changes in LTP.[82] A confound in this type of experiment is that the effects of activity are difficult to disentangle from the effects of the deprivation. A similar neural effect has also been reported by keeping rats in a slowly rotating drum, but, here again, there is a question of how much physical activity and physical stress may have contributed to the suppression of cell proliferation.[83] Nevertheless, sleep restriction by novelty exposure, a more subtle method, prevented the increased survival of new dentate gyrus neurons promoted by spatial training in a Morris water maze.[84] Recently, clear effects of sleep and sleep deprivation on hippocampal function have been demonstrated, showing that hippocampal network activity changes during sleep-dependent memory consolidation, and that sleep deprivation can affect hippocampal synaptic plasticity during defined time frames.[85,86] Work in the visual cortex also shows that sleep affects memory consolidation,[87–89] suggesting these effects are not merely limited to the hippocampus. As always, untangling the contributions of sleep loss from the effects of misalignment of circadian patterns of sleep with the environmental light-dark cycle remains a critical question that should be assessed in both basic research and in the clinic.

INTEGRATION AND SUMMARY

Sleep is thought to be a neural state during which consolidation of declarative memories takes place.[90] Sleep deprivation, even for the course of the active period of the day in diurnal animals, increases the homeostatic drive to sleep, with resulting changes in proinflammatory cytokines and glycogen levels. Relatively brief deprivation of sleep promotes an exacerbation of these processes with progressively more severe physiologic, neurobiological, and behavioral consequences as the sleep deprivation is prolonged.

Circadian disruption is a broader aspect of the problem of sleep disruption, with disruption of the circadian clock contributing to changes in sleep patterns and sleep patterns potentially influencing the circadian clock. Shift work and jet lag are 2 common practices that have measurable effects on the brain and body.[91,92] For instance, long-distance air travel with short turnaround has been reported to be associated with smaller volume of the temporal lobe and impaired performance on a visual-spatial cognitive task.[93]

The long-term consequences of sleep deprivation and circadian disruption constitute a form of allostatic load, with consequences involving hypertension, reduced parasympathetic tone, increased proinflammatory cytokines, increased oxidative stress, and increased evening cortisol and insulin. As noted earlier, reduced sleep and circadian disruption are associated with increased chances of cardiovascular disease and diabetes. Indeed, shorter sleep times have been associated with increased obesity.[44] Moreover, diabetes is associated with impaired hippocampal function,[94] decreased hippocampal volume,[95] and increased risk for Alzheimer disease.[96,97]

In addition to the inflammatory and cardiometabolic changes that are observed, depressive illness is almost universally associated with disturbed sleep.[98] Thus, there are not only linkages between the multiple interacting mediators that are involved in allostasis and allostatic load/overload, as summarized in **Fig. 1**, but also overlaps (ie, comorbidities) between disorders, such as diabetes, hypertension, cardiovascular disease, and depression, that are associated with excessive stress and with the dysregulation of the systems that normally promote allostasis and successful adaptation.

Sleep has important functions in maintaining homeostasis and sleep deprivation. Sleep deprivation or other forms of circadian desynchronization and disruption are stressors that have consequences for the brain as well as many body systems. Whether the sleep deprivation or circadian disruption is due to anxiety, depression, jet lag, shift work, or other aspects of a hectic lifestyle, there are consequences that contribute to allostatic load throughout the body. Taken together, these changes in the brain and body are further evidence that circadian disruption predisposes an individual to altered responses to stressors as well as impaired cognitive function and metabolic dysregulation. Sleep deprivation can be described as a chronic stressor that can cause allostatic overload, including mood and cognitive impairment and autonomic and metabolic dysregulation.

ACKNOWLEDGMENTS

Dr B.S. McEwen sadly passed away in January, 2020, and is posthumously included in this article because he was a trailblazer and thought leader in understanding brain-body interactions in the context of stress and allostasis, who was equally invested in integrating sleep and circadian rhythms into the broader models of adaptive homeostasis. He was a dear mentor to Dr I.N. Karatsoreos who he encouraged to work at the interface of stress, allostatic load, circadian rhythms, sleep, and health.

DISCLOSURE

The authors have nothing to disclose.

REFERENCES

1. Sterling P, Eyer J. Allostasis: a new paradigm to explain arousal pathology. In: Fisher S, Reason J, editors. Handbook of life stress, cognition and health. New York: John Wiley & Sons; 1988. p. 629–49.
2. McEwen BS, Stellar E. Stress and the individual: mechanisms leading to disease. Arch Intern Med 1993;153:2093–101.

3. McEwen BS. Protective and damaging effects of stress mediators. N Engl J Med 1998;338:171–9.

4. Munck A, Guyre PM. Glucocorticoids and immune function. In: Ader R, Felten DL, Cohen N, editors. Psychoneuroimmunology. San Diego (CA): Academic Press; 1991. p. 447–74.

5. Sapolsky RM. Physiological and pathophysiological implications of social stress in mammals. Coping with the environment: neural and endocrine mechanisms. New York: Oxford University Press; 2000. p. 517–32.

6. Borovikova LV, Ivanova S, Zhang M, et al. Vagus nerve stimulation attenuates the systemic inflammatory response to endotoxin. Nature 2000;405:458–62.

7. Bierhaus A, Wolf J, Andrassy M, et al. A mechanism converting psychosocial stress into mononuclear cell activation. Proc Natl Acad Sci U S A 2003;100: 1920–5.

8. Sapolsky RM, Romero LM, Munck AU. How do glucocorticoids influence stress responses? Integrating permissive, suppressive, stimulatory, and preparative actions. Endocr Rev 2000;21:55–89.

9. McEwen BS, Wingfield JC. The concept of allostasis in biology and biomedicine. Horm Behav 2003;43: 2–15.

10. McEwen BS. Structural plasticity of the adult brain: how animal models help us understand brain changes in depression and systemic disorders related to depression. Dialogues Clin Neurosci 2004;6:119–33.

11. McEwen BS. Mood disorders and allostatic load. Biol Psychiatry 2003;54:200–7.

12. Sheline YI. Neuroimaging studies of mood disorder effects on the brain. Biol Psychiatry 2003;54:338–52.

13. Pitman RK. Hippocampal diminution in PTSD: more (or less?) than meets the eye. Hippocampus 2001; 11:73–4.

14. Bremner JD. Neuroimaging studies in posttraumatic stress disorder. Curr Psychiatry Rep 2002;4:254–63.

15. Butler MP, Kriegsfeld LJ, Silver R. Circadian regulation of endocrine functions. In: Pfaff D, Arnold A, Etgen A, et al, editors. Hormones, brain and behavior. 2nd edition. San Diego (CA): Academic Press; 2009. p. 473–505.

16. Cearley C, Churchill L, Krueger JM. Time of day differences in ILIbeta and TNFalpha mRNA levels in specific regions of the rat brain. Neurosci Lett 2003;352:61–3.

17. Lange T, Dimitrov S, Born J. Effects of sleep and circadian rhythm on the human immune system. Ann N Yacad Sci 2010;1193:48–59.

18. Jacobson L, Akana SF, Cascio CS, et al. Circadian variations in plasma corticosterone permit normal termination of adrenocorticotropin responses to stress. Endocrinology 1988;122:1343–8.

19. Boivin DB, Tremblay GM, James FO. Working on atypical schedules. Sleep Med 2007;8:578–89.

20. Knutsson A. Health disorders of shift workers. Occup Med (Lond) 2003;53:103–8.

21. Moore-Ede MC. Physiology of the circadian timing system: predictive versus reactive homeostasis. Am J Phys 1986;250:R735–52.

22. Moore RY, Eichler VB. Loss of a circadian adrenal corticosterone rhythm following suprachiasmatic lesions in the rat. Brain Res 1972;42:201–6.

23. Klein DC, Moore RY, Reppert SM. Suprachiasmatic nucleus: the mind's clock. New York: Oxford University Press; 1991.

24. Balsalobre A, Brown SA, Marcacci L, et al. Resetting of circadian time in peripheral tissues by glucocorticoid signaling. Science 2000;289:2344–7.

25. Segall LA, Perrin JS, Walker CD, et al. Glucocorticoid rhythms control the rhythm of expression of the clock protein, Period2, in oval nucleus of the bed nucleus of the stria terminalis and central nucleus of the amygdala in rats. Neuroscience 2006; 140:753–7.

26. Lamont EW, Robinson B, Stewart J, et al. The central and basolateral nuclei of the amygdala exhibit opposite diurnal rhythms of expression of the clock protein Period2. Proc Natl Acad Sci U S A 2005; 102:4180–4.

27. Karatsoreos IN, McEwen BS. Psychobiological allostasis: resistance, resilience and vulnerability. Trends Cogn Sci 2011;15:576–84.

28. Gilbertson MW, Paulus LA, Williston SK, et al. Neurocognitive function in monozygotic twins discordant for combat exposure: relationship to posttraumatic stress disorder. J Abnorm Psychol 2006;115:484–95.

29. Gilbertson MW, Shenton ME, Ciszewski A, et al. Smaller hippocampal volume predicts pathologic vulnerability to psychological trauma. Nat Neurosci 2002;5:1242–7.

30. Yoo SS, Gujar N, Hu P, et al. The human emotional brain without sleep-a prefrontal amygdala disconnect. Curr Biol 2007;17:R877–8.

31. Gianaros PJ, Jennings JR, Sheu LK, et al. Heightened functional neural activation to psychological stress covaries with exaggerated blood pressure reactivity. Hypertension 2007;49:134–40.

32. Gianaros PJ, Sheu LK. A review of neuroimaging studies of stressor-evoked blood pressure reactivity: emerging evidence for a brain-body pathway to coronary heart disease risk. Neuroimage 2009;47: 922–36.

33. Gianaros PJ, Sheu LK, Matthews KA, et al. Individual differences in stressor-evoked blood pressure reactivity vary with activation, volume, and functional connectivity of the amygdala. J Neurosci 2008;28: 990–9.

34. Karatsoreos IN, Bhagat S, Bloss EB, et al. Disruption of circadian clocks has ramifications for metabolism, brain, and behavior. Proc Natl Acad Sci U S A 2011; 108:1657–62.

35. McEwen BS. Effects of adverse experiences for brain structure and function. Biol Psychiatry 2000; 48:721–31.

36. McEwen BS. Protective and damaging effects of stress mediators: central role of the brain. Dialogues Clin Neurosci 2006;8:367–81.

37. McEwen BS, Coirini H, Westlind-Danielsson A, et al. Steroid hormones as mediators of neural plasticity. J Steroid Biochem Mol Biol 1991;39:223–32.

38. Davis S, Mirick DK, Stevens RG. Night shift work, light at night, and risk of breast cancer. J Natl Cancer Inst 2001;93:1557–62.

39. Suwazono Y, Dochi M, Sakata K, et al. A longitudinal study on the effect of shift work on weight gain in male Japanese workers. Obesity (Silver Spring) 2008;16:1887–93.

40. Lowden A, Moreno C, Holmback U, et al. Eating and shift work - effects on habits, metabolism and performance. Scand J Work Environ Health 2010;36:150–62.

41. Leproult R, Copinschi G, Buxton O, et al. Sleep loss results in an elevation of cortisol levels the next evening. Sleep 1997;20:865–70.

42. Spiegel K, Leproult R, Van Cauter E. Impact of sleep debt on metabolic and endocrine function. Lancet 1999;354:1435–9.

43. Spiegel K, Tasali E, Penev P, et al. Brief communication: sleep curtailment in healthy young men is associated with decreased leptin levels, elevated ghrelin levels, and increased hunger and appetite. Ann Intern Med 2004;141:846–50.

44. Gangwisch JE, Malaspina D, Boden-Albala B, et al. Inadequate sleep as a risk factor for obesity: analyses of the NHANES I. Sleep 2005;28:1289–96.

45. Matthews KA, Dahl RE, Owens JF, et al. Sleep duration and insulin resistance in healthy black and white adolescents. Sleep 2012;35:1353–8.

46. St-Onge MP, O'Keeffe M, Roberts AL, et al. Short sleep duration, glucose dysregulation and hormonal regulation of appetite in men and women. Sleep 2012;35:1503–10.

47. Vetrivelan R, Fuller PM, Yokota S, et al. Metabolic effects of chronic sleep restriction in rats. Sleep 2012; 35:1511–20.

48. Vgontzas AN, Zoumakis E, Bixler EO, et al. Adverse effects of modest sleep restriction on sleepiness, performance, and inflammatory cytokines. J Clin Endocrinol Metab 2004;89:2119–26.

49. Friedman EM, Hayney MS, Love GD, et al. Social relationships, sleep quality, and interleukin-6 in aging women. Proc Natl Acad Sci U S A 2005;102:18757–62.

50. Pearson GL, Savenkova M, Barnwell JJ, et al. Circadian desynchronization alters metabolic and immune responses following lipopolysaccharide inoculation in male mice. Brain Behav Immun 2020;88:220–9. https://doi.org/10.1016/j.bbi.2020.05.033.

51. Phillips DJ, Savenkova MI, Karatsoreos IN. Environmental disruption of the circadian clock leads to altered sleep and immune responses in mouse. Brain Behav Immun 2015;47:14–23. https://doi.org/10.1016/j.bbi.2014.12.008.

52. Lewy AJ, Lefler BJ, Emens JS, et al. The circadian basis of winter depression. Proc Natl Acad Sci U S A 2006;103:7414–9.

53. Karatsoreos IN. Links between circadian rhythms and psychiatric disease. Front Behav Neurosci 2014;8:162.

54. Vogel GW, Thompson FC Jr, Thurmond A, et al. The effect of REM deprivation on depression. Psychosomatics 1973;14:104–7.

55. Wirz-Justice A, Van den Hoofdakker RH. Sleep deprivation in depression: what do we know, where do we go? Biol Psychiatry 1999;46:445–53.

56. Kuhn M, Maier JG, Wolf E, et al. Indices of cortical plasticity after therapeutic sleep deprivation in patients with major depressive disorder. J Affect Disord 2020;277:425–35. https://doi.org/10.1016/j.jad.2020.08.052.

57. Morley-Fletcher S, Mairesse J, Soumier A, et al. Chronic agomelatine treatment corrects behavioral, cellular, and biochemical abnormalities induced by prenatal stress in rats. Psychopharmacology 2011; 217:301–13.

58. Keller J, Flores B, Gomez RG, et al. Cortisol circadian rhythm alterations in psychotic major depression. Biol Psychiatry 2006;60:275–81.

59. Rintamaki R, Grimaldi S, Englund A, et al. Seasonal changes in mood and behavior are linked to metabolic syndrome. PLoS One 2008;3:e1482.

60. Martino TA, OuditGY, Herzenberg AM, et al. Circadian rhythm disorganization produces profound cardiovascular and renal disease in hamsters. Am J Physiol Regul Integr Comp Physiol 2008;294: R1675–83.

61. McEwen BS, Chattarji S. Molecular mechanisms of neuroplasticity and pharmacological implications: the example of tianeptine. Eur Neuropsychopharmacol 2004;14:S497–502.

62. Taishi P, Chen Z, Obal FJ, et al. Sleep-associated changes in interleukin-1beta mRNA in the brain. J Interferon Cytokine Res 1998;18:793–8.

63. Clark RA, Valente AJ. Nuclear factor kappa B activation by NADPH oxidases. Mech Ageing Dev 2004; 125:799–810.

64. Tang J, Liu J, Zhou C, et al. Role of NADPH oxidase in the brain injury of intracerebral hemorrhage. J Neurochem 2005;94:1342–50.

65. Silva RH, Abilio VC, Takatsu AL, et al. Role of hippocampal oxidative stress in memory deficits induced by sleep deprivation in mice. Neuropharmacology 2004;46:895–903.

66. Kong J, Shepel PN, Holden CP, et al. Brain glycogen decreases with increased periods to wakefulness: implications for homeostatic drive to sleep. J Neurosci 2002;22:5581–7.

67. Brown AM. Brain glycogen re-awakened. J Neurochem 2004;89:537–52.

68. Wender R, Brown AM, Fern R, et al. Astrocytic glycogen influences axon function and survival during glucose deprivation in central white matter. J Neurosci 2000;20:6804–10.

69. Youngblood BD, Zhou J, Smagin GN, et al. Sleep deprivation by the "flower pot" technique and spatial reference memory. Physiol Behav 1997;61:249–56.

70. Kim EY, Mahmoud GS, Grover LM. REM sleep deprivation inhibits LTP in vivo in area CA1 of rat hippocampus. Neurosci Lett 2005;388:163–7.

71. Graves LA, Heller EA, Pack AI, et al. Sleep deprivation selectively impairs memory consolidation for contextual fear conditioning. Learn Mem 2003;10: 168–76.

72. Guan Z, Peng X, Fang J. Sleep deprivation impairs spatial memory and decreases extracellular signal-regulated kinase phosphorylation in the hippocampus. Brain Res 2004;1018:38–47.

73. Romcy-Pereira R, Pavlides C. Distinct modulatory effects of sleep on the maintenance of hippocampal and medial prefrontal cortex LTP. Eur J Neurosci 2004;20:3453–62.

74. Lu HJ, Lv J. β-Adrenergic receptor activity in the hippocampal dentate gyrus Participates in spatial learning and memory impairment in sleep-deprived rats. Exp Neurobiol 2021;30(2):144–54.

75. Vecsey CG, Huang T, Abel T. Sleep deprivation impairs synaptic tagging in mouse hippocampal slices. Neurobiol Learn Mem 2018;154:136–40.

76. Wong LW, Chong YS, Wong WLE, et al. Inhibition of Histone Deacetylase Reinstates hippocampus-dependent long-term synaptic plasticity and associative memory in sleep-deprived mice. Cereb Cortex 2020;30(7):4169–82.

77. de Paula HM, Hoshino K. Correlation between the fighting rates of REM sleep-deprived rats and susceptibility to the 'wild running' of audiogenic seizures. Brain Res 2002;926:80–5.

78. Musty RE, Consroe PF. Phencyclidine produces aggressive behavior in rapid eye movement sleep-deprived rats. Life Sci 1982;30:1733–8.

79. Russell JW, Singer G. Relations between muricide, circadian rhythm and consummatory behavior. Physiol Behav 1983;30:23–7.

80. Wood GE, Young LT, Reagan LP, et al. Acute and chronic restraint stress alter the incidence of social conflict in male rats. Horm Behav 2003;43:205–13.

81. Guzman-Marin R, Suntsova N, Stewart DR, et al. Sleep deprivation reduces proliferation of cells in the dentate gyrus of the hippocampus in rats. J Physiol 2003;549(2):563–71.

82. Rajizadeh MA, Esmaeilpour K, Haghparast E, et al. Voluntary exercise modulates learning & memory and synaptic plasticity impairments in sleep deprived female rats. Brain Res 2020;1729:146598. https://doi.org/10.1016/j.brainres.2019.146598.

83. Roman V, Van der Borght K, Leemburg SA, et al. Sleep restriction by forced activity reduces hippocampal cell proliferation. Brain Res 2005;1065:53–9.

84. Hairston IS, Little MT, Scanlon MD, et al. Sleep restriction suppresses neurogenesis induced by hippocampus-dependent learning. J Neurophysiol 2005;94:4224–33.

85. Prince TM, Wimmer M, Choi J, et al. Sleep deprivation during a specific 3-hour time window post-training impairs hippocampal synaptic plasticity and memory. Neurobiol Learn Mem 2014;109:122–30.

86. Ognjanovski N, Maruyama D, Lashner N, et al. CA1 hippocampal network activity changes during sleep-dependent memory consolidation. Front Syst Neurosci 2014;8:61.

87. Aton SJ, Seibt J, Dumoulin M, et al. Mechanisms of sleep-dependent consolidation of cortical plasticity. Neuron 2009;61:454–66.

88. Aton SJ, Broussard C, Dumoulin M, et al. Visual experience and subsequent sleep induce sequential plastic changes in putative inhibitory and excitatory cortical neurons. Proc Natl Acad Sci U S A 2013;110:3101–6.

89. Aton SJ, Suresh A, Broussard C, et al. Sleep promotes cortical response potentiation following visual experience. Sleep 2014;37:1163–70.

90. Gais S, Born J. Declarative memory consolidation: mechanisms acting during human sleep. Learn Mem 2004;11:679–85.

91. Atkinson G, Davenne D. Relationships between sleep, physical activity and human health. Physiol Behav 2007;90:229–36.

92. Karlson B, Eek FC, Hansen AM, et al. Diurnal Cortisol pattern of shift workers on workday and a day off. Scand J Work Environ Health 2006;Suppl(2):27–34.

93. Cho K. Chronic 'jet lag' produces temporal lobe atrophy and spatial cognitive deficits. Nat Neurosci 2001;4:567–8.

94. Hendrickx H, McEwen BS, van der Ouderaa F. Metabolism, mood and cognition in aging: the importance of lifestyle and dietary intervention. Neurobiol Aging 2005;26S:S1–5.

95. Gold SM, Dziobek I, Sweat V, et al. Hippocampal damage and memory impairments as possible early brain complications of type 2 diabetes. Diabetologia 2007;50:711–9.

96. Arvanitakis Z, Wilson RS, Bienias JL, et al. Diabetes mellitus and risk of Alzheimer disease and decline in cognitive function. Arch Neurol 2004;61:661–6.

97. Rasgon N, Jarvik L. Insulin resistance, affective disorders, and Alzheimer's disease: review and hypothesis. J Gerontol 2004;59A:178–83.

98. Tsuno N, Besset A, Ritchie K. Sleep and depression. J Clin Psychiatry 2005;66:1254–69.

Sleep and Athletic Performance

Impacts on Physical Performance, Mental Performance, Injury Risk and Recovery, and Mental Health: An Update

Jonathan Charest, PhD[a,b,c], Michael A. Grandner, PhD, MTR[d,*]

KEYWORDS

• Sleep • Sport • Insomnia • Performance

KEY POINTS

- Insufficient sleep and poor sleep quality are prevalent among athletes, potentially due to time demands, physical demands, and developmental needs.
- Sleep disturbances among athletes have adverse impacts on physical performance, mental performance, injury risk and recovery, medical health, and mental health.
- Sleep interventions among athletes have been shown to improve physical strength and speed, cognitive performance and reaction time, mental health, and other domains.
- Sport organizations should incorporate sleep health promotion programs at individual, team, and system levels.

INTRODUCTION
Scope of the Problem

In recent years, there has been increased attention toward the importance of sleep and its essential role in athletic performance, cognition, health, and mental well-being. Many of these studies examine elite athletes (eg, Olympians, professionals, and/or players recruited to national and varsity teams), and some focus on athletes in general. Despite all the efforts expended, by any definition, numerous athletes still experience inadequate sleep.[1–3] Compared with nonathletes, athletes tend to sleep less on average.[4] Furthermore, athletes' quality of sleep seems lower than their nonathlete peers.[5–7] In addition, it has been suggested that certain types of athletes are more prone to developing sleep difficulties, such as

sleep apnea. For example, according to George and colleagues[8] and Albuquerque and colleagues[9] National Football League (NFL) players have higher rates of obstructive sleep apnea (OSA), which have tremendous deleterious impacts on health and daytime sleepiness. There is increasing evidence that poor sleep is a good predictor for injuries and, more importantly, concussion.[10]

Position Statements

Recently, the International Olympic Committee (IOC) has addressed, for the first time, sleep as a major contributor to athletic performance and as a fundamental feature of athlete mental health.[11,12] In addition, the National Collegiate Athletics Association (NCAA)[13–17] included sleep health as part of their published mental health best practices[18]

This article previously appeared in *Sleep Med Clin* 15 (2020) 41–57.

[a] Department of Psychology, Universite Laval, Quebec City, Quebec, Canada; [b] Centre for Sleep and Human Performance, #106, 51 Sunpark Drive Southeast, Calgary, Alberta T2X 3V4, Canada; [c] Department of Kinesiology, University of Calgary, Calgary, Alberta, Canada; [d] Department of Psychiatry, University of Arizona, 1501 North Campbell Avenue, PO Box 245002, Tucson, AZ 8524-5002, USA
* Corresponding author.
E-mail address: grandner@gmail.com

Sleep Med Clin 17 (2022) 263–282
https://doi.org/10.1016/j.jsmc.2022.03.006
1556-407X/22/© 2022 Elsevier Inc. All rights reserved.

as well as their more recently published official position statement on the importance of sleep health for student-athletes.[18] These position statements from the NCAA and IOC represent the increased awareness of the importance of sleep health among organizations of elite athletes. Both these documents were the result of a literature review, Delphi process of iterative consensus building, and subsequent revision, after exhaustive reviews of the available literature. In addition to the NCAA and IOC position statements, 2 expert consensus documents were also produced that support the importance of sleep in athletes.

The first[19] was the result of a narrative review of sleep in athletes and suggests several recommendations for different challenges faced by athletes and their support team. Alongside 5 key recommendations, the investigators also provide an expert review of athlete sleep assessment tools and a flow diagram for practitioners to optimize and manage sleep for athlete and referral. The second is the result of 26 researchers and/or clinicians who formalized a review and a consensus document on the management of travel fatigue and jet lag in athletes.[20] This document recommends and suggests ways to manage travel fatigue and jet lag in athletes pretravel, during travel, and posttravel. Suggestions include behavioral and pharmacologic management within different possible scenarios faced by athletes.

The IOC mental health document[11] considers sleep health in terms of sufficiency (ie, at least 7 hours for adults), proper circadian alignment, good overall perceived sleep quality, and absence of sleep disorders, including insomnia disorder and sleep apnea. The document recommends that these dimensions of sleep be considered important for mental health as well as physical health and functioning. Furthermore, the document recommends education, proper assessment and screening, and treatment using evidence-based strategies—given the consideration that some treatments may have an impact on safety and/or performance.

The NCAA document focused on sleep as an important aspect of health, performance, and mental functioning in collegiate student-athletes.[18] This document addresses many identified barriers to sleep, including academic, athletic, and social time demands. Similarly, this document defines sleep health in terms of duration (at least 7 hours in adults), timing, overall quality, and absence of disorders, including insomnia and sleep apnea. Particular attention also is paid to the role of tiredness, fatigue, and/or sleepiness as consequences of sleep loss and/or disturbances. The NCAA makes 5 recommendations in this document:

1. Conduct a collegiate athlete time demands survey annually.
2. Ensure that consumer sleep technology, if used, is compliant with Health Insurance Portability and Accountability Act and Family Educational Rights and Privacy Act laws.
3. Incorporate sleep screening into the preparticipation examination.
4. Provide collegiate athletes with evidence-based sleep education that includes (a) information on sleep best practices, (b) information about the role of sleep in optimizing athletic and academic performance and overall well-being, and (c) strategies for addressing sleep barriers.
5. Provide coaches with evidence-based sleep education that includes (a) information on sleep best practices, (b) information about the role of sleep in optimizing athletic and academic performance and overall well-being, and (c) strategies to help optimize collegiate athlete sleep.

These efforts specifically recommend that sleep-related education should be provided, sleep difficulties and disorders should be routinely assessed and screened for, and sleep health promotion should be a goal of athletics programs.

EPIDEMIOLOGY OF SLEEP DISTURBANCES IN ATHLETES
Prevalence of Insufficient Sleep

Insufficient sleep duration can have an impact on metabolism, endocrine function, and athletic and cognitive outcomes, and, furthermore, can increase perceived effort during exercise.[21–23] When athletes are compared with nonathletes, they tend to sleep less and less efficiently. Leeder and colleagues[4] compared the habits of 47 elite athletes over a 4-day period with a group of nonathletes, using actigraphy; ages of participants were not reported, but groups were matched for age and gender. On average, athletes slept 6.55 hours ± 0.43 hours versus nonathletes who slept 7.11 hours ± 0.25 hours ($P = .27$). The investigators did report, however, lower sleep efficiency (80.6 hours ± 6.4 hours vs 88.7 hours ± 3.6 hours; $P < .05$), higher time spent in bed (8:07 hours ± 0:20 hours vs 8:36 hours ± 0.53 hours; $P < .05$), wake after sleep onset (0:50 hours ± 0:16 hours vs 1:17 hours ± 0:31 hours; $P < .05$), sleep-onset latency (5.0 hours ± 2.5 hours vs 18.2 hours ± 16.5 hours; $P < .05$), and sleep fragmentation (29.8 hours ± 9.0 hours vs 36.0 hours ± 12.4 hours; $P < .05$) in athletes. Furthermore, Lastella and colleagues[24] reported insufficient sleep duration among athletes, with

6.8 hours on average. Sargent and colleagues[25,26] also reported that over 14 nights assessed with actigraphy, athletes recorded an average of 6.5 hours of sleep per night.

Taken together, these studies have investigated a total of 241 elite athletes and, documented actigraphically, determined sleep durations of approximately 6.5 hours in most cases. Recently, Mah and colleagues[27] indicated that 39.1% of athletes reported insufficient sleep (<7 hours) by self-report. And, among a large sample of collegiate athletes in the United States (N = 8312), Turner and colleagues[28] reported that the mean number of nights per week that athletes did not think they got enough sleep was 3.8.

A recent review highlighted the insufficient sleep patterns of young athletes and compared them with those of nonathletes, finding conflicting results.[29] Based on 2 studies[30,31] with sleep diaries, young athletes reported sleeping longer than nonathletes by 66 and 25 minutes, respectively. However, a subsequent study with objective sleep measurement (ambulatory polysomnography) showed that young athletes reported a shorter total sleep time by approximately 36 minutes.[32] In addition, training and competition schedules may also decrease the total sleep time, thereby increasing the prevalence of insufficient sleep in athletes. For example, it has been demonstrated that sleep is impacted differently following a day or night game. In elite Australian rugby players, following a day game (15:45–17:45 PM) total sleep time averaged 7.7 ± 0.8 versus 5.3 ± 0.6 hours following an evening game (19:10–21:10 PM).[33] Likewise, in Australian female basketball players, following a double header compared with regular game, total sleep time, measured by actigraphy, was reduced by 11%.[34]

Prevalence of Poor Sleep Quality

Hoshikawa and colleagues[35] investigated the quality of sleep of 817 Japanese elite athletes with the Pittsburgh Sleep Quality Index (PSQI), showing that 28% of the participants exhibited a score greater than 5, suggesting poor quality of sleep. Mah and colleagues[27] reported that 42.2% of the 629 athletes in that study experienced poor sleep quality, also using the PSQI. In 2019, Turner and colleagues[28] examined data from 8312 collegiate student-athletes and found that 19.8% reported that "sleep difficulties" were particularly "traumatic or difficult to handle" over the past 12 months and that 21.8% reported extreme difficulty falling asleep at least 3 nights per week. Bleyer and colleagues[5] reported that 38% of their 452 participants reported poor sleep.

Findings from a study conducted among elite rugby and cricket players (n = 175) showed that 50% of their participants' PSQI score were greater than 5 and that 9% scored greater than 10.[3] Tsunoda and colleagues[7] reported the PSQI scores of 14 wheelchair basketball athletes (mean = 5.8 ± 3.0) and compared their results with those of 103 nonathletes from the general population (mean = 4.51 ± 2.14). Regardless of total sleep time, the wheelchair athletes reported lower sleep quality and lower sleep efficiency than matched nonathletes.

In a cohort of 317 athletes from the Rio de Janeiro 2016 Summer Olympics from 11 different sports, poor sleep quality (as assessed by the PSQI) was prevalent in more than 50% of the athletes after the Olympic Games.[36] This research recapitulates the earlier results with a similar cohort, in which up to 83% of athletes reached the cutoff, indicating poor sleep.[37] The higher proportion with a score greater than 5 occurred in the lead-up to the Olympics and the lower figure was recorded at the games. Consequently, regardless of the type of sports, these results highlight the prevalence of poor sleep quality among athletes.

Prevalence of Daytime Sleepiness

Few studies have examined the prevalence of general fatigue and/or sleepiness among athletes. Turner and colleagues[28] reported that 60.9% of collegiate athletes report that they experience feeling "tired, dragged out, or sleepy during the day" at least 3 days per week (as measured by self-report). Furthermore, 32.75% of these collegiate student-athletes reported an inability to maintain wakefulness at least 3 times per week (by self-report). Mah and colleagues[27] reported that 51% of student-athletes in their study reported high scores (≥10) on the Epworth Sleepiness Scale. Last, among 190 NCAA division 1 student-athletes, 60% reported daytime sleepiness or sleepiness on 2 or more days per month.[10] These findings indicate high levels of sleepiness in elite athletes.

Prevalence of Circadian Preferences and Disruption

Data exploring chronotype among the general population suggest that approximately 25% are morning types, 50% are intermediate types, and approximately 25% are evening types.[38] Few studies have explored the chronotype distribution among athletes. Two studies[2,39] indicated that 51% of athletes were classified as morning types, 40% as intermediate types, and only 9% as evening types. One study examined athletes in wheelchairs, and the other examined school-aged athletes and may not be representative of the elite athlete population. Lastella and colleagues[40] investigated 114 elite athletes emerging from 5 different sports. Their results indicated that 28% were morning types, 65% were intermediate types, and only 6% were evening types, supporting previous findings that athletes tend to pursue and excel in sports that match their chronotype.[41] Circadian rhythms can influence variations in performance, depending on the time of day and typical training schedules, which ultimately can affect competitive performance.[42] When athletes experience disturbances in their environments or routines, such as overnight travel, repetitive time zone changes, evening training, or late-night competition, endogenous circadian rhythms and normal sleep patterns may be out of synchrony.[43,44] Such disruptions in circadian and sleep patterns can increase homeostatic pressure and thus influence the regulation of emotions, body temperature, and circulation of melatonin and cause a significant increase in sleep latency.[45] The sleep/wake behavior of athletes often is governed by their training schedules.[46] Therefore, the role of chronotype among athletes may interact with a training schedule and should be considered to optimize training and performance[42] and reduce the prevalence of chronobiologic disturbances. Circadian variation, such as timing of the day of competition or game have, been demonstrated to have considerable impact on performance.[47] Olympic swim times between 2004 and 2016 have demonstrated that late afternoon competition around 17:12 PM improved performance by 0.32% relative to 8:00 AM competition. Moreover, the time-of-the-day effect exceeded the difference between first and second and second and third places in 40% and 64% of the races, respectively. Despite the elaborate preparation of each Olympic athlete, circadian rhythms and time of the day still represent a major factor in human performance.

Prevalence of Sleep Disorders

Insomnia

Gupta and colleagues[48] demonstrated that the relation between elite sport participation and insomnia symptoms is poorly systematized. Daytime impairment—a key part of insomnia diagnosis—can reflect a wide variety of experiences, including fatigue, emotional fluctuation, and psychomotor and/or neuropsychological performance, which are all important for elite athletes. Given this particular sensitivity to performance impairment and high levels of sleepiness (which

is not common in insomnia), there arise some challenges in insomnia assessment among elite athletes. Traditional insomnia models might poorly discriminate insomnia per se in this nontraditional population.[49] The multifaceted demands of elite sport, including a high level of training volume,[50,51] precompetition anxiety,[24,46,52] and circadian challenges (jet lag),[53] all can predispose and precipitate sleep disturbance, thus leading to or facilitating symptoms of insomnia.

Given the absence of a validated sleep questionnaire specifically for athletes before the creation of the Athlete Sleep Screening Questionnaire (ASSQ),[54] it is difficult to precisely indicate the insomnia prevalence in elite athletes. The systematic review conducted by Gupta and colleagues,[48] however, reported that sleep disturbance complaints range from 13% to 70% of the athletes and that overall, on average, 26% of the athletes significantly scored for insomnia symptoms using the Insomnia Severity Index and PSQI. Supporting the previous review, of 111 professional soccer players in Qatar, 27% reported subthreshold insomnia based on an Insomnia Severity Index (ISI) score of greater than 11 and 68.5% reported poor sleep.[55] Notwithstanding the popularity of these 2 questionnaires, neither of them is specifically validated in an elite athlete population. Elite athletes are selected primarily based on not only physiologic predisposition but also psychological attributes.[56,57] It is possible that personality traits that include a focus on success (eg, perfectionism) also may predispose an elite athlete to insomnia.[58] Furthermore, the demands of elite sports, including an elevated frequency, intensity, and volume of activity and scheduling challenges,[25,51] coupled with precompetition anxiety[52] and jet lag/travel,[59,60] may all lead an individual toward sleep difficulties. Given that these challenges are uncommon among the general population and the relationship between risk factors and sleep may be fundamentally different in this group (eg, distribution of muscle mass), tools not specifically validated in athletic populations should be used somewhat cautiously.

Sleep apnea

The prevalence of sleep apnea may be high in certain type of sports, such as strength, power, and high-contact sports, where athletes often present with a large body mass and neck circumference.[3,61,62] In the NFL and National Hockey League, 2 high-speed and high-contact sports, an elevated body mass index and a large neck circumference are considered protective assets, making athletes less injury prone.[3] These specific body traits, however, unfortunately, also predispose these athletes to an increased risk of OSA.[62–64] Two studies carried out among NFL players illustrated that players with these specific physical traits seemed to have a higher incidence of OSA.[8,65] In addition, in line with the previous football studies, Dobrosielski and colleagues[66] illustrated that approximately 8% of the NCAA division I football players were at risk for OSA. Moreover, in professional hockey players, OSA was present in approximately 10% of athletes.[67] It is reported that, in most cases, the OSA severity was mild but even mild OSA might cause major disturbances in sleep,[68] potentially having an impact on athletic performance. In a study involving 25 elite rugby union players, 24% were diagnosed with sleep apnea after an overnight polysomnography.[69] These results demonstrate that sleep apnea is a prevalent disorder in certain types of sports and, given its potentially harmful impact on health,[70,71] it would justify a process for identifying those at risk and a plan for care.

Other disorders

Few studies have been conducted on restless legs syndrome (RLS) among athletes. Findings from a study assessing a population of runners indicate that prevalence is suggested at approximately 13%.[72] Among hockey players, prevalence is suggested at approximately 5%[67]; finally, within a sample of rugby players, no participants reported RLS but 12% reported periodic limb movements (PLMs).[69] These 2 studies have shown that sleep disorders, such as RLS and PLMs, are relatively common among elite athletes from a variety of sports.

IMPACT OF SLEEP ON PHYSICAL PERFORMANCE

Adverse effects of sleep restriction on athletic performance have been documented for many years, including cardiorespiratory and psychomotor effects, which require sustained and stable performance over time.[73–78] Mougin and colleagues[78] observed 7 participants on a cycle ergometer, in a study that included a 10-minute warm-up and then a 20-minute steady exercise corresponding to 75% of the predetermined maximal oxygen consumption and was followed by an increased-intensity exercise until exhaustion; this was done along with sleep restriction (3 hours of wakefulness in the middle of the night). In this study, physiologic demands were significantly higher during the submaximal effort compared with a baseline night (10:30 PM to 7:00 AM).[78] Heart rate was significantly higher when measured after 9 minutes (167.1 ± 2.0 bpm vs 171.3 ± 2.5 bpm) and after

20 minutes (176.0 ± 2.6 bpm vs 179.1 ± 2.4 bpm). Also, ventilation (141.0 ± 5.7 bpm vs 157.5 ± 6.4 bpm) and respiratory frequency (43.0 ± 1.6 bpm vs 44.7 ± 1.7 bpm) were both altered after a sleep restriction compared with baseline. Similarly, these same variables were significantly higher after the sleep restriction condition when performing a graded exercise stress test, until exhaustion, whereas the volume of maximal oxygen uptake decreased. Lactate accumulation was also greater at the ninth minute ($P < .01$), at the twentieth minute ($P < .05$) of the steady power exercise, and at maximal exercise ($P < .05$) after sleep restriction. These results from Mougin and colleagues[78] elegantly demonstrated that after a sleep restriction, physical performances require a higher physiologic demand, ultimately leading the athletes to exhaustion faster than he should have been. In a separate study, however, there was no significant change in mean or maximal power in anaerobic tests after a 3:00 AM bedtime compared with a 10:30 PM bedtime.[79] Subsequent studies by Mougin and colleagues[80] showed that after 4-hour sleep restriction, the maximum work rate developed by the participants was reduced by 15 W for cyclists in a 30-minute exercise at 75% of maximum power. In agreement with some of the previous results, the average and maximum powers of an anaerobic test decrease among students,[81] football players,[82] and judokas[83] after a single 4-hour sleep restriction. The reasoning behind the decrease in resistance to exercise is the alteration of the aerobic pathways[77] or in the perceptual change (impression of a longer effort), because the physiologic aspects remain predominantly unchanged.[75,76] The increase in perceived effort accompanied by a reduction in generated power supports the theory of neuromuscular fatigue,[84] possibly indicating a combination of central nervous system response and neural theory of sleep.[75,85,86]

Other studies also have shown adverse impacts of sleep restriction on athletes' anaerobic power,[87] tennis serving accuracy,[88] isometric force,[89] and cortisol levels.[90] In addition, the average distance traveled by elite runners decreases (6.224–6.037 miles) in a treadmill exercise (30 minutes) at their own pace.[91] Skein and colleagues[92] reported lower average sprint times, reduced glycogen concentration in the muscles, and decreased strength and activation during an isometric force test after a 30-hour total sleep deprivation, with 10 athletes from team sports, compared with a normal 8 hours of sleep. Submaximal-effort sports, such as running, might be more likely affected by total sleep deprivation than maximum-effort sports, such as weightlifting, because they require more time and, therefore, have a negative impact on the perception of effort throughout time perhaps due to the higher physiologic demand required.[78] After sleep restriction, the perception of effort increases exponentially increased completion time of the test.[91] The differences in muscle contraction results (voluntary activation), however, can probably be explained by the sensitivity and accuracy of the electromyography equipment used. For example, previous studies probably have been limited in this aspect contrary to recent studies due to the technological advancement of equipment.[92,93] In summary, although the effects of sleep deprivation on exercise are not completely understood, many converging results imply adverse effects of sleep deprivation on athletic performance.

Moreover, the balance of the energy substrate seems vulnerable to sleep deprivation. For instance, a 30-hour sleep deprivation compared with an 8-hour sleep opportunity demonstrated the inability of the human body to fully recover (24 hours) muscle glycogen in an athletic population, as shown by the muscle glycogen concentration before exercise (310 mmol·kg^{-1} dry weight [dw] $\pm$ 67 mmol·kg^{-1} dw vs 209 mmol·kg^{-1} dw $\pm$ 60 mmol·kg^{-1} dw).[92] Inadequate glucose intake would hinder athletes' ability to compete for extended periods, because glycogen shortage is known to reduce muscle function and athletic stamina.[94,95] It seems that a large energy imbalance leads to a deterioration in both aerobic and anaerobic power production when activity is sustained over several days and sleep is reduced.[93–100] Prolonged periods of sleep deprivation are associated with increased sympathetic nervous system activity and decreases in parasympathetic nervous system activity as well as altered spontaneous baroreflex sensitivity during vigilance testing in healthy adults.[101] Because disturbances of sympathetic and parasympathetic equilibrium are associated with overtraining,[102] it is possible that these disturbances of the autonomic nervous system after sleep deprivation may promote the development of a state of overtraining in athletes.[95,103] Despite these nervous system disturbances, several studies have reported that sleep deprivation has minimal impact on the cardiorespiratory variables during exercise,[75,79,104] as opposed to the previous finding of Mougin and colleagues.[78] Differences probably are more attributable to the protocols administered and the exercise mode used (running, cycling, and time of exhaustion) throughout these different studies. In addition to these results, there were no significant effects on cardiorespiratory or thermoregulatory function in athletes despite a

reduction in the distance run for 30 minutes on a treadmill after sleep deprivation.[91] Oliver and colleagues[91] hypothesized that the minimal effects on cardiorespiratory function could be due to the influence of perceived effort during the final stages of prolonged high-intensity exercise (described previously).

Furthermore, several performance aspects also lie in tactical and technical outcomes.[105] In 10 elite rugby players, 10 single-passing skill trials were investigated under normal sleep (7–9 hours) and restricted sleep (3–5 hours).[106] Following a period of familiarization with the dominant and nondominant side for passing, the players performed significantly worse under sleep restriction compared with normal sleep. In 11 collegiate athlete basketball players, following a sleep extension, shooting accuracy improved by 9.0% in free throw and by 9.2% for 3-point attempts.[27] Similarly, in 12 collegiate athlete tennis players, following a sleep extension to at least 9 hours, participants improved their serving accuracy compared with their normal sleep from 35.7% to 41.8%.[107] Last, the sleep of 17 elite Australian female basketball players was monitored with actigraphy over the course of 2 seasons.[34] The study investigated the sleep patterns of their players for game at home, on the road, and double headers alongside basketball efficiency statistic (EFF). Results reported a small correlation between total sleep time at prematch for regular game ($r = -0.25$; $P = .430$; n = 12) and double header ($r = -0.22$; $P = .484$; n = 12).

IMPACT OF SLEEP ON INJURY RISK AND RECOVERY
Sleep and Concussions

It is estimated that as many as 3.8 million concussions are sustained in the United States during competitive sports per year.[108] Regrettably, approximately 50% of concussions may go unreported.[108] As many as 1 million student-athletes reported having 2 or more concussions during a period of 12 months.[109] A study indicated that 40% of athletes with a concussion reported that their coaches were not aware of their symptoms.[110] Moreover, it is suggested that athletes involved in team sports have significantly higher risk for 1 or more concussions than athletes in individual sports.[109]

Sleep may play an important role as a risk factor for concussions. Participants were given sleep screening questionnaires and followed over a 1-year period. Predictors of incident concussions included clinically moderate to severe insomnia (relative risk [RR], 3.13; 95% confidence interval

[CI], 1.320–7.424; $P = .015$) and excessive daytime sleepiness (RR, 2.856; 95% CI, 0.681–11.977; $P = .037$), in a study of 190 NCAA athletes,[10] and these risk factors outperformed more traditional risk factors (eg, high-risk sport and history of concussions) as predictors.

Postconcussion sleep also is important. Recently, a meta-analysis reported that sleep disturbances were reported after a concussion approximately 50% of the time.[111] The most common sleep disturbances reported after a concussion are daytime sleepiness and insomnia, 50% and 25%, respectively.[112] In addition, sleep disturbance may be a prominent contributor to exacerbate comorbid features of depression, fatigue, and pain after a concussion[111] and worsen recovery because normal recuperative functions of sleep are altered.[113]

A return to baseline cognition and self-reported symptoms are key priorities that could be adopted to ensure player safety.[114,115] It has been demonstrated, however, that athletes sleeping fewer than 7 hours the previous night of testing would perform worse.[116] Considering that the decision of allowing a player back to play results from a comparison of preconcussion and postconcussion performances, a valid neurocognitive baseline is needed. In that sense, sleep should be monitored throughout the year to obtain an adequate neurocognitive performance and, therefore, a valid baseline. Moreover, the difference in symptomatic presentation after a concussion is highly divergent between male and female athletes,[117] which highlights the existing gap between the type of athletes and the consideration that should be directed toward an individualized baseline assessment to better detect the symptoms of a concussion.

Concussion, regardless of severity, is an injury to the brain, and athletes who are suspected of such an injury should be monitored carefully.[118,119]

An increase in awareness has directly led to more interest into postconcussion symptoms.[120,121] Research has specifically pointed out that the continuation of poor sleep symptoms after a concussion was a reliable predictor of prolonged recovery.[122–124] In addition, Kostyun and colleagues[125] demonstrated that during recovery, adolescents who reported greater sleep disturbance performed worse on neurocognitive testing.

Insufficient Sleep as a Risk Factor for Injury

Athletes aim to achieve peak performance for as long as possible, given typically short careers with high stakes. An online study of adolescent students (12–18 years old) reported that students sleeping less than 8.1 hours a night were 1.7 times more likely to have had an injury than their peers who slept more than 8.1 hours.[126,127] Furthermore, the same study also indicated that for each additional grade in school, students were 1.4 times more likely to have had an injury. Taken together, insufficient sleep duration may increase the risk of injury. In addition, the summation of years of (accumulated) sleep debt may play a role in risk injury outcomes.

Nutrition plays a fundamental role in recovery and injury prevention,[37,128–130] and nutrition and sleep have a bidirectional relationship.[131–135] There is an association between the number of hours slept and the intake of dietary nutriment categories.[133] Furthermore, individuals who have a later bedtime tend to consume a higher percentage of carbohydrates, fat, and protein than the average sleepers.[136] On the other hand, some nutriment categories may have a positive effect on sleep, such as tart cherries and kiwis, which are believed to reduce the number of awakening and increasing the sleep time.[137] Although nutritional knowledge is assumed to be high among athletes,[138] data are sparse on the number of athletes who are following their diets on a regular basis, and this may be impacted by poor sleep, which influences food intake.[139]

Adolescents sleeping fewer than 8 hours per night were more likely to sustain an injury[140] compared with students sleeping greater than 8 hours. These results are in line with the conclusions of Milewski and colleagues,[127] which is interesting given that the results are replicated in a population of athletes. In additional, Von Rosen and colleagues[140] found that the recommended intake of fruits, vegetables, and fish was not met for 20%, 39%, and 43% of their athletes, respectively. Therefore, the hypothesis of combined effect of poor sleep and a poor nutrition needs to be further explored to better understand the mechanisms underlying injuries in athletes.

Moreover, lack of sleep and poor sleep quality exacerbate depression and anxiety symptoms,[141] which also may increase injury risk. In a study of 958 athletes, 40.6% experienced an injury of various nature.[142] At preseason, 28.8% of the 958 enrolled athletes in this study reported anxiety symptoms and 21.7% reported depressive symptoms. Those with anxiety symptoms were 2.3 times more likely to have had an injury.[142] Given the strong association between poor sleep, anxiety, and depression symptoms,[143,144] it can be speculated that insufficient sleep may indirectly lead to an injury.

Insufficient Sleep and Recovery

Poor sleep quality and sleep deprivation impair brain functions that affect a wide array of cognitive functions,[145] which may directly or indirectly facilitate recovery from mental effort and/or physical injury. Furthermore, sleep-deprived individuals might increase their intake of unhealthy foods, which ultimately impairs glycogen repletion and protein synthesis,[146] which are critical for recovery in athletes. In addition, impaired sleep directly affects growth hormone release and alters cortisol secretion,[80] having an impact on recovery from exercise and stress. Sleep deprivation also increases proinflammatory cytokines, such as interleukin-6 and C-reactive protein levels, which are pain-facilitating agents,[147] ultimately affecting the immune system; hinders muscle recovery and repair from damages sustained in high-intensity training; and leads toward an imbalance of the autonomic nervous system.[148,149] Moreover, athletes who feel the need to push the boundaries of their capabilities may tend to develop poor sleep patterns, increasing their chances of illness (ie, medical symptoms), and this has an impact on their performance and recovery.[97] In addition to the aforementioned studies, others have also pointed out the association of insufficient sleep with higher symptoms both subjectively and objectively. In 545 adolescent athletes treated for sports-related concussion, Kostyun and colleagues[125] reported that subjectively sleeping fewer than 7 hours per night correlated with higher complaints of concussion symptoms during their recovery. In another study, Sufrinko and colleagues[150] investigated 670 student-athletes with a diagnosis of sport-related concussion. Those with a history of sleep disturbance before the injury performed worse on the Post-Concussion Symptom Scale and Verbal Memory and reported a higher number of total symptoms.[150] Ultimately, preinjury sleep disturbances may exacerbate neurocognitive symptoms and alter the recovery trajectory following a sports-related concussion.

IMPACT OF SLEEP ON MENTAL AND COGNITIVE PERFORMANCE
Vigilance and Reaction Time

Sleep restriction has been demonstrated to have a negative impact on attention and reaction times.[151–154] Furthermore, it has been demonstrated that reaction times are adversely impacted after only a 1-night, complete sleep deprivation.[87] In 12 healthy handball goalkeepers, it was demonstrated that following a partial sleep restriction, athletes were significantly slower on the reaction time test compared with normal sleep.[155]

Sleep extension, conversely, has been shown to improve reaction times by 15% and also improve objective daytime sleepiness,[156] in a study of student-athletes. Mah and colleagues[157]

extended the sleep of a college basketball team during a 5- to 7-week period. The average total sleep time increased from 7.50 hours to 10.25 hours of sleep over this period. Student-athletes improved their reaction time scores ($P < .001$) in morning and evening testing sessions. Given that athletes often experience at least mild sleep restriction (especially during intense periods of training or competition), sleep management becomes a priority to maximize reaction time. Consistent with the findings on sleep extension, there is evidence that sleep can be banked to optimize vigilance and reaction time.[158–160]

Executive Function and Decision Making

Executive functions are one of the cornerstones of athletic performance.[161,162] These functions include the highest levels of thinking required to engineer a strategy, make a fast decision, demonstrate cognitive flexibility, and manage the prioritization of attention. Deep sleep/slow wave sleep seems to have different restorative functions both at the neurophysiologic and phenomenological levels. Deep sleep seems to have a beneficial impact on the prefrontal cortex, which also has a positive impact on the functions directed by this cerebral region.[163,164] Prioritization or inhibitory control ensures the control of the athlete's concentration, attention, and thoughts and suppresses the cognitive and behavioral external and internal distractions.[165,166] Cognitive flexibility is vital for athletes by ensuring efficiency and adaptation in changing tasks.[165,167] Adaptation is key in athletics; it prevents athletes from making a bad or a risky decision, and this inhibitory control is highly linked to sleep deprivation.[168,169] As sleep restriction is a common feature and reflects of the reality of the athletic population, studies have focused on its impact on decision making.[170,171] Demos and colleagues[171] demonstrated that sleep restriction had no impact statistically on decision making. However, participants were 30% more likely to make inhibition errors.[171] Officials represent a crucial part of sport, and they are subject to the same sleep challenges as athletes.[172] Although they may have a direct impact on the outcome of certain sports, the effect of sleep on decision making has yet to be adequately investigated among the population of sports officials.[172]

These studies underscore the deleterious effects of lack of sleep on executive functions. Too little sleep may alter an athlete's ability to make a good decision versus a risky one in a split second, during the course of a game or event. Caffeine has been suggested as a countermeasure to protect against effects on risk taking or poor decision making.[173] It has been demonstrated, however, that caffeine does not replace a proper night of sleep for these functions.[88,174–176]

Learning and Memory

Learning new skills is crucial for every athlete. The roots of memory consolidations are found in sleep.[85,177–179] The ability to recall information[180] is inevitably of interest for athletes. For example, the NFL requires emphasis on the playbook, and the ability to recall complex plays is essential for participation in football. Moreover, learning and improving a motor skill are known to continue 24 hours after training.[181] In healthy young adults, non–rapid eye movement (NREM) stage 2 sleep typically represents approximately 45% to 55% of total sleep time.[182] It has been demonstrated that the duration of sleep stage 2 (NREM) is strongly correlated with the consolidation of motor skills.[183–185] Arguably, the sleep period following learning a new skill is crucial, and it has been shown that sleep restriction can have an adverse impact on the memory consolidation.[186]

Although it is true to a certain point that practice makes perfect, the results of several studies indicated that sleep after learning improves performance significantly, relative to sleep deprivation.[187–189] So perhaps sleep makes perfect. Also, sleep restriction also has a negative impact on the academic performance of student-athletes.[190] Fifty-six students were either assigned to a 5 hours' or 9 hours' time in bed for 14 consecutive days, in which participants had to study for the Graduate Record Examination. Results showed that the sleep-restricted group was significantly impacted for the recall of massed item, which is fundamental in academic success.

Another group of elite athletes, student-athletes, need to be prepared not only for their competitions but also for academics. Turner and colleagues[28] found that general sleep difficulty, initial insomnia, daytime tiredness, daytime sleepiness, and insufficient sleep all were associated with decreased academic performance among student-athletes. It is partially a coach's responsibility to mentor the student-athletes to be ready for any kind of test, either athletic or academic. Ultimately, assessing sleep on a regular basis could provide crucial information for the coaching members and the athletes.[191] Furthermore, having a clear idea of how an athlete sleeps may help a team medical specialist prevent injuries, such as concussion.[10]

Creativity and Thinking

Through sleep, the consolidation theory suggests that learning and memory consolidation benefit creativity.[192] The relationship between sleep and creativity stems from the direct influence of sleep on learning and formation of new concepts, ideas, solutions, and, ultimately, the genesis of creativity.[193] It was demonstrated that rapid eye movement (REM) sleep can improve creative problem solving.[194] REM sleep, according to Cai and colleagues,[194] enhanced creativity for items that are primed before sleep by more than 40%. Another study showed that stage 1 sleep was associated with fluency and flexibility, and slow wave sleep and REM sleep were associated with originality and global measure of figural creativity.[195] Furthermore, in a Remote Associates Test study, participants were faced with different levels of difficulty and the unsolved problems were presented again after a period of sufficient sleep, wake, or no delay.[196] The sleep group solved a greater number of difficult Remote Associates Test items than the other groups. These findings suggest that sleep facilitates creative thinking for harder problems. Creative problem solving is essential for elite athletes. During every game and every competition, elite athletes are faced with decisions that either can improve or lessen their chances of winning. Therefore, it is essential to investigate how sleep can enhance problem solving within an environment filled with distractions, coupled with the rapidity of execution, which is more typical for elite athletes than nonathletes.

IMPACT OF SLEEP ON MENTAL HEALTH

Previous studies have pointed out the bidirectional associations between sleep, daily stressors, and poor mood states.[197,198] Moreover, poor sleep quality and short sleep duration were significantly associated with cognitive interferences related to stress the next day, such as the experience of intrusive, unwanted, off-task, and potentially ruminated thoughts.[144] In addition, associations in the opposite direction were found, such as stressful and cognitive interferences throughout the day, which would lead to an earlier bedtime and earlier wake time.[144]

Prevalence of anxiety symptoms in adult athletes ranges from 7.1% to 26%.[199,200] Student-athletes report higher rates of anxiety, up to 37%.[142,201] In a study by Lastella and colleageus,[202,203] 21% of the athletes reported that anxiety was the primary reason for their awakening during the night. Additionally, Savis and colleagues[204] reported, among student-athletes, a lower sleep quality the night before a competition. Student-athletes reported that the primary reason for their sleep difficulty was anxiety and that this greatly affected their performance the following day.[144,205,206] Moreover, Davenne[207] reported that continuously being in a new sleep environment exacerbated the anxiety, thus having a negative impact on sleep and therefore performance.

Worldwide, depression may affect close to 300 million individuals across all ages.[208] Sleep and depression are interrelated, because sleep represents a core component of depression.[209] Awareness of mental health issues among high-performance athletes has grown. However, the evidence varies considerably regarding the prevalence of depression in the athletic population. In 2016, a systematic review indicated that more than 1 in 3 athletes (34%) had reported symptoms of depression based on a clinical interview.[210] A subsequent systematic review in 2020 reported a prevalence of depression ranging from 6.7% and 34% among high-performance athletes aged 17 years and older.[211] In the pursuit to investigate the prevalence of mental health problems, including depressive disorder, eating disorders, and stress-related disorders, among elite athletes, another study found that women (37.8%) were more likely than men (16.8%) to seek for help.[212] The lifetime prevalence of mental health problems is reported by almost half of the elite athlete population,[212] which coincides with the reported prevalence of insufficient sleep and poor sleep quality. To support the closely knitted relationship between sleep difficulties and mental health problems, a study with outpatient polysomnography showed that athletes with clinical sleep difficulties were more likely to report depressive symptoms.[213] Last, a large study reported that 7.4% had had suicide ideation within the past year,[214] which was significantly associated with sleep distress, sleep onset insomnia, as well as insufficient sleep.

Athletes not getting sufficient sleep consistently show higher rates of anxiety and depression, leading to increased difficulty in coping with new environmental challenges and stressors, a key component of performance for every athlete.[184,185] Altogether, these studies underlined the crucial role of sleep in mental health, and adequate sleep has always been recognized to positively influence mental health and well-being in different populations, including athletes. Further studies are needed to clarify this bidirectional relation in athletes to develop appropriate plans of action and adaptative strategies to optimize performance and mental health.

INTERVENTIONS AT THE TEAM LEVEL
Promoting a Culture of Healthy Sleep

Prioritizing sleep in athletes' preparation and recovery routines is not an easy task. There is an omnipresent attitude in society toward sleep that has been put forward where being able to tolerate insufficient sleep is a sign of mental strength and a badge of honor.[215] This attitude may influence young elite athletes who are trying to reach the highest-level performance in their respective sports. To counter this, teams can promote a culture of healthy sleep as a performance enhancer. This culture includes embracing the idea that sleep is essential to athletic performance and recovery and counteracting the perception that getting sufficient sleep should produce a feeling of guilt. Several high-profile athletes have now publicly discussed the importance of sleep in their preparation and recovery.[216] Unfortunately, these athletes' habits are not yet the norm and, throughout the sports literature and culture, sleep is not yet a priority among elite athletes and professional team sports, although this may be changing.

Systematically Screening for Sleep Problems

Systematically screening for sleep problems is required to understand the scope of a problem, identify areas that need improvement, and identify individuals at risk for sleep problems.[18,19] Ideally, teams need to screen athletes at the beginning of a season and follow-up with prospective sleep assessment. Challenges include integrating sleep assessments into existing programs, decisions about what tools to use, implementing sleep assessment at multiple time points, and strategies for assessing sleep disorders. In addition, developing collaborative relationships with sleep providers should be a priority.[217,218] It should be noted that if athletes are not adequately screened for sleep disturbances, most sleep recommendations would be undermined and ineffective.[19] The recent expert consensus on sleep and athletes recommends a sleep toolbox for practitioners that includes screening sleep disturbances in all types of sports with the appropriate tools.

To date, only 1 sleep questionnaire has been validated in athletes, the ASSQ.[54] Another promising tool is the Athlete Sleep Behavioral Questionnaire,[219] which addresses mainly poor sleep behavior.

Treating Sleep Disorders

To treat sleep disorders among elite athletes, proper sleep screening is essential. Different types of athletes may be differently susceptible to certain types of sleep disorders. For example, American football players may have a higher prevalence of sleep apnea due to their physical attributes,[220,221] and swimmers may experience circadian rhythm problems due to their early practice schedules.[51]

Sports medicine teams should be educated on diagnosing and treating sleep disorders and referring to sleep specialists when appropriate,[22] and education about sleep disorders should be provided to both athletes and staff.[18,19] Furthermore, the sports medicine specialist also should be the provider and the promoter of good sleep behavior and its beneficial effects on athletic and academic performance.

When sleep disorders are identified, appropriate evidence-based treatments should be applied, just as in nonathletes,[11,18,19] including positive airway pressure therapy and oral appliances for sleep apnea and cognitive behavioral therapy for insomnia. Sometimes, however, evidence-based treatments of sleep disorders in athletes can be problematic. For example, sedating medications may be clinically indicated but may impede athletic performance, and some empirically supported treatments actually may be banned substances in sport.[11] For this reason, clinical providers may need to be sensitive to these issues and may need to consider whether sedating treatments impair performance or whether stimulating treatments are restricted because they are performance enhancing.

Managing Training and Travel Schedules

The relationship between training loads, timing, intensity, sleep, and performance is likely complex and not entirely understood. An increase in training load and training intensity, and decrease in hours of sleep, is associated with increased injury risk.[222,223] Therefore, training more efficiently may be preferable to training longer or harder; this would be more preferable to the accumulation of training load without a profitable recovery, accompanied by a decrease in performance and need for an extended period of recovery.[224,225]

Traveling represents a crucial component of an athlete's reality. Despite considerable evidence of the inevitable impact of travel fatigue and jet lag on performance, optimal management strategies remain unclear. As mentioned earlier, a consensus statement was produced by several researchers/clinicians.[20] The consensus includes information including definitions of circadian physiology terminology, a comprehensive explanation of the human circadian system, and how time-givers affect it, and ultimately provides consensus on recommendations for the management of travel fatigue and jet lag in athletes. Similarly, another group produced an outline on how to manage travel fatigue and jet lag in athletes with 3 distinct categories[226]; they provide recommendations pretravel, during travel, and last, posttravel. These practical tips are encouraged to be implemented to reduce the potential impact of travel on performance.

SUMMARY AND FUTURE DIRECTIONS

Sleep health is an important consideration for athletic performance. Athletes are at high risk of insufficient sleep duration (ie, less than 7–8 hours per night), poor sleep quality (eg, difficulty initiating or maintaining sleep or other sleep difficulties), daytime sleepiness and fatigue, suboptimal sleep schedules (eg, too early or too late), irregular sleep schedules, and sleep and circadian disorders (especially insomnia and sleep apnea). These issues, individually and in combination, likely have an impact on athletic performance via several domains. Sleep loss and/or poor sleep quality can impair muscular strength, speed, and other aspects of physical performance. Sleep issues also can increase risk of concussions and other injuries and impair recovery after injury. Cognitive performance is also impacted in several domains, including vigilance, learning and memory, decision making, and creativity. Sleep also plays important roles in mental health, which is important not only for athletic performance but also for the well-being of athletes in general. **Fig. 1** depicts a summary of these findings. These relationships have begun to be formally incorporated into athletics organizations, with official position statements that address sleep health published by the NCAA and the IOC.[11,18]

Much future research on sleep in athletes is needed because athletes represent a diverse group of individuals, and most studies in athletes are small, confined to a single team and/or sport, and include inconsistent measurement approaches. In particular, it is not clear what the best strategy is for assessing sleep parameters in athletes, and it likely may depend on factors intrinsic to the sport or activity. In addition, it is not known if standard approaches should be adapted. There also is a lack of trials of sleep interventions thought to have a positive impact on sleep and still an insufficient number of studies describing how improving sleep can improve performance. Despite that, there is a large and growing body of evidence that clearly establishes sleep health as an important factor in sport.

Improving sleep in athletes through sleep education at every level of sports organizations has significant implications for health, athletic performance, academic performance, and beyond, given the influence each athlete has on the general

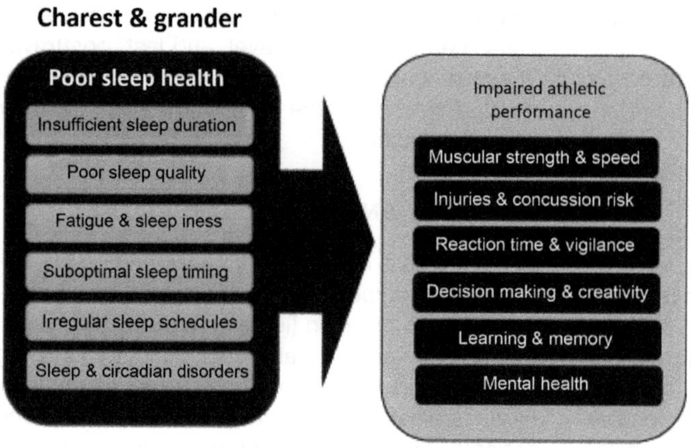

Charest & grander

Fig. 1. Relationships between sleep health and athletic performance.

population as a role model; this not only will provide an opportunity to explore a crucial aspect of mental and physical health but also will pave the way for new interventions in the area of mental well-being. Tracking sleep through questionnaires, wearables, and other objective devices is promising, but there still are a lot of question marks remaining. It is, therefore, crucial to develop strategies to mitigate sleep difficulties, not only for physical performance but also for mental well-being, which will require additional data for a better understanding of the science of sleep.

CLINICS CARE POINTS

- Systematically screening for insufficient sleep and sleep disorder at key points during the season.
- When incorporating a plan of action to enhance sleep, consider other factors that may weight in insufficient sleep and sleep disorder (type of sports, gender, ongoing injury).
- Use adequate and validated screening tool in athletes (Athlete Sleep Screening Questionnaire - ASSQ).
- Identifiy athletes' chronotype to implement an adequate traveling plan and reduce the impact of time zone differences/jetlag.

DISCLOSURE

Dr M.A. Grandner has received grants from Jazz Pharmaceuticals, National Institutes of Health, Nexalin Technology, and Kemin Foods. He has performed consulting activities for Fitbit, Natrol, Casper, Curaegis, Thrive, Pharmavite, SPV, Nightfood, and Merck. This work was supported by R01MD011600 and an Innovation Grant from the National Collegiate Athletic Association.

REFERENCES

1. Lucidi F, Lombardo C, Russo PM, et al. Sleep complaints in Italian Olympic and recreational athletes. J Clin Sport Psychol 2007;1(2):121–9.
2. Samuels C. Sleep, recovery, and performance: the new frontier in high-performance athletics. Neurol Clin 2008;26(1):169–80.
3. Swinbourne R, Gill N, Vaile J, et al. Prevalence of poor sleep quality, sleepiness and obstructive sleep apnea risk factors in athletes. Eur J Sport Sci 2016;16(7):850–8.
4. Leeder J, Glaister M, Pizzoferro K, et al. Sleep duration and quality in elite athletes measured using wristwatch actigraphy. J Sports Sci 2012; 30(6):541–5.
5. Bleyer F, Barbosa D, Andrade R, et al. Sleep and musculoskeletal complaints among elite athletes of Santa Catarina. Rev Dor Sao Paulo 2015;16(2):102–8.
6. Bonnet MH, Arand DL. Hyperarousal and insomnia: state of the science. Sleep Med Rev 2010;14(1):9–15.
7. Tsunoda K, Hotta K, Mutsuzaki H, et al. Sleep status in male wheelchair basketball players on a Japanese national team. J Sleep Disord Ther 2015;4(4):1–4.
8. George CF, Kab V, Kab P, et al. Sleep and breathing in professional football players. Sleep Med 2003;4(4):317–25.
9. Albuquerque FN, Kuniyoshi FHS, Calvin AD, et al. Sleep-disordered breathing, hypertension, and obesity in retired National Football League players. J Am Coll Cardiol 2010;56(17):1432–3.

10. Raikes AC, Athey A, Alfonso-Miller P, et al. Insomnia and daytime sleepiness: risk factors for sports- related concussion. Sleep Med 2019;58: 66–74.

11. Reardon CL, Hainline B, Aron CM, et al. Mental health in elite athletes: international Olympic Committee consensus statement. Br J Sports Med 2019;53(11):667–99.

12. Reilly T, Waterhouse J. Sport, exercise and environmental physiology. Edinburgh: Elsevier; 2005. p. 89–115.

13. NCAA. The student-athlete perspective of the college experience findings from the NCAA GOALS and SCORE studies. 2008. Available at: https://www.ncaa.org/sites/default/files/The%20Student%20Athlete%20Perspective%20of%20the%20College%20Experience.pdf.

14. NCAA. Defining countable athletically related activities. 2009. Available at: https://www.ncaa.org/sites/default/files/Charts.pdf.

15. NCAA. How student-athletes feel about time demands. 2017. Available at: https://www.ncaa.org/sites/default/files/2017GOALS_Time_demands_20170628.pdf.

16. NCAA. NCAA sports sponshirship and participation rates report. 2018. Available at: https://ncaaorg.s3.amazonaws.com/research/sportpart/Oct2018RES_2017-18SportsSponsorshipParticipationRatesReport.pdf.

17. Nixdorf I, Frank R, Hautzinger M, et al. Prevalence of depressive symptoms and correlating variables among German elite athletes. J Clin Sport Psychol 2013;7(4):313–26.

18. Kroshus E, Wagner J, Wyrick D, et al. Wake up call for collegiate athlete sleep: narrative review and consensus recommendations from the NCAA Inter-association Task Force on Sleep and Wellness. Br J Sports Med 2019;53(12):731–6.

19. Walsh NP, Halson SL, Sargent C, et al. Sleep and the athlete: narrative review and 2021 expert consensus recommendations. Br J Sports Med 2021;55:356–68.

20. Janse van Rensburg DC, Jansen van Rensburg A, Fowler PM, et al. Managing travel fatigue and jet lag in athletes: a review and consensus statement. Sports Med 2021;51(10):2029–50.

21. Chase JD, Roberson PA, Saunders MJ, et al. One night of sleep restriction following heavy exercise impairs 3-km cycling time-trial performance in the morning. Appl Physiol Nutr Metab 2017;42(9): 909–15.

22. Spiegel K, Leproult R, Van Cauter E. Impact of sleep debt on metabolic and endocrine function. Lancet 1999;354(9188):1435–9.

23. Spiegel K, Leproult R, L'hermite-Balériaux M, et al. Leptin levels are dependent on sleep duration: relationships with sympathovagal balance, carbohydrate regulation, cortisol, and thyrotropin. J Clin Endocrinol Metab 2004;89(11):5762–71.

24. Lastella M, Roach GD, Halson SL, et al. Sleep/wake behaviours of elite athletes from individual and team sports. Eur J Sport Sci 2015;15(2): 94–100.

25. Sargent C, Lastella M, Halson SL, et al. The impact of training schedules on the sleep and fatigue of elite athletes. Chronobiol Int 2014;31(10):1160–8.

26. Sargent C, Lastella M, Romyn G, et al. How well does a commercially available wearable device measure sleep in young athletes? Chronobiol Int 2018;35(6):754–8.

27. Mah CD, Kezirian EJ, Marcello BM, et al. Poor sleep quality and insufficient sleep of a collegiate student-athlete population. Sleep Health 2018; 4(3):251–7.

28. Turner RW, Vissa K, Hall C, et al. Sleep problems are associated with academic performance in a national sample of collegiate athletes. J Am Coll Health 2019;1–8.

29. Fox JL, Scanlan AT, Stanton R, Sargent C. Insufficient sleep in young athletes? Causes, consequences, and potential treatments. Sports Med 2020;50(3):461–70.

30. Brand S, Beck J, Gerber M, Hatzinger M, Holsboer-Trachsler E. Football is good for your sleep": favorable sleep patterns and psychological functioning of adolescent male intense football players compared to controls: favorable sleep patterns and psychological functioning of adolescent male intense football players compared to controls. J Health Psychol 2009;14(8):1144–55.

31. Whitworth-Turner C, Di Michele R, Muir I, Gregson W, Drust B. A comparison of sleep patterns in youth soccer players and non-athletes. Sci Med Footb 2018;2(1):3–8.

32. Brand S, Beck J, Gerber M, Hatzinger M, Holsboer-Trachsler E. Evidence of favorable sleep-EEG patterns in adolescent male vigorous football players compared to controls. World J Biol Psychiatry 2010;11(2–2):465–75.

33. Sargent C, Roach GD. Sleep duration is reduced in elite athletes following night-time competition. Chronobiol Int 2016;33(6):667–70.

34. Staunton C, Gordon B, Custovic E, Stanger J, Kingsley M. Sleep patterns and match performance in elite Australian basketball athletes. J Sci Med Sport 2017;20(8):786–9.

35. Hoshikawa M, Uchida S, Hirano Y. A subjective assessment of the prevalence and factors associated with poor sleep quality amongst elite Japanese athletes. Sports Med Open 2018; 4(1):10.

36. Drew M, Vlahovich N, Hughes D, et al. Prevalence of illness, poor mental health and sleep quality and low energy availability prior to the 2016 summer

Olympic games. Br J Sports Med 2018;52(1): 47–53.

37. Drew MK, Vlahovich N, Hughes D, et al. A multifactorial evaluation of illness risk factors in athletes preparing for the Summer Olympic Games. J Sci Med Sport 2017;20(8):745–50.

38. Fischer D, Lombardi DA, Marucci-Wellman H, et al. Chronotypes in the US-influence of age and sex. PLoS One 2017;12(6):e0178782.

39. Silva A, Queiroz SS, Winckler C, et al. Sleep quality evaluation, chronotype, sleepiness and anxiety of Paralympic Brazilian athletes: Beijing 2008 Paralympic Games. Br J Sports Med 2012;46(2): 150–4.

40. Lastella M, Roach GD, Halson SL, et al. The chronotype of elite athletes. J Hum Kinet 2016;54(1): 219–25.

41. Lastella M, Roach GD, Hurem DC, et al. Does chronotype affect elite athletes' capacity to cope with the training demands of elite triathlon?. In: Sargent C, Darwent D, Roach GD, editors. Living in a 24/7 world: the impact of circadian disruption on sleep. Adelaide: Australasian Chronobiology Society Press; 2018. p. 25–8.

42. Drust B, Waterhouse J, Atkinson G, et al. Circadian rhythms in sports performance—an update. Chronobiol Int 2005;22(1):21–44.

43. Beersma DG, Gordijn MC. Circadian control of the sleep-wake cycle. Physiol Behav 2007;90(2–3): 190–5.

44. Reilly T, Edwards B. Altered sleep-wake cycles and physical performance in athletes. Physiol Behav 2007;90(2–3):274–84.

45. Lack LC, Wright HR. Chronobiology of sleep in humans. Cell Mol Life Sci 2007;64(10):1205.

46. Lastella M, Roach GD, Halson SL, et al. Sleep/wake behaviour of endurance cyclists before and during competition. J Sports Sci 2015;33(3):293–9.

47. Lok R, Zerbini G, Gordijn MCM, Beersma DGM, Hut RA. Gold, silver or bronze: circadian variation strongly affects performance in Olympic athletes. Sci Rep 2020;10(1):16088.

48. Gupta L, Morgan K, Gilchrist S. Does elite sport degrade sleep quality? A systematic review. Sports Med 2017;47(7):1317–33.

49. Samuels C, James L, Lawson D, et al. The Athlete Sleep Screening Questionnaire: a new tool for assessing and managing sleep in elite athletes. Br J Sports Med 2016;50(7):418–22.

50. Collette R, Kellmann M, Ferrauti A, et al. Relation between training load and recovery-stress state in high-performance swimming. Front Physiol 2018; 9:845.

51. Sargent C, Halson S, Roach GD. Sleep or swim? Early-morning training severely restricts the amount of sleep obtained by elite swimmers. Eur J Sport Sci 2014;14(sup1):S310–5.

52. Erlacher D, Ehrlenspiel F, Adegbesan OA, et al. Sleep habits in German athletes before important competitions or games. J Sports Sci 2011;29(8): 859–66.

53. Samuels CH. Jet lag and travel fatigue: a comprehensive management plan for sport medicine physicians and high-performance support teams. Clin J Sport Med 2012;22(3):268–73.

54. Bender AM, Lawson D, Werthner P, et al. The clinical validation of the athlete sleep screening questionnaire: an instrument to identify athletes that need further sleep assessment. Sports Med Open 2018;4(1):23.

55. Khalladi K, Farooq A, Souissi S, et al. Inter-relationship between sleep quality, insomnia and sleep disorders in professional soccer players. BMJ Open Sport Exerc Med 2019;5(1):e000498.

56. Allen MS, Greenlees I, Jones M. Personality in sport: a comprehensive review. Int Rev Sport Exerc Psychol 2013;6(1):184–208.

57. American College Health Association. American college health association-national college health assessment, Fall 2015, spring 2016, Fall 2016, Spring 2017, Fall 2017 [data file]. Hanover (MD): American College Health Association. [producer and distributor] 2018-11-15.

58. Harvey CJ, Gehrman P, Espie CA. Who is predisposed to insomnia: a review of familial aggregation, stress-reactivity, personality and coping style. Sleep Med Rev 2014;18(3):237–47.

59. Fowler P, Duffield R, Howle K, et al. Effects of north bound long-haul international air travel on sleep quantity and subjective jet lag and wellness in professional Australian soccer players. Int J Sports Physiol Perform 2015; 10(5):648–54.

60. Fowler PM, Duffield R, Lu D, et al. Effects of long-haul transmeridian travel on subjective jet-lag and self-reported sleep and upper respiratory symptoms in professional rugby league players. Int J Sports Physiol Perform 2016; 11(7):876–84.

61. Dunican IC, Martin DT, Halson SL, et al. The effects of the removal of electronic devices for 48 hours on sleep in elite judo athletes. J Strength Cond Res 2017;31(10):2832–9.

62. Emsellem HA, Murtagh KE. Sleep apnea and sports performance. Clin Sports Med 2005;24(2): 329–41.

63. Ahbab S, Ataoğlu HE, Tuna M, et al. Neck circumference, metabolic syndrome and obstructive sleep apnea syndrome; evaluation of possible link age. Med Sci Monit 2013;19:111.

64. Mihaere KM, Harris R, Gander PH, et al. Obstructive sleep apnea in New Zealand adults: prevalence and risk factors among Maori and non-Māori. Sleep 2009;32(7):949–56.

65. Rice TB, Dunn RE, Lincoln AE, et al. Sleep-disordered breathing in the national football league. Sleep 2010;33(6):819–24.

66. Dobrosielski DA, Nichols D, Ford J, et al. Estimating the prevalence of sleep-disordered breathing among collegiate football players. Respir Care 2016;61(9):1144–50.

67. Tuomilehto H, Vuorinen VP, Penttila E, et al. Sleep of professional athletes: underexploited potential to improve health and performance. J Sports Sci 2017;35(7):704–10.

68. Jackson ML, Howard ME, Barnes M. Cognition and daytime functioning in sleep-related breathing dis orders. Brain Res 2011;190:53–68. Elsevier.

69. Dunican IC, Walsh J, Higgins CC, et al. Prevalence of sleep disorders and sleep problems in an elite super rugby union team. J Sports Sci 2019;37(8):950–7.

70. Santos I, Rocha I, Gozal D, Meira E Cruz M. Obstructive sleep apnea, shift work and cardiometabolic risk. Sleep Med 2020;74:132–40.

71. Hoyos CM, Drager LF, Patel SR. OSA and cardiometabolic risk: what's the bottom line? Respirology 2017;22(3):420–9.

72. Fagundes SB, Fagundes DJ, Carvalho LB, et al. Prevalence of restless legs syndrome in runners. Sleep Med 2010;33:A252. One Westbrook Corporate CTR, STE 920, Westchester, IL 60154 USA: Amer Acad Sleep Medicine.

73. Englund CE, et al. Cognitive performance during successive sustained physical work episodes. Behav Res Methods Instrum Comput 1985;17(1):75–85.

74. Edwards BJ, Waterhouse J. Effects of one night of partial sleep deprivation upon diurnal rhythms of accuracy and consistency in throwing darts. Chronobiol Int 2009;26(4):756–68.

75. Horne JA, Pettitt AN. Sleep deprivation and the physiological response to exercise under steady-state conditions in untrained subjects. Sleep 1984;7(2):168–79.

76. Martin BJ. Effect of sleep deprivation on tolerance of prolonged exercise. Eur J Appl Physiol Occup Physiol 1981;47(4):345–54.

77. Mougin F, Davenne D, Simon-Rigaud ML, et al. Disturbance of sports performance after partial sleep deprivation. C R Seances Soc Biol Fil 1989;183(5):461–6.

78. Mougin F, Simon-Rigaud ML, Davenne D, et al. Effects of sleep disturbances on subsequent physical performance. Eur J Appl Physiol Occup Physiol 1991;63(2):77–82.

79. Mougin F, Bourdin H, Simon-Rigaud ML, et al. Effects of a selective sleep deprivation on subsequent anaerobic performance. Int J Sports Med 1996;17(02):115–9.

80. Mougin F, Bourdin H, Simon-Rigaud ML, et al. Hormonal responses to exercise after partial sleep deprivation and after a hypnotic drug-induced sleep. J Sports Sci 2001;19(2):89–97.

81. Souissi N, Souissi M, Souissi H, et al. Effect of time of day and partial sleep deprivation on short-term, high-power output. Chronobiol Int 2008;25(6):1062–76.

82. Abedelmalek S, Souissi N, Chtourou H, et al. Effects of partial sleep deprivation on proinflammatory cytokines, growth hormone, and steroid hormone concentrations during repeated brief sprint interval exercise. Chronobiol Int 2013;30(4):502–9.

83. Souissi N, Chtourou H, Aloui A, et al. Effects of time-of-day and partial sleep deprivation on short-term maximal performances of judo competitors. J Strength Cond Res 2013;27(9):2473–80.

84. Abbiss CR, Laursen PB. Models to explain fatigue during prolonged endurance cycling. Sports Med 2005;35(10):865–98.

85. Stickgold R. Sleep-dependent memory consolidation. Nature 2005;437(7063):1272.

86. Walker MP, Stickgold R. It's practice, with sleep, that makes perfect: implications of sleep- dependent learning and plasticity for skill performance. Clin Sports Med 2005;24(2):301–17.

87. Taheri M, Arabameri E. The effect of sleep deprivation on choice reaction time and anaerobic power of college student athletes. Asian J Sports Med 2012;3(1):15.

88. Reyner LA, Horne JA. Sleep restriction and serving accuracy in performance tennis players, and effects of caffeine. Physiol Behav 2013;120:93–6.

89. Ben RC, Latiri I, Dogui M, et al. Effects of one-night sleep deprivation on selective attention and isometric force in adolescent karate athletes. J Sports Med Phys Fitness 2017;57(6):752–9.

90. Omisade A, Buxton OM, Rusak B. Impact of acute sleep restriction on cortisol and leptin levels in young women. Physiol Behav 2010;99(5):651–6.

91. Oliver SJ, Costa RJ, Laing SJ, et al. One night of sleep deprivation decreases treadmill endurance performance. Eur J Appl Physiol 2009;107(2):155–61.

92. Skein M, Duffield R, Edge J, et al. Intermittent-sprint performance and muscle glycogen after 30 h of sleep deprivation. Med Sci Sports Exerc 2011;43(7):1301–11.

93. Katirji B. Clinical neurophysiology: clinical electromyography. Philadelphia: Saunders Elsevier; 2012.

94. Costill DL, Flynn MG, Kirwan JP, et al. Effects of repeated days of intensified training on muscle glycogen and swimming performance. Med Sci Sports Exerc 1988;20(3):249–54.

95. Le Meur Y, Duffield R, Skein M. Sleep. In: Hausswirth C, Mujika I, editors. Recovery for

performance in sport. Champaign (IL): Human Kinetics; 2012. p. 99–107.

96. Guezennec CY, Satabin P, Legrand H, et al. Physical performance and metabolic changes induced by combined prolonged exercise and different energy intakes in humans. Eur J Appl Physiol Occup Physiol 1994;68(6):525–30.

97. Hausswirth C, Louis J, Aubry A, et al. Evidence of disturbed sleep and increased illness in over reached endurance athletes. Med Sci Sports Exerc 2014;46(5):1036–45.

98. Jung CM, Melanson EL, Frydendall EJ, et al. Energy expenditure during sleep, sleep deprivation and sleep following sleep deprivation in adult humans. J Physiol 2011;589(1):235–44.

99. Markwald RR, Melanson EL, Smith MR, et al. Impact of insufficient sleep on total daily energy expenditure, food intake, and weight gain. Proc Natl Acad Sci U S A 2013;110(14):5695–700.

100. Waterhouse J, Atkinson G, Edwards B, et al. The role of a short post-lunch nap in improving cognitive, motor, and sprint performance in participants with partial sleep deprivation. J Sports Sci 2007; 25(14):1557–66.

101. Zhong X, Hilton HJ, Gates GJ, et al. Increased sympathetic and decreased parasympathetic cardiovascular modulation in normal humans with acute sleep deprivation. J Appl Physiol (1985) 2005;98(6):2024–32.

102. Achten J, Jeukendrup AE. Heart rate monitoring. Sports Med 2003;33(7):517–38.

103. Hynynen ESA, Uusitalo A, Konttinen N, et al. Heart rate variability during night sleep and after awakening in overtrained athletes. Med Sci Sports Exerc 2006;38(2):313.

104. Azboy O, Kaygisiz Z. Effects of sleep deprivation on cardiorespiratory functions of the runners and volleyball players during rest and exercise. Acta Physiol Hung 2009;96(1):29–36.

105. Kirschen GW, Jones JJ, Hale L. The impact of sleep duration on performance among competitive athletes: a systematic literature review. Clin J Sport Med 2020;30:503–12.

106. Cook CJ, Crewther BT, Kilduff LP, Drawer S, Gaviglio CM. Skill execution and sleep deprivation: effects of acute caffeine or creatine supplementation - a randomized placebo-controlled trial. J Int Soc Sports Nutr 2011;8(1):2.

107. Schwartz J, Simon RD Jr. Sleep extension improves serving accuracy: a study with college varsity tennis players. Physiol Behav 2015;151:541–4.

108. Harmon KG, Drezner JA, Gammons M, et al. American Medical Society for Sports Medicine position statement: concussion in sport. Br J Sports Med 2013;47(1):15–26.

109. Depadilla L, Miller GF, Jones SE, et al. Self-reported concussions from playing a sport or being

physically active among high school students—United States, 2017. MMWR Morb Mortal Wkly Rep 2018;67(24):682.

110. Rivara FP, Schiff MA, Chrisman SP, et al. The effect of coach education on reporting of concussions among high school athletes after passage of a concussion law. Am J Sports Med 2014;42(5): 1197–203.

111. Mathias JL, Alvaro PK. Prevalence of sleep disturbances, disorders, and problems following traumatic brain injury: a meta-analysis. Sleep Med 2012;13(7):898–905.

112. Verma A, Anand V, Verma NP. Sleep disorders in chronic traumatic brain injury. J Clin Sleep Med 2007;3(04):357–62.

113. Weber M, Webb CA, Killgore WDS. A brief and selective review of treatment approaches for sleep disturbance following traumatic brain injury. J Sleep Disord Ther 2013;2:110.

114. McCrory P, Meeuwisse WH, Aubry M, et al. Consensus statement on concussion in sport—the 4th international conference on concussion in sport held in Zurich, November 2012. PMR 2013; 5(4):255–79.

115. McCrory P, Meeuwisse W, Dvorak J, et al. Consensus statement on concussion in sport—the 5th international conference on concussion in sport held in Berlin, October 2016. Br J Sports Med 2017;51(11):838–47.

116. McClure DJ, Zuckerman SL, Kutscher SJ, et al. Baseline neurocognitive testing in sports-related concussions: the importance of a prior night's sleep. Am J Sports Med 2014;42(2):472–8.

117. Brown DA, Elsass JA, Miller AJ, et al. Differences in symptom reporting between males and females at baseline and after a sports-related concussion: a systematic review and meta-analysis. Sports Med 2015;45(7):1027–40.

118. Graham R, Rivara FP, Ford MA, et al. Sports-related concussion in youth: improving the science, changing the culture. Washington, DC: The National Acadamies Press; 2014.

119. McCrory P, Meeuwisse WH, Echemendia RJ, et al. What is the lowest threshold to make a diagnosis of concussion? Br J Sports Med 2013;47(5):268–71.

120. Eisenberg MA, Meehan WP, Mannix R. Duration and course of post-concussive symptoms. Pediatrics 2014;133(6):999–1006.

121. Lau BC, Collins MW, Lovell MR. Cutoff scores in neurocognitive testing and symptom clusters that predict protracted recovery from concussions in high school athletes. Neurosurgery 2011;70(2):371–9.

122. Gosselin N, Lassonde M, Petit D, et al. Sleep following sport-related concussions. Sleep Med 2009;10(1):35–46.

123. Lau BC, Collins MW, Lovell MR. Sensitivity and specificity of subacute computerized

neurocognitive testing and symptom evaluation in predicting outcomes after sports-related concussion. Am J Sports Med 2011;39(6):1209–16.

124. Sufrinko AM, Howie EK, Elbin RJ, et al. A preliminary investigation of accelerometer-derived sleep and physical activity following sport-related concussion. J Head Trauma Rehabil 2018;33(5):E64–74.

125. Kostyun RO, Milewski MD, Hafeez I. Sleep disturbance and neurocognitive function during the recovery from a sport-related concussion in adolescents. Am J Sports Med 2015;43(3):633–40.

126. Jones C, Griffiths P, Towers P, et al. Pre-season injury and illness associations with perceptual well- ness, neuromuscular fatigue, sleep and training load in elite rugby union. Australian Journal of Strength and Conditioning; 2018.

127. Milewski MD, Skaggs DL, Bishop GA, et al. Chronic lack of sleep is associated with increased sports injuries in adolescent athletes. J Pediatr Orthop 2014;34(2):129–33.

128. Mountjoy M, Sundgot-Borgen JK, Burke LM, et al. IOC consensus statement on relative energy deficiency in sport (RED-S): 2018 update. Br J Sports Med 2018;52(11):687–97.

129. Smyth EA, Newman P, Waddington G, et al. Injury prevention strategies specific to pre-elite athletes competing in Olympic and professional sports - a systematic review. J Sci Med Sport 2019;22(8): 887–901.

130. Pyne DB, Verhagen EA, Mountjoy M. Nutrition, illness, and injury in aquatic sports. Int J Sport Nutr Exerc Metab 2014;24(4):460–9.

131. ChaputJP Dutil C. Lack of sleep as a contributor to obesity in adolescents: impacts on eating and activity behaviors. Int J Behav Nutr Phys Act 2016; 13(1):103.

132. Grandner MA, Jackson N, Gerstner JR, et al. Dietary nutrients associated with short and long sleep duration. Data from a nationally representative sample. Appetite 2013;64:71–80.

133. Grandner MA, Jackson N, Gerstner JR, et al. Sleep symptoms associated with intake of specific dietary nutrients. J Sleep Res 2014;23(1):22–34.

134. Halson SL. Monitoring training load to understand fatigue in athletes. Sports Med 2014;44(2):139–47.

135. Ordonez FM, Oliver AJS, Bastos PC, et al. Sleep improvement in athletes: use of nutritional supplements. Am J Sports Med 2017;34:93–9.

136. Baron KG, Reid KJ, Van Horn L, et al. Contribution of evening macronutrient intake to total caloric intake and body mass index. Appetite 2013;60: 246–51.

137. Lin HH, Tsai PS, Fang SC, et al. Effect of kiwifruit consumption on sleep quality in adults with sleep problems. Asia Pac J Clin Nutr 2011;20(2):169.

138. Heaney S, O'Connor H, Michael S, et al. Nutrition knowledge in athletes: a systematic review. Int J Sport Nutr Exerc Metab 2011;21(3):248–61.

139. Shechter A, Grandner MA, St-Onge MP. The role of sleep in the control of food intake. Am J Lifestyle Med 2014;8(6):371–4.

140. Von Rosen P, Frohm A, Kottorp A, et al. Too little sleep and an unhealthy diet could increase the risk of sustaining a new injury in adolescent elite athletes. Scand J Med Sci Sports 2017;27(11): 1364–71.

141. Owens J, Adolescent Sleep Working Group. Insufficient sleep in adolescents and young adults: an update on causes and consequences. Pediatrics 2014;134(3):e921–32.

142. Li H, Moreland JJ, Peek-Asa C, et al. Preseason anxiety and depressive symptoms and prospective injury risk in collegiate athletes. Am J Sports Med 2017;45(9):2148–55.

143. Baglioni C, Battagliese G, Feige B, et al. Insomnia as a predictor of depression: a meta-analytic evaluation of longitudinal epidemiological studies. J Affect Disord 2011;135(1–3):10–9.

144. Lee S, Buxton OM, Andel R, et al. Bidirectional associations of sleep with cognitive interference in employees' work days. Sleep Health 2019;5(3): 298–308.

145. Killgore WD. Effects of sleep deprivation on cognition. Prog Brain Res 2010;185:105–29. Elsevier.

146. Morselli L, Leproult R, Balbo M, et al. Role of sleep duration in the regulation of glucose metabolism and appetite. Best Pract Res Clin Endocrinol Metab 2010;24(5):687–702.

147. McMahon SB, Cafferty WB, Marchand F. Immune and glial cell factors as pain mediators and modulators. Exp Neurol 2005;192(2):444–62.

148. Haack M, Sanchez E, Mullington JM. Elevated inflammatory markers in response to prolonged sleep restriction are associated with increased pain experience in healthy volunteers. Sleep 2007;30(9):1145–52.

149. Haack M, Lee E, Cohen DA, et al. Activation of the prostaglandin system in response to sleep loss in healthy humans: potential mediator of increased spontaneous pain. Pain 2009;145(1- 2):136–41.

150. Sufrinko A, Pearce K, Elbin RJ, et al. The effect of preinjury sleep difficulties on neurocognitive impairment and symptoms after sport-related concussion. Am J Sports Med 2015;43(4):830–8.

151. Basner M, Dinges DF. Maximizing sensitivity of the psychomotor vigilance test (PVT) to sleep loss. Sleep 2011;34(5):581–91.

152. Dinges DF, Pack F, Williams K, et al. Cumulative sleepiness, mood disturbance, and psychomotor vigilance performance decrements during a week of sleep restricted to 4-5 hours per night. Sleep 1997;20(4):267–77.

153. Wlodarczyk D, Jaskowski P, Nowik A. Influence of sleep deprivation and auditory intensity on reaction time and response force. Percept Mot Skills 2002; 94(3_suppl):1101–12.

154. Wolanin A, Hong E, Marks D, et al. Prevalence of clinically elevated depressive symptoms in college athletes and differences by gender and sport. Br J Sports Med 2016;50(3):167–71.

155. Jarraya S, Jarraya M, Chtourou H, Souissi N. Effect of time of day and partial sleep deprivation on the reaction time and the attentional capacities of the handball goalkeeper. Biol Rhythm Res 2014; 45(2):183–91.

156. Kamdar BB, Kaplan KA, Kezirian EJ, et al. The impact of extended sleep on daytime alertness, vigilance, and mood. Sleep Med 2004;5(5): 441–8.

157. Mah CD, Mah KE, Kezirian EJ, et al. The effects of sleep extension on the athletic performance of collegiate basketball players. Sleep 2011;34(7): 943–50.

158. Arnal PJ, Sauvet F, Leger D, et al. Benefits of sleep extension on sustained attention and sleep pressure before and during total sleep deprivation and recovery. Sleep 2015;38(12):1935–43.

159. Arnal PJ, Lapole T, Erblang M, et al. Sleep extension before sleep loss: effects on performance and neuromuscular function. Med Sci Sports Exerc 2016;48(8):1595–603.

160. Rupp TL, Wesensten NJ, Bliese PD, et al. Banking sleep: realization of benefits during subsequent sleep restriction and recovery. Sleep 2009;32(3): 311–21.

161. Marchetti R, Forte R, Borzacchini M, et al. Physical and motor fitness, sport skills and executive function in adolescents: a moderated prediction model. Psychology 2015;6(14):1915.

162. Micai M, Kavussanu M, Ring C. Executive function is associated with antisocial behavior and aggression in athletes. J Sport Exerc Psychol 2015;37(5): 469–76.

163. Goel N, Rao H, Durmer JS, et al. Neurocognitive consequences of sleep deprivation. Semin Neurol 2009;29(04):320–39. © Thieme Medical Publishers.

164. Wilckens KA, Erickson KI, Wheeler ME. Age-related decline in controlled retrieval: the role of the PFC and sleep. Neural Plast 2012;2012: 624795.

165. Diamond A. Executive functions. Annu Rev Psychol 2013;64:135–68.

166. Lehto JE, Juujarvi P, Kooistra L, et al. Dimensions of executive functioning: evidence from children. Br J Dev Psychol 2003;21(1):59–80.

167. Kiesel A, Steinhauser M, Wendt M, et al. Control and interference in task switching—a review. Psy Chol Bull 2010;136(5):849.

168. Killgore WD, Balkin TJ, Wesensten NJ. Impaired decision making following 49 h of sleep deprivation. J Sleep Res 2006;15(1):7–13.

169. Rossa KR, Smith SS, Allan AC, et al. The effects of sleep restriction on executive inhibitory control and affect in young adults. J Adolesc Health 2014; 55(2):287–92.

170. Vitale KC, Owens R, Hopkins SR, Malhotra A. Sleep hygiene for optimizing recovery in athletes: review and recommendations. Int J Sports Med 2019; 40(8):535–43.

171. Demos KE, Hart CN, Sweet LH, et al. Partial sleep deprivation impacts impulsive action but not impulsive decision-making. Physiol Behav 2016;164(Pt A):214–9.

172. Lastella M, Onay Z, Scanlan AT, Elsworthy N, Pitchford NW, Vincent GE. Wakeup call: Reviewing the effects of sleep on decision-making in athletes and implications for sports officials. Montenegrin J Sports Sci Med 2020;9(2):65–71.

173. Killgore WD, Kamimori GH, Balkin TJ. Caffeine protects against increased risk-taking propensity during severe sleep deprivation. J Sleep Res 2011; 20(3):395–403.

174. Clark I, Landolt HP. Coffee, caffeine, and sleep: a systematic review of epidemiological studies and randomized controlled trials. Sleep Med Rev 2017;31:70–8.

175. Drake C, Roehrs T, Shambroom J, et al. Caffeine effects on sleep taken 0, 3, or 6 hours before going to bed. J Clin Sleep Med 2013;9(11):1195–200.

176. Dunican IC, Higgins CC, Jones MJ, et al. Caffeine use in a super rugby game and its relationship to post-game sleep. Eur J Sport Sci 2018;18(4): 513–23.

177. Huber R, Ghilardi MF, Massimini M, et al. Local sleep and learning. Nature 2004;430(6995):78.

178. Maquet P. The role of sleep in learning and memory. Science 2001;294(5544):1048–52.

179. Stickgold R, Hobson JA, Fosse R, et al. Sleep, learning, and dreams: off-line memory reprocessing. Science 2001;294(5544):1052–7.

180. Gais S, Lucas B, Born J. Sleep after learning aids memory recall. Learn Mem 2006;13(3):259–62.

181. Karni A, Meyer G, Rey-Hipolito C, et al. The acquisition of skilled motor performance: fast and slow experience-driven changes in primary motor cortex. Proc Natl Acad Sci U S A 1998;95(3):861–8.

182. Carskadon MA, Dement WC. Normal human sleep: an overview. In: Kryger MH, Roth T, Dement WC, editors. Principles and practice of sleep medicine. St Louis (MO): Saunders/Elsevier; 2011. p. 16–26.

183. Albouy G, King BR, Maquet P, et al. Hippocampus and striatum: dynamics and interaction during acquisition and sleep-related motor sequence memory consolidation. Hippocampus 2013; 23(11):985–1004.

184. Doyon J, Gabitov E, Vahdat S, et al. Current issues related to motor sequence learning in humans. Curr Opin Behav Sci 2018;20:89–97.

185. Walker MP, Brakefield T, Morgan A, et al. Practice with sleep makes perfect: sleep-dependent motor skill learning. Neuron 2002;35(1):205–11.

186. Curcio G, Ferrara M, De Gennaro L. Sleep loss, learning capacity and academic performance. Sleep Med Rev 2006;10(5):323–37.

187. Albouy G, Vandewalle G, Sterpenich V, et al. Sleep stabilizes visuomotor adaptation memory: a functional magnetic resonance imaging study. J Sleep Res 2013;22(2):144–54.

188. Ashworth A, Hill CM, Karmiloff-Smith A, et al. Sleep enhances memory consolidation in children. J Sleep Res 2014;23(3):304–10.

189. Walker MP, Stickgold R. Sleep, memory, and plasticity. Annu Rev Psychol 2006;57:139–66.

190. Huang S, Deshpande A, Yeo SC, et al. Sleep restriction impairs vocabulary learning when adolescents cram for exams: the need for sleep study. Sleep 2016;39(9):1681–90.

191. Okano K, Kaczmaryk J, Dave N, et al. Sleep quality, duration, and consistency are associated with better academic performance in college students. NPJ Sci Learn 2019;4(1):16.

192. Oudiette D, Constantinescu I, Leclair-Visonneau L, et al. Evidence for the re-enactment of a recently learned behavior during sleepwalking. PLoS One 2011;6(3):e18056.

193. Marguilho R, Jesus SN, Viseu J, et al. Sleep and creativity: a quantitative review. In: Milcu M, Krall H, Dan P, editors. Prospecting interdisciplinary in health, education and social sciences. Bucharest: Editura Universitara; 2014. p. 117–26.

194. Cai DJ, Mednick SA, Harrison EM, et al. REM, not incubation, improves creativity by priming associative networks. *Proc Natl Acad Sci* U S A 2009; 106(25):10130–4.

195. Drago V, Foster PS, Heilman KM, et al. Cyclic alternating pattern in sleep and its relationship to creativity. Sleep Med 2011;12(4):361–6.

196. Sio UN, Monaghan P, Ormerod T. Sleep on it, but only if it is difficult: effects of sleep on problem solving. Mem Cognit 2013;41(2):159–66.

197. Lee S, Crain TL, McHale SM, et al. Daily antecedents and consequences of nightly sleep. J Sleep Res 2017;26(4):498–509.

198. Sin NL, Almeida DM, Crain TL, et al. Bidirectional, temporal associations of sleep with positive events, affect, and stressors in daily life across a week. Ann Behav Med 2017;51(3):402–15.

199. Gouttebarge V, Frings-Dresen MHW, Sluiter JK. Mental and psychosocial health among current and former professional footballers. Occup Med 2015;65(3):190–6.

200. Gulliver A, Griffiths KM, Mackinnon A, et al. The mental health of Australian elite athletes. J Sci Med Sport 2015;18(3):255–61.

201. Storch EA, Storch JB, Killiany EM, et al. Self-reported psychopathology in athletes: a comparison of intercollegiate student-athletes and non-athletes. J Sport Behav 2005;28(1):86–97.

202. Lastella M, Lovell GP, Sargent C. Athletes' precompetitive sleep behaviour and its relationship with subsequent precompetitive mood and performance. Eur J Sport Sci 2014;14(sup1):S123–30.

203. Lastella M, Roach GD, Halson SL, et al. The effects of transmeridian travel and altitude on sleep: preparation for football competition. J Sports Sci Med 2014;13(3):718.

204. Savis JC, Eliot JF, Gansneder B, et al. A subjective means of assessing college athletes' sleep: a modification of the morningness/eveningness questionnaire. Int J Sport Psychol 1997;28(2): 157–70.

205. Brassington GS. Sleep problems. In: Mostofsky DL, Zaichkowsky LD, editors. Medical and psychological aspects of sport and exercise. Morgantown (WV). Fitness Information Technology; 2002. p. 193–204.

206. Walters PH. Sleep, the athlete, and performance. Strength Condit J 2002;24(2):17–24.

207. Davenne D. Sleep of athletes-problems and possible solutions. Biol Rhythm Res 2009;40(1): 45–52.

208. World Health Organization [Internet]. Depression. Geneva, Switzerland: World Health Organization; 2021 [cited 2021 Sept 13]. Available at: https://www.who.int/news-room/fact-sheets/detail/depression.

209. American Psychiatric Association. Diagnostic and statistical manual of mental disorders. 5th edition. Washington, DC: APA; 2013.

210. Hammond T, Gialloreto C, Kubas H, et al. The prevalence of failure-based depression among elite athletes. Clin J Sport Med 2013;23(4):273–7.

211. Golding L, Gillingham RG, Perera NKP. The prevalence of depressive symptoms in high-performance athletes: a systematic review. Phys Sportsmed 2020;48(3):247–58.

212. Åkesdotter C, Kenttä G, Eloranta S, Franck J. The prevalence of mental health problems in elite athletes. J Sci Med Sport 2020;23(4):329–35.

213. Gerber M, Best S, Meerstetter F, et al. Cross-sectional and longitudinal associations between athlete burnout, insomnia, and polysomnographic indices in young elite athletes. J Sport Exerc Psychol 2018;40(6):312–24.

214. Khader WS, Tubbs AS, Haghighi A, et al. Onset insomnia and insufficient sleep duration are associated with suicide ideation in university students and athletes. J Affect Disord 2020;274:1161–4.

215. Adler M. In today's world, the well-rested lose respect. Morning edition. Washington, DC: National Public Radio; 2009.

216. Schultz J. These famous athletes rely on sleep for peak performance, Huffington Post. 2014. Available at: http://www.huffingtonpost.com/2014/08/13/these-famous-athletes-rely-on-sleep_n_5659345.html. Accessed October 1, 2019.

217. Grandner MA, Alfonso-Miller P, Fernandez-Mendoza J, et al. Sleep: important considerations for the prevention of cardiovascular disease. Curr Opin Cardiol 2016;31(5):551.

218. Grandner MA. Healthy sleep for student-athletes: a guide for athletics departments and coaches. NCAA Sport Sci Inst Newsl 4(2).

219. Driller MW, Mah CD, Halson SL. Development of the athlete sleep behavior questionnaire: a tool for identifying maladaptive sleep practices in elite athletes. *Sleep* Sci 2018;11(1):37.

220. George CF, Kab V. Sleep-disordered breathing in the National Football League is not a trivial matter. Sleep 2011;34(3):245.

221. Rogers AJ, Xia K, Soe K, et al. Obstructive sleep apnea among players in the National Football League: a scoping review. J Sleep Disord Ther 2017;6(5) [pii:278].

222. Brown GT, Hainline B, Kroshus E, et al. Mind, body and sport: understanding and supporting student-athlete mental wellness. Indianapolis: NCAA; 2014.

223. Von Rosen P, Frohm A, Kottorp A, et al. Multiple factors explain injury risk in adolescent elite athletes: applying a biopsychosocial perspective. Scand J Med Sci Sports 2017;27(12):2059–69.

224. Meeusen R, Duclos M, Foster C, et al. Prevention, diagnosis, and treatment of the overtraining syndrome: joint consensus statement of the European College of Sport Science and the American College of Sports Medicine. Med Sci Sports Exerc 2013;45(1):186–205.

225. Halson SL, Jeukendrup AE. Does overtraining exist? Sports Med 2004;34(14):967–81.

226. Janse van Rensburg DCC, Fowler P, Racinais S. Practical tips to manage travel fatigue and jet lag in athletes. Br J Sports Med 2021;55(15):821–2.

Menstrual Cycle Effects on Sleep

Fiona C. Baker, PhD[a,b],*, Kathryn Aldrich Lee, RN, PhD, CBSM[c]

KEYWORDS

- Menstrual cycle • Follicular • Luteal • Estrogen • Premenstrual syndrome • Dysmenorrhea
- Polycystic ovary syndrome • Sleep spindles

KEY POINTS

- Self-reported sleep disturbance increases during premenstrual and menstruation phases of the menstrual cycle, particularly in women with premenstrual symptoms or painful menstrual cramps (dysmenorrhea).
- Sleep spindles increase in the luteal phase relative to the follicular phase, possibly due to an effect of progesterone and/or its metabolites.
- Women with polycystic ovary syndrome (PCOS), particularly if obese, are at risk of sleep-disordered breathing (SDB), partly due to hyperandrogenism that characterizes this syndrome.
- Poorer sleep quality is apparent in the premenstrual phase in women with severe premenstrual syndrome, yet polysomnographic measures show more trait-like sleep alterations that may be related to altered melatonin rhythms. Light therapy shows efficacy in improving mood symptoms.
- Sleep and reproductive function have a bidirectional relationship such that disrupted sleep is associated with altered menstrual cycles, which could impact reproductive function.

INTRODUCTION

From menarche, or the first menstrual period, to menopause that signals the end of reproduction, women experience monthly variations in hormones that regulate reproduction. These hormones have widespread effects outside their direct reproductive functions, including influences on regulating mood, body temperature, respiration, autonomic nervous system, and sleep. This review highlights the effects of the menstrual cycle on sleep, considering both physiologic changes in homeostatic and circadian sleep regulation as well as perceived changes in sleep quality. The authors discuss sleep disturbances in the context of young women and menstrual-associated disorders, including polycystic ovary syndrome (PCOS), dysmenorrhea, and premenstrual dysphoric

disorder. They also consider reverse relationships: how sleep and circadian disturbances impact women's reproductive physiology.

DEFINITIONS AND MENSTRUAL CYCLE PHYSIOLOGY

Most women have menstrual cycle lengths between 21 and 30 days, with menses lasting less than 7 days.[1] The menstrual cycle is divided into a preovulatory follicular phase and postovulatory luteal phase, with the onset of menstrual flow marking the beginning of a new cycle (day 1) (**Fig. 1**).

During the follicular phase, follicle-stimulating hormone and luteinizing hormone (LH) are released from the anterior pituitary and act on the ovaries to initiate the development of several

Sleep Med Clin 13 (2018) 283-294 https://doi.org/10.1016/j.jsmc.2018.04.002 1556-407X/18/© 2018 Elsevier Inc. All rights reserved.

[a] Human Sleep Research Program, SRI International, 333 Ravenswood Avenue, Menlo Park, CA 94025, USA; [b] Brain Function Research Group, School of Physiology, University of the Witwatersrand, 7 York Road, Parktown, Johannesburg 2193, South Africa; [c] Department of Family Health Care Nursing, UCSF School of Nursing, University of California, San Francisco, Box 0606, San Francisco, CA 94143, USA

* Corresponding author. SRI International, 333 Ravenswood Avenue, Menlo Park, CA 94025.
E-mail address: Fiona.baker@sri.com

Sleep Med Clin 17 (2022) 283–294
https://doi.org/10.1016/j.jsmc.2022.02.004
1556-407X/22/© 2022 Elsevier Inc. All rights reserved.

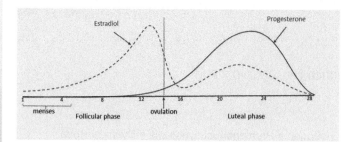

Fig. 1. Changes in estradiol and progesterone across a typical 28-day ovulatory menstrual cycle, where day 1 represents the first day of bleeding.

primary follicles, which produce estrogens, principally estradiol. At the end of the follicular phase, estrogen levels increase, triggering a peak in LH. Ovulation occurs 12 to 16 hours later, around day 14. Following ovulation, the corpus luteum develops, producing progesterone and estrogen, which peak 5 to 7 days after ovulation before declining (in the absence of implantation), resulting in endometrial breakdown and menstruation.

Estrogen and progesterone receptors are widely distributed throughout the central nervous system (CNS), including the basal forebrain, hypothalamus, dorsal raphe nucleus, and locus coeruleus.[2,3] These areas are also involved in sleep regulation, and fluctuations in ovarian steroids across the menstrual cycle can modulate sleep. Indeed, work in rodents shows that sleep patterns fluctuate in concert with natural fluctuations of ovarian steroids; ovariectomy eliminates these fluctuations in sleep, with effects depending on the time of day.[4,5] Although ovarian steroids' mechanisms of action on sleep regulation are not completely clear, both sleep- and wake-promoting areas of the CNS are sensitive to the effects of estrogen. Ovarian steroids could also influence circadian rhythms, including sleep–wake activity, through direct or indirect effects on the master pacemaker: the suprachiasmatic nucleus. The mechanistic framework is, therefore, in place for menstrual cycle-related changes in reproductive hormones to influence sleep and circadian rhythms.

SLEEP AND CIRCADIAN RHYTHMS ACROSS THE MENSTRUAL CYCLE
Self-reported Sleep Quality

Collectively, studies show that sleep disturbances are more commonly reported by women around the time of menstruation, encompassing the last few premenstrual days (late-luteal phase) and the first few days of menstrual bleeding (early follicular phase).[6–9] However, not all studies find a menstrual cycle effect on sleep quality[10] or find only small effects,[11] possibly reflecting between-individual variability in the relationship between sleep and menstrual cycle phase. Van Reen and Kiesner[12] identified 3 patterns: some women show no relationship, others show a midcycle increase in difficulty sleeping, and others show a premenstrual increase in difficulty sleeping. The extent that ovarian hormones directly contribute to perceived sleep disturbance, versus other factors that vary with the menstrual cycle, remains unclear. Changes in progesterone and estrogen, rather than absolute levels, in the late-luteal phase, may be a critical factor for sleep quality. Further, symptoms that vary across the menstrual cycle in some women, such as anxiety, depression, headaches, cramps, and breast tenderness, are also associated with difficulty sleeping.[12] Menstrual cycle characteristics are also relevant: women with irregular cycles report more sleep difficulties than women with regular cycles, even when controlling for age, body mass index (BMI), dysmenorrhea, and premenstrual complaints.[13]

Objectively Measured Sleep Quality

Sleep across the menstrual cycle has been studied objectively with actigraphy and polysomnography (PSG). Actigraphy can be easily used to track changes in daily sleep–wake activity in many participants; however, few studies have investigated menstrual cycle-related patterns in sleep. In a actigraphy study of 163 late-reproductive-aged women, there was a significant decline in sleep efficiency (SE) and total sleep time (TST) in the premenstrual week relative to the prior week, with greater effects associated with obesity, financial strain, smoking, and greater apnea–hypopnea index,[14] corresponding with studies showing poorer self-reported sleep quality in the premenstrual phase. In a smaller study of 19 women (1843 years of age), actigraphy SE was positively associated with 1-day lagged estrogen metabolites and negatively with 1-day lagged progesterone metabolites, although effects were weak and self-reported sleep was unassociated with hormone metabolites.[10]

PSG has been used in small numbers of women to compare sleep between discrete menstrual cycle phases, such as midfollicular versus midluteal phase. An exception is a seminal study by Driver and colleagues.[15] Although the sample size was small, sleep was recorded with PSG every second night across an entire menstrual cycle in 9 young women, with phases carefully characterized. They found stable sleep-onset latency (SOL), wakefulness after sleep onset (WASO), and SE across the menstrual cycle.[16] N2 sleep was increased and REM sleep tended to decline in the absence of any change in the amount of slow-wave sleep (SWS) or slow-wave activity (SWA) averaged for the whole night in the luteal phase relative to follicular phase,[15] indicating no change in this marker of sleep homeostasis across the menstrual cycle. Analysis of SWA by sleep cycle, did reveal subtle changes; however, higher activity in the first non-REM (NREM) sleep episode and lower activity in the second NREM episode in the midluteal phase compared with the midfollicular phase.[16]

Other studies have mostly confirmed no difference in SWS or SWA between the follicular and luteal phases in young women, although inconsistencies remain (see reviews[16,17]). Others have also found variability in REM sleep with the menstrual cycle phase: REM sleep had an earlier onset[18] and REM sleep episodes were shorter,[16,19] with the amount of REM sleep negatively correlating with progesterone and estradiol levels in the luteal phase.[19] Using a careful ultrarapid sleep–wake cycle procedure, Shechter and Boivin[17] also found that REM sleep was decreased (at circadian phase 0° and 30°) in the luteal phase compared with the follicular phase. This reduction in REM sleep may relate to raised body temperature in the luteal phase.

Finally, most studies support Driver and colleagues'[15] findings of no menstrual cycle variability in sleep continuity PSG measures in young women, although 2 studies found more wakefulness/awakenings in the late-luteal phase[20,21] and one study found a steeper increase in progesterone from the follicular to the early to midluteal phase associated with WASO in the luteal phase.[22] Inconsistencies between studies reflect methodologic challenges, such as small sample sizes, variable cycle length, differences in sampling times across the menstrual cycle, and age-related variability.[16] For example, one study found that women seemed to be more vulnerable to physiologic changes associated with the luteal phase in midlife.[23]

The most dramatic menstrual cycle change in sleep is an electroencephalogram (EEG) activity in the 14.25 to 15.0 Hz (sigma) band corresponding to the upper frequency range of sleep spindles, which is significantly increased in the luteal compared with the follicular phase[15,19,24,25] associated with increased spindle density and duration.[23] Interestingly, midlife women with insomnia showed a blunted increase in sigma EEG activity in the luteal phase, possibly reflecting a weaker influence of the menstrual cycle on sleep EEG in the presence of insomnia.[23] The mechanism for luteal phase increases in spindle activity is unknown; however, it may involve the modulation of g-aminobutyric acid A receptors by progesterone metabolites.[15] Given the supposed sleep-protective function of spindles,[26] increased spindles may function to maintain sleep quality in the presence of luteal phase hormonal changes.[17] Work has begun to explore implications for menstrual cycle variation in sleep spindles, with findings suggesting that spindles could mediate menstrual cycle changes in sleep-dependent memory consolidation.[27,28]

Major findings for PSG measures are summarized in **Table 1**. Upper airway resistance also varies across the menstrual cycle, being lower in the luteal phase in healthy women.[29] The severity of sleep-disordered breathing (SDB) may also vary by menstrual phase, which could impact a sleep apnea diagnosis in women. Surprisingly, however, women evaluated for sleep apnea in their self-reported follicular phase had a lower apnea–hypopnea index than women evaluated in their self-reported luteal phase.[30] Further studies using a within-subject design are needed.

Circadian Rhythms

Hormonal variations across the menstrual cycle are also associated with changes in circadian rhythms. Body temperature is increased by about 0.4°C[31] due to the thermogenic action of progesterone and has a smaller amplitude due to a blunted nocturnal decline, in the luteal phase compared with the follicular phase.[20] Using an ultrashort sleep–wake cycle procedure to control for light, posture, and food intake, Shechter and colleagues[32] confirmed a reduced amplitude and found no difference in phase for core temperature rhythm in the luteal phase. Melatonin did not differ in acrophase, onset, or offset, similar to previous studies that also used controlled conditions.[33,34] Two of these studies also found no menstrual cycle differences in the amplitude of the melatonin rhythm.[32,34] In one study with controlled conditions, the amplitude of cortisol and thyroid-stimulating hormone rhythms were blunted in the

Table 1
Summary of evidence comparing objective sleep and related measures during the luteal phase relative to the follicular phase of the menstrual cycle

Variable	Luteal Phase (Relative to Follicular Phase)
SOL	No change
SE	No change
WASO	Most studies in young women show no change Midlife women have more awakenings[3]
SWS and slow-wave EEG activity	No change in all-night measures in young women Decreased in midlife women[a]
REM sleep	Decrease in the duration of REM sleep episodes
Sigma EEG activity (spindle frequency range)	Increased activity, associated with increased spindle density and duration
Stage 2 sleep	Studies find either increased or no change
Body temperature	Reduced amplitude due to blunted nocturnal decline; no circadian phase shift
Melatonin	No change in phase; 2 of 3 controlled studies find no change in amplitude
Heart rate	Increased ($\sim$4 bpm) during sleep, associated with decreased vagal activity
Upper airway resistance	Lower[b]

[a] Data available from only one study.[23].
[b] Data available from only one study.[29].

luteal phase[33]; but this finding remains to be replicated.

There are also reports of a raised heart rate (about 4 beats per minute), particularly at night, in the luteal compared with the follicular phase,[16,35–37] although controlled conditions were not used to investigate the rhythms.

In summary, studies using controlled conditions consistently show blunted amplitude of the body temperature rhythm in the luteal phase compared with the follicular phase. Available evidence suggests that melatonin's rhythm is not influenced by the menstrual cycle phase to the same extent as body temperature; however, this remains to be confirmed with additional controlled studies.

SLEEP AND OVARIAN DYSFUNCTION AND ANDROGEN EXCESS (POLYCYSTIC OVARY SYNDROME)
Prevalence, Cause, and Symptoms

The most common endocrine disorder for reproductive-age women is PCOS. PCOS affects 5% to 20% of women, depending on age, type of epidemiologic survey, and diagnostic criteria. There are likely different phenotypes for this syndrome; because polycystic ovaries may or may not be present, discussion about the misleading label of PCOS is leaning toward 3 types: androgen

excess with ovarian dysfunction, androgen excess with polycystic ovary morphology, and ovarian dysfunction with polycystic ovarian morphology. The National Institutes of Health estimate that PCOS affects about 5 million women of reproductive age in the United States.[38] High testosterone levels, clinical signs of hyperandrogenism, and irregular menstrual cycles may occur; polycystic ovaries may or may not be present. It is often first diagnosed when a young woman presents clinically with a chief complaint of infertility and laboratory results indicate high serum testosterone or ultrasound reveals an accumulation of cystic, dysfunctional follicles in the ovary.[39] The National Institutes of Health[38] and the Rotterdam Consensus Panel[40] have similar diagnostic criteria (**Box 1**). Long-term health consequences typically result from obesity-related issues and include hyperlipidemia, type 2 diabetes, SDB, and cardiovascular disease.

Although the exact cause of PCOS remains unknown, the abnormal ovarian morphology seen on ultrasound results in the absence of ovarian sources of estrogen and progesterone and leads to irregular menstrual cycles that are likely anovulatory. Theca cells within the ovary continue to secret androgens; the high, unopposed testosterone level is thought to be responsible for clinical manifestations, including acne,

Box 1	
Diagnostic criteria for polycystic ovary syndrome	
National Institutes of Health[38] **(Both of These Criteria Must** **Be Present)**	**Rotterdam[40] (Any 2 of These 3** **Criteria Must Be Present)**
• Presence of oligomenorrhea (fewer than 6 menstrual cycles per year)	• Chronic oligomenorrhea (6 or fewer episodes of spontaneous menses per year)
• Presence of hyperandrogenism (elevated testosterone >2 standard deviations greater than the mean value for the particular laboratory assay)	• Evidence of hyperandrogenism (either clinical or biochemical)
	• Polycystic ovaries on ultrasonography

From National Institutes of Health. Final report: evidence-based methodology workshop on polycystic ovary syndrome. December 3–5, 2012; and Rotterdam ESHRE/ASRM-sponsored PCOS consensus workshop group. Revised 2003 consensus on diagnostic criteria and long-term health risks related to polycystic ovary syndrome (PCOS). Hum Reprod 2004;19(1):41–7; with permission.

hirsutism (excessive hair growth on face and body), and alopecia (thinning scalp hair). Excessive weight gain, insulin resistance, snoring, and SDB are also likely to develop; but the time course for these aspects of the syndrome is unknown. Between 50% and 60% of women with PCOS are obese,[41] but adolescents with PCOS are less likely to have SDB than older women with PCOS.[42,43]

Perceived Sleep Quality

Women diagnosed with PCOS often experience sleep problems. Franik and colleagues[41] used self-report measures to compare insomnia in women with and without PCOS. The 95 women with PCOS were 17 to 43 years old and just more than half (53.6%) were normal weight. The prevalence of insomnia was higher in women with PCOS (12.6% scored >10 on the Athens Insomnia Scale and 10.5% scored >14 on the Insomnia Severity Index) compared with controls (3% and 1%, respectively). Although there was no difference in the percentage of women in each group with poor sleep quality on the Pittsburgh Sleep Quality Index (PSQI), 25% of the PCOS group reported sleeping less than 6 hours, whereas all controls slept greater than 6 hours per night. It is thought that sleep complaints in women with PCOS are associated with obesity; however, it is not clear that BMI was controlled in this analysis.

Daytime Sleepiness

Daytime sleepiness would be an expected outcome of poor sleep, but findings are mixed when women with PCOS are compared with controls. Franik and colleagues[41] found no difference in the rate of daytime sleepiness (PCOS 7.4%; controls 6.4%), but the cut point for the Epworth Sleepiness Scale (ESS) was not mentioned. Suri and colleagues[44] reported a significant difference in mean ESS scores between PCOS cases (12.5) and controls who self-reported snoring (9.3). They did not control for BMI or SDB and did not report rates of daytime sleepiness based on ESS cut points. The highest rate for daytime sleepiness was reported by Vgontzas and colleagues[45] who used a 4-point scale (none, mild, moderate, severe) and found a high prevalence of daytime sleepiness in women with PCOS (80.4%) compared with controls (27%).

Objective Polysomnography Sleep Comparisons

Two studies that compared PCOS and healthy women's sleep based on one night of PSG had different results. Suri and colleagues[44] compared 50 women with untreated PCOS to controls all studied on the second or third day of the menstrual cycle. The Berlin Sleep Questionnaire was used to screen for SDB, and 58% of the 50 patients with PCOS reported snoring compared with 16% of

100 controls. Based on PSG, only 4% of the 16 controls had SBD, whereas 78% of the patients with PCOS snored and 66% had SDB. After adjusting for BMI and waist circumference, there was no difference in SDB between the 2 groups. Without adjusting for BMI or SDB, the 2 groups differed significantly on WASO; patients averaged 55 minutes, whereas controls averaged 38 minutes. SE was similar for patients (84.6%) and controls (87.8%), and they did not differ on SOL (18–23 minutes). REM sleep approached significance, with 56 minutes for patients and 38 minutes for controls $(P = .063)$. In contrast, Vgontzas and colleagues[45] also compared women with PCOS with controls in a one-night PSG study without the mention of the menstrual cycle phase. The 53 patients with PCOS were 16 to 45 year old, with BMIs ranging from 24 to 67 kg/m^2. After adjusting for BMI, both patients and controls had similar REM (percentage of TST), but the PCOS group had longer SOL (44 minutes) compared with controls (30 minutes; $P < .05$). Both groups had longer SOL and less variance[45] compared with the Suri and colleagues' sample.[44]

Sleep-disordered Breathing

It is likely that excessive weight, specifically central obesity, contributes to a high risk for obstructive sleep apnea (OSA) in women with PCOS. In a study of 44 racially/ethnically diverse women (18–40 year old) with PCOS based on the National Institutes of Health's criteria, Mokhlesi and colleagues[46] divided the group into obese (BMI >30; n = 27) and nonobese (n = 17), compared with 34 controls. PSG was not used, and the risk of OSA was based on the Berlin Questionnaire. BMI was the strongest predictor of risk for OSA based on self-reports, but BMI is also a major risk factor in the Berlin Questionnaire. Age was not a significant predictor; when controlling for BMI, neither testosterone level nor PCOS diagnosis was associated with the risk for OSA.[46]

In a recent report of a longitudinal population study in Taiwan, Lin and colleagues[43] noted prevalence for PCOS of less than 1% of the population. Over time, this group had a higher incidence of OSA than healthy controls after adjusting for age and comorbidities, such as obesity. As shown elsewhere, once BMI is controlled, however, the rates of snoring and SDB are similar to controls[44]; an elevated testosterone level was associated with SDB regardless of PCOS or control group.[44] In contrast, testosterone was not associated with SDB in the 9 patients of PCOS in the Vgontzas and colleagues study[45] but rather with insulin resistance and BMI; however, the BMI cut point

was high (32 kg/m^2). Of note with implications for treatment, oral contraceptives were used by only 7% of the patients with PCOS with SDB, compared with 20% of patients with PCOS who did not have SDB.

Summary

Few studies have been conducted using PSG; when there are objective sleep data, it is typically based on one night of PSG with no control for age or menstrual cycle phase. Most sleep research on women with PCOS is focused on SDB, whereby efforts have been made to determine if there is a direct effect of PCOS on SDB or an indirect effect of excess testosterone on central obesity. Despite their relatively young age, women with ovarian dysfunction, androgen excess, and polycystic ovaries are at higher risk of SDB; this risk continues as they age and as their BMI increases. Treatment includes hormonal efforts to lower testosterone levels, which has some evidence of efficacy.[45] Treatment depends on age and phenotype of the syndrome; but oral contraceptives are effective in managing menstrual cycle irregularity, acne, and hirsutism. Metformin is indicated for weight reduction and insulin resistance as well as hirsutism.[47] If present, OSA would be treated with similar protocols for other adults with OSA.

SLEEP AND PREMENSTRUAL SYNDROME
Prevalence, Cause, and Symptoms

Premenstrual syndrome (PMS) is characterized by emotional, behavioral, and physical symptoms that manifest almost exclusively in the late-luteal (premenstrual) phase, with the resolution soon after the onset of menses. Although many women experience some symptoms premenstrually, up to 18% have severe symptoms that impact daily function.[48] Premenstrual dysphoric disorder (PMDD) is a severe form of PMS evident in 3% to 8% and classified as a depressive disorder in the American Psychiatric Association's *Diagnostic and Statistical Manual of Mental Disorders,* Fifth Edition (DSM-5).[48] A PMDD diagnosis requires the occurrence of 5 specified symptoms, of which at least one must be a mood-related symptom experienced in the late-luteal phase, documented for at least 2 consecutive cycles. One of these symptoms is sleep disturbance (insomnia or hypersomnia). The cause of PMDD remains unclear, although symptoms are effectively managed with selective serotonin reuptake inhibitors, anxiolytics, and ovulation-suppressing agents.[49,50]

Perceived Sleep Quality

Women with severe PMS frequently report late-luteal phase sleep symptoms, including insomnia, disturbing dreams, poor sleep quality, daytime sleepiness, and fatigue.[51,52] A recent study used the PSQI to evaluate sleep quality in the past month, not considering the menstrual phase, in a sample of female university students (67 with severe PMS/PMDD symptoms and 195 controls).[53] The PMS/PMDD group was more likely than controls to have PSQI scores greater than 5, reflecting poor sleep quality (80.5% vs 56.4%) and higher PSQI scores overall (8.2 ± 3.4 vs 6.5 ± 3.1).[53] PSQI components of sleep duration, SOL, and SE did not differ between groups; however, sleep disturbance, daytime dysfunction, use of sleep medications, and rating sleep quality as poor or very poor were all more prevalent in the PMS/PMDD group.

There may be both trait (across the menstrual cycle) and state (in conjunction with other symptoms) differences in women with PMS/PMDD compared with controls.[51] Trait-like symptoms may then magnify when an additional stressor (eg, hormonal changes associated with menstruation) is present.

Indeed, in one laboratory-based study, women with PMS/PMDD reported more awakenings and felt less refreshed on awakening compared with controls in both the follicular and late-luteal phases and also reported worse sleep quality in their late-luteal phase relative to their own follicular phase.[19]

Objective Polysomnography Sleep Comparisons

Despite evidence of perceived poor sleep quality in the late-luteal phase in women with PMS/PMDD, laboratory studies show little evidence of disturbed PSG sleep parameters specific to this phase. Most studies show no change in SE, arousals, SOL, or sleep EEG in the late-luteal phase relative to the follicular phase.[17,19,51] Perception of poor sleep quality in late-luteal phase may be a component of the symptom profile of PMS in the absence of actual sleep disruption, as sleep quality correlated with anxiety in women with PMS/PMDD in the late-luteal phase.[19]

Some studies found differences in PSG measures at both phases of the menstrual cycle, suggesting trait differences in sleep, although the nature of these differences varies between studies.[17,51] Age may influence the severity of sleep disruption in association with symptoms; findings indicate that women more than 40 years old with PMS report more frequent awakenings than younger women[54]; however, PSG studies

have not been powered to investigate age-PMS interactions.

Daytime Sleepiness

A few researchers have investigated the second type of sleep disturbance (hypersomnia) listed in the *DSM-5* for diagnosis of PMDD. Mauri[55] found that PMS clinic patients reported greater daytime sleepiness in luteal and menstruation phases than other times of the menstrual cycle. Similarly, women with PMS symptoms were sleepier and less alert in the late-luteal phase than in the follicular phase, an effect not found in controls in another study.[56] In a survey of 269 young women, women with PMS were more likely to report daytime sleepiness and fatigue premenstrually than controls.[52] Based on objective measures, women with PMS showed psychomotor slowing, with increased lapses and slower reaction times, corresponding with their perceived greater late-luteal levels of sleepiness and fatigue compared with their follicular phase and compared with controls.[57] However, waking EEG measures of alertness and cognitive processing, as well as SOL on the maintenance of wakefulness task, did not differentiate women with PMS when symptomatic, although there were some trait differences.[57]

Altered Circadian Rhythms

Parry and colleagues[58] have conducted several studies to investigate rhythm disturbances under normal sleep and sleep deprivation conditions in PMDD. Although no differences were evident in temperature rhythm between women with and without PMDD during normal sleep, group differences emerged during partial sleep deprivation in the late-luteal phase. Women with PMDD had higher temperature maxima and mesors (rhythm-adjusted mean) than controls. Also, during early sleep deprivation (only sleep 03:0007:00) compared with baseline in the late-luteal phase, women with PMDD had a delayed acrophase (later time at which temperature peaked), whereas controls had an advanced acrophase.[58] Parry and colleagues[59] also found disturbances in melatonin rhythms and timing of rhythms for cortisol and thyroid-stimulating hormone, suggesting that circadian regulation disturbances may be a factor in PMDD.

In one pilot study on melatonin rhythms in PMDD, the PMDD group had lower nocturnal melatonin levels under controlled conditions at both menstrual phases compared with controls, suggesting a trait difference.[60] A decreased melatonin amplitude in the symptomatic luteal phase was also evident, suggesting an additional sensitivity to the altered ovarian hormone environment (ie, state difference) in PMDD.[60] Women with PMDD also had increased SWS in both follicular and luteal phases compared with controls (similar to other findings[19]), which the investigators hypothesized to be functionally linked to decreased melatonin secretion.[61]

Parry and colleagues[62] have extended their work to investigate differences in response to light between women with and without PMDD. They found that women with PMDD have a blunted phase-shift response to morning bright light in the luteal phase but not in the follicular phase, suggesting less ability to entrain internal rhythms to the external environment and to synchronize other internal circadian rhythms with each other, possibly contributing to mood disturbances that characterize the luteal phase. Given the disturbed melatonin rhythms seen in PMDD, Parry and colleagues[63] have tested appropriately timed light therapy with positive outcomes for mood, although further trials are needed to confirm these effects in larger samples.[50,64]

Summary

Women with severe PMS/PMDD are likely to report poor sleep quality and daytime sleepiness in association with other symptoms in the late-luteal phase. However, PSG sleep disruption specific to the symptomatic late-luteal phase is minimal, suggesting that perceived poor sleep and sleepiness may be associated with non–sleepiness-related factors, such as depressed mood or anxiety. Overall, PSG studies indicate trait-like differences in sleep measures; however, the effects are not consistent across studies. A clear disturbance in the circadian rhythm of melatonin is evident in PMDD, both across the menstrual cycle, and specific to the symptomatic phase, which could contribute to the cause of the disorder, and suggests that nonpharmacologic chronotherapies may be effective, with evidence supporting benefit with light therapy.

SLEEP AND DYSMENORRHEA

Dysmenorrhea, defined as painful menstrual cramps of uterine origin, is either primary (menstrual pain without organic disease that typically emerges in adolescence) or secondary (associated with conditions such as endometriosis and pelvic inflammatory disease). The relationship between primary dysmenorrhea and sleep is detailed elsewhere in this special issue (Joan L. Shaver and Stella Iacovides' article, "Sleep in Women with Chronic Pain and Autoimmune Conditions: A Narrative Review," in this issue, 2018). Briefly,

evidence indicates that when severe, dysmenorrhea negatively impacts sleep, daytime function, and mood[65–68]; PSG studies also indicate sleep disturbances (lower SE) in association with painful menses.[69,70] Sleep and pain share a reciprocal relationship.[71] Breaking this pain-sleep cycle could be critical for the long-term health of women with primary dysmenorrhea who show increased pain sensitization.[72] One study showed promising effects of a nonsteroidal anti-inflammatory drug that alleviated nocturnal pain and restored sleep quality in women with primary dysmenorrhea.[70]

SLEEP AND HORMONAL CONTRACEPTIVES

Combined oral contraceptives (OCs) contain ethinyl estradiol and synthetic progestin taken for 21 days and a placebo taken for 7 days. During the 21-day period, hypothalamic–pituitary–ovarian axis activity is suppressed and endogenous estradiol and progesterone levels are low, similar to levels in the follicular phase for nonusers.[73] Across most of the 7-day placebo period, estrogen levels remain suppressed. New formulations contain the minimum steroid doses necessary to inhibit ovulation.[74] Therefore, levels of estrogen and progestin in today's OCs are lower than in older formulations, which need to be considered when comparing studies.

The few studies that have examined PSG measures in women taking OCs have not found increased sleep disruption or poorer sleep quality; however, sleep architecture is altered. Women had about 12% more N2 sleep on a night during the 21-day period of active pill compared with a night in the 7-day placebo period.[75] They also have more N2 sleep and less N3 (SWS) than naturally cycling women in the luteal phase[75–77] and possibly a shorter REM onset latency.[77] Hachul and colleagues[13] found that women using OCs experienced less snoring, a lower apnea–hypopnea index, shorter latency to REM sleep, and fewer arousals. Finally, the use of synthetic progestin (medroxyprogesterone) was associated with increased upper spindle frequency activity and greater sleep spindle density in women,[78] similar to natural luteal phase effects.

Women taking OCs have increased 24-h body temperature profiles, similar to the natural luteal phase, probably due to progestin. This increased temperature profile persists during the 7-day placebo period,[76] which contrasts with the rapid decline in temperature, as progesterone levels decline before menstruation in ovulatory cycles. OCs may also influence the melatonin profile, although findings are inconsistent.[20] In one study using a modified constant routine procedure, melatonin levels did not differ between naturally cycling women and women taking OCs, although there was a trend for increased melatonin in the latter part of the night in the OC group.[34]

In summary, OCs alter aspects of sleep architecture as well as body temperature, although their impact on sleep quality seems to be minimal. Given the lower doses of hormones in current OCs, it would be interesting to investigate whether sleep architecture and body temperature changes are still evident.

IMPACT OF SLEEP ON REPRODUCTIVE FUNCTION

Not only does the reproductive cycle influence sleep but sleep can also influence reproductive function.[79] Sleep duration, timing, and quality can influence the reproductive system, with effects depending on reproductive maturity. During puberty, LH is released in a pulsatile fashion during N3, playing a critical role in reproductive regulation.[80,81] In adulthood, the direction of the relationship changes in the early follicular phase, with sleep inhibiting pulsatile LH secretion, thought to be critical for the recruitment of ovarian follicles.[82]

There are reports of associations between short sleep duration and altered menstrual cycles in both adolescents and adults. Women reporting less than 6-h sleep were more likely to report abnormal (short or long) menstrual cycle lengths[83]; in a survey of adolescents, short sleep duration (<5 hours) was significantly associated with an increased likelihood of menstrual cycle irregularity, even after adjusting for confounding variables.[84] There has been a larger body of work investigating the impact of shiftwork on reproductive function in women, given the typical disrupted sleep and circadian patterns in this group. This work is described in detail elsewhere in this special issue (Kervezee and colleagues' article, "Impact of Shift Work on the Circadian Timing System and Health in Women," in this issue, 2018).

DISCLOSURE STATEMENT

Authors declare no conflict of interest related to the current work. F.C. Baker has received research funding unrelated to this work from Noctrix Health, Inc., Verily Life Sciences LLC., and Lisa Health Inc., and has ownership of shares in Lisa Health.

REFERENCES

1. Wood C, Larsen L, Williams R. Menstrual characteristics of 2,343 women attending the Shepherd Foundation. Aust N Z J Obstet Gynaecol 1979;19(2): 107–10.

2. Shughrue PJ, Lane MV, Merchenthaler I. Comparative distribution of estrogen receptor-alpha and -beta mRNA in the rat central nervous system. J Comp Neurol 1997;388(4):507–25.

3. Curran-Rauhut MA, Petersen SL. The distribution of progestin receptor mRNA in rat brainstem. Brain Res Gene Expr Patterns 2002;1(3–4):151–7.

4. Mong JA, Baker FC, Mahoney MM, et al. Sleep, rhythms, and the endocrine brain: influence of sex and gonadal hormones. J Neurosci 2011;31(45): 16107–16.

5. Mong JA, Cusmano DM. Sex differences in sleep: impact of biological sex and sex steroids. Philos Trans R Soc Lond B Biol Sci 2016;371(1688): 20150110.

6. Baker FC, Driver HS. Self-reported sleep across the menstrual cycle in young, healthy women. J Psychosom Res 2004;56(2):239–43.

7. Kravitz HM, Janssen I, Santoro N, et al. Relationship of day-to-day reproductive hormone levels to sleep in midlife women. Arch Intern Med 2005;165(20): 2370–6.

8. Manber R, Baker FC, Gress JL. Sex differences in sleep and sleep disorders: a focus on women's sleep. Int J Sleep Disord 2006;1:7–15.

9. National Sleep Foundation NSF. Sleep in America 2008 poll. 2008. Available at: http://www. sleepfoundation.org/atf/cf/%7Bf6bf2668-a1b4-4fe8-8d 1a-a5d39340d9cb%7D/2008%20POLL%20SOF. PDF. Accessed August 20, 2008.

10. Li DX, Romans S, De Souza MJ, et al. Actigraphic and self-reported sleep quality in women: associations with ovarian hormones and mood. Sleep Med 2015;16(10):1217–24.

11. Romans SE, Kreindler D, Einstein G, et al. Sleep quality and the menstrual cycle. Sleep Med 2015; 16(4):489–95.

12. Van Reen E, Kiesner J. Individual differences in self-reported difficulty sleeping across the menstrual cycle. Arch Womens Ment Health 2016;19(4):599–608.

13. Hachul H, Andersen ML, Bittencourt LR, et al. Does the reproductive cycle influence sleep patterns in women with sleep complaints? Climacteric 2010; 13(6):594–603.

14. Zheng H, Harlow SD, Kravitz HM, et al. Actigraphy-defined measures of sleep and movement across the menstrual cycle in midlife menstruating women: study of Women's Health across the Nation Sleep Study. Menopause 2015;22(1):66–74.

15. Driver HS, Dijk DJ, Werth E, et al. Sleep and the sleep electroencephalogram across the menstrual cycle in young healthy women. J Clin Endocrinol Metab 1996;81(2):728–35.

16. Driver HS, Werth E, Dijk D, et al. The menstrual cycle effects on sleep. Sleep Med Clin 2008;3:1–11.

17. Shechter A, Boivin DB. Sleep, hormones, and circadian rhythms throughout the menstrual cycle in

healthy women and women with premenstrual dysphoric disorder. Int J Endocrinol 2010;2010: 259345.

18. Lee KA, Shaver JF, Giblin EC, et al. Sleep patterns related to menstrual cycle phase and premenstrual affective symptoms. Sleep 1990;13(5):403–9.

19. Baker FC, Sassoon SA, Kahan T, et al. Perceived poor sleep quality in the absence of polysomnographic sleep disturbance in women with severe premenstrual syndrome. J Sleep Res 2012;21(5): 535–45.

20. Baker FC, Driver HS. Circadian rhythms, sleep, and the menstrual cycle. Sleep Med 2007;8(6):613–22.

21. Parry BL, Berga SL, Mostofi N, et al. Morning versus evening bright light treatment of late luteal phase dysphoric disorder. Am J Psychiatry 1989;146(9): 1215–7.

22. Sharkey KM, Crawford SL, Kim S, et al. Objective sleep interruption and reproductive hormone dynamics in the menstrual cycle. Sleep Med 2014;15(6): 688–93.

23. de Zambotti M, Willoughby AR, Sassoon SA, et al. Menstrual cycle-related variation in physiological sleep in women in the early menopausal transition. J Clin Endocrinol Metab 2015;100(8):2918–26.

24. Baker FC, Kahan TL, Trinder J, et al. Sleep quality and the sleep electroencephalogram in women with severe premenstrual syndrome. Sleep 2007; 30(10):1283–91.

25. Ishizuka Y, Pollak CP, Shirakawa S, et al. Sleep spindle frequency changes during the menstrual cycle. J Sleep Res 1994;3(1):26–9.

26. Steriade M, McCormick DA, Sejnowski TJ. Thalamo cortical oscillations in the sleeping and aroused brain. Science 1993;262(5134):679–85.

27. Genzel L, Kiefer T, Renner L, et al. Sex and modulatory menstrual cycle effects on sleep related memory consolidation. Psychoneuroendocrinology 2012;37(7):987–98.

28. Sattari N, McDevitt EA, Panas D, et al. The effect of sex and menstrual phase on memory formation during a nap. Neurobiol Learn Mem 2017;145: 119–28.

29. Driver HS, McLean H, Kumar DV, et al. The influence of the menstrual cycle on upper airway resistance and breathing during sleep. Sleep 2005; 28(4):449–56.

30. Spector AR, Loriaux D, Alexandru D, et al. The influence of the menstrual phases on polysomnography. Cureus 2016;8(11):e871.

31. de Mouzon J, Testart J, Lefevre B, et al. Time relationships between basal body temperature and ovulation or plasma progestins. Fertil Steril 1984; 41(2):254–9.

32. Shechter A, Varin F, Boivin DB. Circadian variation of sleep during the follicular and luteal phases of the menstrual cycle. Sleep 2010;33(5):647–56.

33. Shibui K, Uchiyama M, Okawa M, et al. Diurnal fluctuation of sleep propensity and hormonal secretion across the menstrual cycle. Biol Psychiatry 2000; 48(11):1062–8.

34. Wright KP Jr, Badia P. Effects of menstrual cycle phase and oral contraceptives on alertness, cognitive performance, and circadian rhythms during sleep deprivation. Behav Brain Res 1999;103(2): 185–94.

35. Baker FC, Colrain IM, TrinderJ. Reduced parasympa- thetic activity during sleep in the symptomatic phase of severe premenstrual syndrome. J Psychosom Res 2008;65(1):13–22.

36. de Zambotti M, Nicholas CL, Colrain IM, et al. Autonomic regulation across phases of the menstrual cycle and sleep stages in women with premenstrual syndrome and healthy controls. Psychoneuroendocrinology 2013;38(11):2618–27.

37. de Zambotti M, Trinder J, Colrain IM, et al. Menstrual cycle-related variation in autonomic nervous system functioning in women in the early menopausal transition with and without insomnia disorder. Psychoneuroendocrinology 2017;75:44–51.

38. National Institutes of Health. Final Report: evidence-based methodology workshop on polycystic ovary syndrome. December 2012;3-5.

39. Legro RS, Arslanian SA, Ehrmann DA, et al. Diagnosis and treatment of polycystic ovary syndrome: an Endocrine Society clinical practice guideline. J Clin Endocrinol Metab 2013;98(12):4565–92.

40. Rotterdam ESHRE/ASRM-Sponsored PCOS Consensus Workshop Group. Revised 2003 consensus on diagnostic criteria and long-term health risks related to polycystic ovary syndrome (PCOS). Hum Reprod 2004;19(1):41–7.

41. Franik G, Krysta K, Madej P, et al. Sleep disturbances in women with polycystic ovary syndrome. Gynecol Endocrinol 2016;32(12):1014–7.

42. Helvaci N, Karabulut E, Demir AU, et al. Polycystic ovary syndrome and the risk of obstructive sleep apnea: a meta-analysis and review of the literature. Endocr Connect 2017;6(7):437–45.

43. Lin TY, Lin PY, Su TP, et al. Risk of developing obstructive sleep apnea among women with polycystic ovarian syndrome: a nationwide longitudinal follow-up study. Sleep Med 2017;36:165–9.

44. Suri J, Suri JC, Chatterjee B, et al. Obesity may be the common pathway for sleep-disordered breathing in women with polycystic ovary syndrome. Sleep Med 2016;24:32–9.

45. Vgontzas AN, Legro RS, Bixler EO, et al. Polycystic ovary syndrome is associated with obstructive sleep apnea and daytime sleepiness: role of insulin resistance. J Clin Endocrinol Metab 2001;86(2):517–20.

46. Mokhlesi B, Scoccia B, Mazzone T, et al. Risk of obstructive sleep apnea in obese and nonobese women with polycystic ovary syndrome and healthy

reproductively normal women. Fertil Steril 2012; 97(3):786–91.

47. Kamboj MK, Bonny AE. Polycystic ovary syndrome in adolescence: diagnostic and therapeutic strategies. Transl Pediatr 2017;6(4):248–55.

48. Halbreich U. The etiology, biology, and evolving pathology of premenstrual syndromes. Psychoneuroendocrinology 2003;28(Suppl 3):55–99.

49. Rapkin A. A review of treatment of premenstrual syndrome and premenstrual dysphoric disorder. Psychoneuroendocrinology 2003;28(Suppl 3):39–53.

50. Sepede G, Sarchione F, Matarazzo I, et al. Premenstrual dysphoric disorder without comorbid psychiatric conditions: a systematic review of therapeutic options. Clin Neuropharmacol 2016;39(5):241–61.

51. Baker FC, Lamarche LJ, Iacovides S, et al. Sleep and menstrual-related disorders. Sleep Med Clin 2008;3:25–35.

52. Gupta R, Lahan V, Bansal S. Subjective sleep problems in young women suffering from premenstrual dysphoric disorder. N Am J Med Sci 2012;4(11): 593–5.

53. Khazaie H, Ghadami MR, Khaledi-Paveh B, et al. Sleep quality in university students with premenstrual dysphoric disorder. Shanghai Arch Psychiatry 2016;28(3):131–8.

54. Kuan AJ, Carter DM, Ott FJ. Premenstrual complaints before and after 40 years of age. Can J Psychiatry 2004;49(3):215.

55. Mauri M. Sleep and the reproductive cycle: a review. Health Care Women Int 1990;11(4):409–21.

56. Lamarche LJ, Driver HS, Wiebe S, et al. Nocturnal sleep, daytime sleepiness, and napping among women with significant emotional/behavioral premenstrual symptoms. J Sleep Res 2007;16(3): 262–8.

57. Baker FC, Colrain IM. Daytime sleepiness, psychomotor performance, waking EEG spectra and evoked potentials in women with severe premenstrual syndrome. J Sleep Res 2010;19(1 Pt 2): 214–27.

58. Parry BL, LeVeau B, Mostofi N, et al. Temperature circadian rhythms during the menstrual cycle and sleep deprivation in premenstrual dysphoric disorder and normal comparison subjects. J Biol Rhythms 1997;12(1):34–46.

59. Parry BL, Martinez LF, Maurer EL, et al. Sleep, rhythms and women's mood. Part I. Menstrual cycle, pregnancy and postpartum. Sleep Med Rev 2006; 10(2):129–44.

60. Shechter A, Lesperance P, Ng Ying Kin NM, et al. Pilot investigation of the circadian plasma melatonin rhythm across the menstrual cycle in a small group of women with premenstrual dysphoric disorder. PLoS One 2012;7(12):e51929.

61. Shechter A, Lesperance P, Ng Ying Kin NM, et al. Nocturnal polysomnographic sleep across the menstrual cycle in premenstrual dysphoric disorder. Sleep Med 2012;13(8):1071–8.

62. Parry BL, Meliska CJ, Sorenson DL, et al. Reduced phase-advance of plasma melatonin after bright morning light in the luteal, but not follicular, menstrual cycle phase in premenstrual dysphoric disorder: an extended study. Chronobiol Int 2011;28(5): 415–24.

63. Parry BL, Berga SL, Mostofi N, et al. Plasma melatonin circadian rhythms during the menstrual cycle disorder and normal control subjects. J Biol Rhythms 1997;12(1):47–64.

64. Krasnik C, Montori VM, Guyatt GH, et al. The effect of bright light therapy on depression associated with premenstrual dysphoric disorder. Am J Obstet Gynecol 2005;193(3 Pt 1):658–61.

65. (NSF) NSF. Women and sleep poll. 1998. Available at: www.sleepfoundation.org. Accessed February 24, 2006.

66. Davis S, Mirick DK. Circadian disruption, shift work and the risk of cancer: a summary of the evidence and studies in Seattle. Cancer Causes Control 2006;17(4):539–45.

67. Woosley JA, Lichstein KL. Dysmenorrhea, the menstrual cycle, and sleep. Behav Med 2014;40(1): 14–21.

68. Liu X, Chen H, Liu ZZ, et al. Early menarche and menstrual problems are associated with sleep disturbance in a large sample of Chinese adolescent girls. Sleep 2017;40(9).

69. Baker FC, Driver HS, Rogers GG, et al. High nocturnal body temperatures and disturbed sleep in women with primary dysmenorrhea. Am J Physiol 1999;277(6 Pt 1):E1013–21.

70. Iacovides S, Avidon I, Bentley A, et al. Diclofenac potassium restores objective and subjective measures of sleep quality in women with primary dysmenorrhea. Sleep 2009;32(8):1019–26.

71. Iacovides S, George K, Kamerman P, et al. Sleep fragmentation hypersensitizes healthy young women to deep and superficial experimental pain. J Pain 2017;18(7):844–54.

72. Iacovides S, Avidon I, Baker FC. What we know about primary dysmenorrhea today: a critical review. Hum Reprod Update 2015;21(6):762–78.

73. Gogos A, Wu YC, Williams AS, et al. The effects of ethinylestradiol and progestins ("the pill") on cognitive function in pre-menopausal women. Neurochem Res 2014;39(12):2288–300.

74. Cedars MI. Triphasic oral contraceptives: review and comparison of various regimens. Fertil Steril 2002; 77(1):1–14.

75. Baker FC, Waner JI, Vieira EF, et al. Sleep and 24 hour body temperatures: a comparison in young men, naturally cycling women and women taking hormonal contraceptives. J Physiol 2001;530(Pt 3): 565–74.

76. Baker FC, Mitchell D, Driver HS. Oral contra- ceptives alter sleep and raise body temperature in young women. Pflugers Arch 2001;442(5):729–37.

77. Shine-Burdick R, Hoffmann R, Armitage R. Short note: oral contraceptives and sleep in depressed and healthy women. Sleep 2002;25(3):347–9.

78. Plante DT, Goldstein MR. Medroxyprogesterone acetate is associated with increased sleep spindles during non-rapid eye movement sleep in women referred for polysomnography. Psychoneuroendocrinology 2013;38(12):3160–6.

79. Kloss JD, Perlis ML, Zamzow JA, et al. Sleep, sleep disturbance, and fertility in women. Sleep Med Rev 2015;22:78–87.

80. Boyar R, Finkelstein J, Roffwarg H, et al. Synchronization of augmented luteinizing hormone secretion with sleep during puberty. N Engl J Med 1972; 287(12):582–6.

81. Shaw ND, Butler JP, McKinney SM, et al. Insights into puberty: the relationship between sleep stages and pulsatile LH secretion. J Clin Endocrinol Metab 2012;97(11):E2055–62.

82. Hall JE, Sullivan JP, Richardson GS. Brief wake epi sodes modulate sleep-inhibited luteinizing hormone secretion in the early follicular phase. J Clin Endocri Nol Metab 2005;90(4):2050–5.

83. Lim AJ, Huang Z, Chua SE, et al. Sleep duration, exercise, shiftwork and polycystic ovarian syndrome-related outcomes in a healthy population: a cross-sectional study. PLoS One 2016;11(11):e0167048.

84. Nam GE, Han K, Lee G. Association between sleep duration and menstrual cycle irregularity in Korean female adolescents. Sleep Med 2017;35:62–6.

Parasomnias and Sleep-Related Movement Disorders in Older Adults

Alex Iranzo, MD, PhD

KEYWORDS

- Sleep paralysis • Disorders of arousal • Idiopathic REM sleep Behavior disorder
- Anti-IgLON5 disease • Restless legs syndrome • Periodic limb movement disorder

KEY POINTS

- Sleepwalking and night terrors may persist in the older adult.
- Zolpidem may induce sleepwalking and sleep-related eating syndrome.
- Patients with idiopathic rapid eye movement sleep (REM) sleep behavior represent the prodromal stage of Parkinson disease and related synucleinopathies and should be enrolled in disease-modifying trials to stop the neurodegenerative process.
- Anti-IgLON5 disease is a novel condition characterized by abnormal sleep architecture, abnormal behaviors in nonrapid eye movement sleep, REM sleep behavior disorder (RBD), antibodies against the protein IgLON5, HLA-DQB1*05:01, and a tau deposits involving the brainstem and the hypothalamus.
- Patients with a severe form of periodic limb movements in sleep involving the whole body and severe obstrtive sleep apnea may present with dream-enacting behaviors and unpleasant dreams. In these cases, video-polysomnography is capable of excluding RBD and identifying periodic limb movements and apneic events.

Parasomnias are defined as undesirable physic events or experiences that occur during entry into sleep, within sleep, or during arousal from sleep.[1] Parasomnias may occur during nonrapid eye movement (NREM) sleep, rapid eye movement (REM) sleep, or during transitions from and to sleep.[1] In this article, we will review the parasomnias and other sleep-related disorders that can occur in older people.

SLEEP PARALYSIS

Sleep paralysis (SP) is the inability to perform voluntary movements at sleep onset or waking from sleep, with a duration ranging from seconds to few minutes.[1] Individuals experience SP as an unpleasant phenomenon where they are completely aware that they cannot move, open their eyes, or speak, usually linked to the feeling of suffocation, chest pressure and, in extreme cases, to the fear of dying. The events end abruptly and spontaneously or after tactile stimulation. The association with vivid visual, auditory, and tactile hallucinations is common. SP represents a dissociated state where REM sleep atonia coexists with the full consciousness of wakefulness. Sleep deprivation and irregular sleep–wake schedule are predisposing factors. SP is common among healthy people with a prevalence of 15% to 40% of at least one episode with onset usually in adolescence. Episodes may be recurrent and some subjects report a familial aggregation of the phenomenon. SP is very common in adolescents and young adults. However, in a few cases, SP may persist in the elderly, particularly in families suffering from this phenomenon. In most cases, including those occurring in the elderly, small doses of REM sleep suppressants such as

Published: November 15, 2017 DOI: https://doi.org/10.1016/j.jsmc.2017.09.005.
Neurology Service, Hospital Clinic de Barcelona, C/ Villarroel 180, Barcelona 08036, Spain
E-mail address: airanzo@clinic.cat

Sleep Med Clin 17 (2022) 295–305
https://doi.org/10.1016/j.jsmc.2022.02.005

clomipramine can reduce dramatically the frequency and intensity of the episodes.

DISORDERS OF AROUSALS

Disorders of arousal are parasomnias occurring in NREM sleep and comprise confusional arousals, sleepwalking, and sleep terrors. Clinically, patients present brief recurrent episodes of confused, complex and bizarre behaviors, frightening screams, and walking. They develop as a result of incomplete and partial awakenings from deep sleep. Most of the cases are benign and idiopathic. A familial pattern is common, but a genetic signature has not been found. A positive correlation with the HLA-DQB1*05 subtype has been reported.[2,3] In contrast to popular belief, individuals with sleepwalking and sleep terrors usually have nightmares that are related to aggression, misfortune, and apprehension, and their sleep behaviors seem to involve fear and unpleasant confusion.[4] In severe cases, episodes may result in broken sleep, daytime fatigue, psychological problems, social effects, injuries, and medico-legal issues. Predisposing factors are those that result in deep sleep (eg, sleep deprivation, night shifts, fever) and in sleep fragmentation (eg, noise, touch, psychological stress). Alcohol is another trigger.[4] Obstructive sleep apnea and periodic leg movements in sleep are not associated with disorders of arousals, but they can coexist by chance and then trigger some events when apneic episodes and limb movements cause arousals.

Disorders of arousal usually start during childhood, but they can persist into adulthood up to the age of 60 years, and even they can arise de novo in adults.[5] When disorders of arousal start in the adulthood or elderly one has to suspect the effect of a medication (particularly zolpidem) as the cause.

Disorders of arousal have been related to the effect of some medications. In most reports, the disorder of arousal has not been documented by polysomnography (PSG). The assumption of drug-induced sleepwalking is based on the temporal association between the introduction of the drug and the onset of the abnormal sleep behaviors and their cessation after it was stopped. The most common drugs inducing sleepwalking are zolpidem (used at therapeutic doses for insomnia) and sodium oxybate (at high doses within the normal range for narcolepsy). Postmarketing studies of zolpidem reported sleepwalking between 0.3% and 1% of the patients taking this medication. Besides sleepwalking, zolpidem can also cause the sleepwalking variants sleep-related eating disorder, sleep driving, and sleep

sex in the same patient. There are few case reports and small series of other medications such as lithium carbonate, typical and atypical neuroleptics, zaleplon, stimulants, antihistamines, antidepressants including paroxetine, bupropion and reboxetine, sedative hypnotics, statins, and topiramate that have induced or precipitated disorders of arousals (mainly sleepwalking). These medications may disturb sleep architecture and precipitate some events in predisposed individuals with and without past medical history of disorders of arousal. These medications usually induce sleepwalking and its variants. These variants include eating with consumption of peculiar forms or combinations of food (sleep-related eating disorder), smoking (sleep smoking), driving (sleep driving), and having sex (sleep sex or sexsomnia).

REM SLEEP BEHAVIOR DISORDER

REM sleep behavior disorder (RBD) is a REM sleep parasomnia characterized by dream-enacting behaviors and nightmares linked to REM sleep without muscle atonia. The diagnosis of RBD requires confirmation with video-PSG because other sleep disorders (eg, severe obstructive sleep apnea, periodic limb movement disorder (PLMD), nocturnal frontal lobe epilepsy, and sleepwalking) may also present with nightmares and abnormal sleep behaviors. RBD can be classified into an idiopathic form (REM sleep behavior disorder [IRBD]) and a secondary form. Available data indicate that most patients with IRBD will eventually be diagnosed with the neurodegenerative disorders Parkinson disease (PD), dementia with Lewy bodies (DLB), and multiple system atrophy (MSA).[6,7] Patients with IRBD represent the prodromal stage of these synucleinopathies. The secondary form of RBD is related to neurodegenerative diseases, autoimmune diseases, focal structural lesions in the brainstem, and the use of some medications. Psychiatric disorders are not linked to RBD.[6,7] In IRBD and RBD secondary to the synucleinopathies, RBD occurs in people aged older than 50 years, usually between the ages of 60 and 75. Herein, we will review IRBD and RBD secondary to the synucleinopathies PD, MSA, and DLB.

Idiopathic REM Sleep Behavior Disorder

The diagnosis of IRBD requires a history of dream-enacting behaviors, video-PSG detection of REM sleep with increased muscular activity associated with abnormal behaviors, absence of known neurodegenerative diseases, lack of motor and cognitive complaints, normal neurologic examination, normal brain magnetic resonance imaging, and RBD not explained by a brain lesion (eg, stroke, demyelinating plaque, encephalitis) or by the introduction or withdrawal of any medication or substance (eg, antidepressants, beta-blockers).[1,6] In many patients with IRBD, subclinical abnormalities such as olfactory deficits, cognitive deficits on neuropsychological tests, and decreased dopamine transporters imaging in the striatum on functional neuroimaging can be detected. These findings suggest that when IRBD is diagnosed, a neurodegenerative process is already widespread in the nervous system. Of these abnormalities, hyposmia, color vision impairment, substantia nigra hyperechogenicity, and decreased striatal dopamine transporter uptake identify those patients with IRBD who are at increased short-term risk (2.5–5 years) for being diagnosed with a synucleinopathy according to accepted clinical criteria.[8,9] Prospective studies have further shown that the echogenic size of the substantia nigra,[10] color vision, olfactory dysfunction,[9] and dysautonomic changes[11] remain stable over time. In contrast, dopamine transporter imaging shows progressive decline in striatal tracer uptake.[12] Thus, dopamine transporter imaging, serve better as a marker of subclinical progression in IRBD. The same happens with cognitive testing that shows worsening in executive, visuospatial, and memory domains with time.[13]

It has been shown that PD, DLB, and MSA frequently develop in patients with IRBD who are followed at sleep centers. In the seminal study, Schenck and colleagues[14] found that parkinsonism developed in 11 of 29 (38%) IRBD subjects nearly 4 years after the diagnosis of IRBD and almost 13 years after the onset of RBD. After 16 additional years of follow-up, 21 (72.4%) patients with IRBD from the original cohort were diagnosed with PD in 13 cases, DLB in 3, MSA in 2, unspecified dementia in 1, and Alzheimer disease (with autopsy-confirmed combined Alzheimer disease pathologic condition plus Lewy pathologic condition) in 2. Three IRBD subjects were lost during the follow-up period.[15] In a second series, we reported that 20 of 44 (45%) patients with IRBD developed a neurologic disorder after a mean interval of 11.5 years estimated from RBD onset and after a mean follow-up of 5.1 years from the diagnosis of IRBD. Emerging disorders were PD in 9 patients (2 with associated dementia), DLB in 6, MSA with predominant cerebellar syndrome in 1, and mild cognitive impairment (MCI) in 4 in whom visuospatial dysfunction was prominent. The finding that patients who developed a disorder were those with longer follow-up suggested that conversion rate (45%) could increase with the passage of time.[16] This was confirmed after 7 additional years of follow-up of this original cohort. We found that after a median follow-up of 10.5 years, 82% were diagnosed with PD ($n = 16$), DLB ($n = 14$), MSA ($n = 1$), and MCI ($n = 5$). The estimated risk of defined neurodegenerative syndrome from the diagnosis of IRBD was 34.8% at 5 years, 73.4% at 10 years, and 92.5% at 14 years.[17] These findings, in a group of 44 individuals with long and close follow-up, indicate that most patients with IRBD develop a synucleinopathy with time. Because additional patients with IRBD were diagnosed and followed in our sleep center, we aimed to confirm our initial observation in a larger cohort of subjects that comprised all the 174 consecutive IRBD patients diagnosed up to July 2013 in our sleep center. The risk of a defined neurodegenerative syndrome from the time of IRBD diagnosis was 33.1% at 5 years, 75.7% at 10 years, and 90.9% at 14 years. Emerging diagnoses (37.4%) were DLB in 29 patients, PD in 22, MSA in 2, and MCI in 12. In 6 patients who were diagnosed with PD, DLB, and MCI, neuropathological examination disclosed neuronal loss and widespread Lewy-type pathologic condition in the brain in each case.[18] Similar findings were observed in other series.[19–22] In a large multicenter study involving 1280 polysomnographically confirmed patients with IRBD from 24 centers, the overall conversion rate from IRBD diagnosis to an overt neurodegenerative syndrome was 6.3% per year, with 73.5% converting after 12-year follow-up.[22bis] Predictors of conversion were abnormal quantitative motor testing, hyposmia, MCI, erectile dysfunction, abnormal DAT-SPECT, color vision deficits, constipation, REM muscle atonia loss and age. Perhaps, the most relevant evidence that IRBD represents a neurodegenerative condition is that in vivo biopsy of the colon, submandibular gland, minor salivary glands, parotid, and skin shows deposits of synuclein in patients with IRBD but not in controls.[23–28] In IRBD, the RT-QuIC method can detect misfolded synuclein in the olfactory mucosa and cerebrospinal fluid. Interestingly, the sensitivity and specificity in the cerebrospinal fluid are both 90%.[24,29,30]

Taken together, IRBD is an optimal population to test disease-modifying strategies to stop the neurodegenerative disease and prevent the clinical appearance of the cardinal manifestations of the synucleinopathies, namely parkinsonism and dementia.

The Transition Between IRBD and Clinical Diagnosis of PD, DLB, and MSA

PD has a prodromal period of several years where progressive neuronal loss occurs before parkinsonism becomes clinically manifest and the disease can be clinically diagnosed. Olfactory loss, depression, constipation, and RBD may be present during the prodromal period of PD.[31] It is thought that DLB and MSA have also a prodromal phase before the clinical onset of their cardinal symptoms that define the disease (eg, dementia, parkinsonism, dysautonomia, and cerebellar syndrome). We reported the case of a 63-year-old man who presented with IRBD, and a 10-year clinical follow-up showed the serial development of constipation, hyposmia, depression, and MCI. The patient died without clinical parkinsonism and without dementia, and postmortem examination showed neuronal loss and Lewy bodies in the brainstem including the substantia nigra, olfactory bulb, hippocampus, limbic system, and synuclein aggregates in the peripheral autonomic nervous system.[32]

One study evaluated the presence of motor signs in patients with IRBD.[33] In those patients with IRBD who developed PD with time, voice and face akinesia emerged earliest (estimated prodromal interval of nearly 10 years), followed by rigidity (4.4 years), gait abnormalities (4.4 years), and limb bradykinesia (4.2 years). In another prospective study following clinically 44 patients with IRBD, 16 (13 men and 3 women) were diagnosed with PD.[17] The mean age at PD diagnosis was 75 years, estimated RBD duration at the time of the diagnosis of PD was 13 years, and the interval between diagnosis of IRBD and diagnosis of PD was 5.5 years. Five PD patients developed dementia. In these 5 patients, the median interval between the diagnosis of PD and the development of dementia was 6 years. Patients with IRBD seen at sleep centers who later develop PD, present a progressive parkinsonian syndrome where rigidity, bradykinesia, and hypomimia are prominent. This rigid-akinetic syndrome responds to levodopa. Resting tremor is not usually the presenting sign, but this may emerge at later stages of the disease. In these patients, constipation and self-reported loss of smell is common before the emergence of parkinsonian signs. In some patients, parkinsonism emerges in parallel with MCI onset.

In patients with IRBD who later develop DLB, the first presentation may be 1) severe acute episodes of agitation, hallucinations, and delirium after elective surgery (eg, knee, hip, abdominal) that resolve spontaneously or with small doses of neuroleptics after 1 or 2 weeks, 2) subacute episodes of paranoid delusions and visual hallucinations, 3) isolated visual hallucinations such as bugs running on the floor or the sensation of having someone or a shadow behind his or her back, and 4) MCI. MCI is an intermediate stage between normal cognitive function and dementia where individuals have cognitive complains, objective cognitive deficits are detected in neuropsychological tests, and daily living activities are preserved. In the particular setting of IRBD, MCI can be considered an abnormal condition that evolves into DLB and sometimes into PD. This is based on the following data. First, MCI occurs in nearly 20% of untreated PD patients at the time of initial diagnosis, and predicts conversion to dementia. Second, most patients with IRBD seen in sleep centers who develop MCI are eventually diagnosed with DLB. Third, patients with IRBD who develop MCI but no dementia show markers of a synucleinopathy such as decreased striatal dopamine transporter, hyperechogenicity of the substantia nigra, and hyposmia. Finally, in patients with MCI with co-morbid RBD who later develop dementia, postmortem examination shows Lewy-body pathologic condition.[32]

In our cohort of 44 patients with IRBD, 14 were eventually diagnosed with DLB.[17] All 14 subjects diagnosed with DLB were men. In these subjects with DLB, recurrent visual hallucinations occurred in 13 (93%), parkinsonism in 11 (79%), and fluctuating cognition in 9 (65%). Dementia was preceded by a recognized period of MCI characterized by executive, visuospatial, and memory dysfunction. The median interval between the diagnosis of MCI and the diagnosis of DLB was 2 years. The median age at DLB diagnosis was 76 years, the median estimated RBD duration at the time of the diagnosis of DLB was 12 years, and the median interval between diagnosis of RBD with video-PSG and clinical diagnosis of DLB was 7 years.

In patients with IRBD who later developed MSA with cerebellar signs, brain MRI may show atrophy of the pons and cerebellum before the emergence of a cerebellar syndrome. In these patients, urinary problems and falls due to cerebellar ataxia may be one of the initial manifestations of the disease. Nocturnal stridor may also appear before the appearance of parkinsonism or ataxia in MSA.

RBD in Patients Already Diagnosed with Parkinson Disease

PD is a neurodegenerative disorder characterized by parkinsonism and neuronal loss and Lewy bodies in the substantia nigra and many other central and peripheral structures of the nervous system. RBD is common among PD, because cell loss is common within the neuronal structures that regulate REM sleep atonia, namely the subcoeruleus nucleus and magnocellularis nucleus in the brainstem, and the amygdala. RBD occurs in

PD patients weather treated or untreated with dopaminergic agents. RBD is more common in MSA (90%–100%) and DLB (50%–70%) than in PD (25%–58%). Type of RBD-related unpleasant dreams, dream-enacting behaviors, and polysomnographic abnormalities are similar among sporadic PD, MSA, and IRBD.[34] RBD has also been described in small series involving other neurodegenerative disorders such as progressive supranuclear palsy and Machado-Joseph disease.

RBD occurs in 25% to 58% of the patients with sporadic PD, antedating the onset of parkinsonism by several years in about 20% of them with RBD.[35–38] RBD may precede parkinsonism or may develop concomitant or after the onset of parkinsonism. RBD confirmed by PSG may also occur in patients with PD linked to Parkin 2 mutations, but in this condition, RBD-related clinical manifestations are usually mild. RBD was not detected in one PARK 6 family, an autosomal recessive disorder that manifests as early-onset PD with a particularly mild progression. RBD occurs in PD associated with LRRK2 G2019S mutations where parkinsonism onset precedes RBD onset.[39] One study showed that in subjects with sporadic PD, the report of sleep-related falling out of bed was clinically suggestive of RBD.[40] In a study involving nondemented PD patients with RBD, video-PSG analysis and bed partners' reports demonstrated alleviation of parkinsonism during elaborated and complex RBD episodes. Movements during RBD episodes were faster, stronger, and smoother than those seen when the PD patient was awake. In the same manner, speech during RBD was more intelligible, better articulated, and louder than during wakefulness.[41]

RBD in manifested PD is associated with cognitive impairment, the rigid-akinetic motor subtype, older age, predominance in men, autonomic dysfunction, and an increased risk to develop dementia over time. This suggests that the presence of RBD in PD predicts the development of widespread neuropathological changes in the brain. Most studies have shown that in nondemented, nonhallucinator sporadic PD patients, the presence of RBD in PD is neither associated with hypersomnia, sleep benefit, sleep architecture disruption, olfactory dysfunction, or lower daily levodopa equivalent dose. When sporadic PD patients exhibit RBD, this parasomnia precedes the onset of parkinsonism in 18% to 22% of the patients.

RBD in Patients Already Diagnosed with Multiple System Atrophy

MSA is a neurodegenerative disease clinically characterized by parkinsonism, dysautonomia,

and cerebellar syndrome in any combination. Most patients with MSA have RBD.[42–44] The finding that in MSA brainstem cell loss is consistently widespread and severe may explain the high prevalence of RBD in this disease. RBD is currently considered a red flag for the diagnosis of MSA. In one study, 21 consecutive patients with MSA without sleep behavioral complaints underwent video-PSG that demonstrated RBD in 19 (90.5%).[43] In another study, video-PSG showed RBD in 35 out of 37 (95%) consecutive patients.[42]

Self-awareness of abnormal sleep behaviors and unpleasant dream recall is variable among MSA patients with RBD. In one study, 27 of 39 (69%) consecutive MSA patients with RBD or their relatives reported dream-enacting behaviors. Interestingly, most of the 12 that did not report dream-enacting behaviors were sleeping alone at their home.[42] In another study, only 7 of 21 (33%) MSA patients with RBD recalled vivid dreams.[43] In our first published case series comprising 26 consecutive MSA patients with RBD free of psychoactive drugs, 77% of the patients were unaware of their abnormal behaviors, which were only noticed by bed partners. Recall of unpleasant dreams was absent in 35% of the patients.[34] Like in PD, RBD-related movements are faster, stronger, and smother than during wakefulness.[43]

RBD may be the first symptom of MSA.[45,46] In one study of 27 RBD patients aware of their dream-enacting behaviors, RBD preceded the waking motor symptoms in 12 (44%).[43] In another study with 19 patients, RBD features were reported by the patients or their relatives as the first manifestation of the disease in 3, concomitant with other symptoms in 9, and developed after the onset of waking symptoms in the remaining 7. In our series, RBD onset antedated parkinsonian, cerebellar and dysautonomic onset in 35 of 67 (52%) patients by a mean of 7 years (range, 1–38 years).[34] MSA is eventually diagnosed in only a few subjects with the initial diagnosis of idiopathic RBD (most of them are diagnosed with PD and DLB), probably because in the general population MSA is much more rare than PD and DLB. We reported a patient presenting with dysautonomia, stridor during sleep, and RBD without parkinsonism or cerebellar syndrome in whom brain pathologic condition disclosed MSA after sudden death during wakefulness.[45]

RBD in Patients Already Diagnosed with Dementia with Lewy Bodies

DLB is the second most common cause of neurodegenerative dementia after Alzheimer disease. It is characterized by parkinsonism, recurrent visual hallucinations, and fluctuations in cognition and alertness. DLB is diagnosed if dementia precedes or appears within 1 year before the onset of parkinsonism. Neuronal loss and Lewy bodies are found in the brainstem, limbic system, and neocortex.[47]

The most studied sleep disturbance in DLB is RBD. Available data indicate that in patients with DLB, RBD is common, may be the first symptom of the disease, is associated with less Alzheimer disease pathologic condition in the brain, and can be considered a red flag of the disease. RBD is very rare in Alzheimer disease and other forms of dementia with the exception of PD associated with dementia. A retrospective study involving 37 consecutive patients with dementia plus RBD showed that 34 (92%) were men.[48] In 35 (96%) patients, RBD symptoms preceded or occurred simultaneously with the cognitive complaints. The diagnosis of DLB was confirmed in the 3 patients that underwent autopsy and supported the notion that the combination of dementia and RBD most often reflects DLB. This is in agreement with neuropathological studies in patients with antemortem diagnosis of DLB plus RBD showing cell loss and Lewy bodies in the brainstem, limbic system, and neocortex.[49,50] In a cohort of 234 autopsy-confirmed dementia patients followed longitudinally, a history suggestive of RBD was present in 76% of 98 with autopsy confirmed DLB, indicating that RBD is a common feature of DLB. In contrast, only 6 of the 136 patients without autopsy-confirmed DLB exhibited RBD.[50] Thus, the inclusion of RBD improves the diagnostic accuracy of DLB. Dugger and colleagues compared the clinical characteristics of 71 DLB patients with RBD and 19 without RBD. Those with RBD were predominantly men, had shorter duration of dementia, earlier onset of parkinsonism and visual hallucinations, and less Alzheimer disease-related pathologic condition on autopsy.[51] In 54 of the 71 (76%) patients with RBD, this parasomnia coincided or developed before dementia onset. This group of patients in whom RBD developed before the cognitive impairment were characterized by an earlier onset of visual hallucinations and parkinsonism, more severe baseline parkinsonism, and shorter duration of dementia.

In a retrospective study, Pao and colleagues[52] reviewed the polysomnographic findings of 78 patients with DLB (71 men, the mean age of 71 years) with sleep-related complaints. Seventy-five (96%) patients had histories of dream-enactment behaviors with 65 (83%) showing confirmation of RBD during PSG. The remaining 13 subjects did not attain any REM sleep, and hence RBD could not be confirmed by PSG.

Terzaghi and colleagues[53] evaluated the clinical and video-PSG findings of 29 consecutive DLB patients. Patients were taking levodopa but no dopamine agonists, benzodiazepines, cholinergics, neuroleptics, or antidepressants. Patients were 21 men, their mean age was 75 years, and the mean disease duration was 3 years. Dissociated or ambiguous sleep was found in 6 patients who had severe dementia. Disruptive motor behaviors during sleep were found in 70% and consisted in RBD in 11 subjects, confusional episodes from NREM sleep in 7 cases, and arousal-related episodes from REM or NREM sleep mimicking RBD in 2.

Ferman and colleagues evaluated with PSG 61 DLB patients with a mean estimated duration of cognitive impairment of 4 years and a mean estimated duration of RBD of 10 years. PSG showed REM sleep without atonia in 71% and 19% did not achieve REM sleep.[54]

Ratti and colleagues[55] evaluated by PSG a group of DLB patients and showed that those who reported sleep-related motor events corresponded either to RBD or to awakenings from sleep.

PARASOMNIA OVERLAP DISORDER

This term describes patients who have coexistent non-REM sleep disorder of arousal and RBD. Parasomnia overlap diosrder can be idiopathic or associated with conditions such as narcolepsy, Moebius syndrome and brain structural lesions.[56] The link between these 2 types of parasomnia can be by chance in a subject who had a disorder of arousal during childhood and decades later developed RBD. In some cases, this may explain the fact that subjects with IRBD who are older than 60 years and may report that their abnormal behaviors started 30 or 50 years earlier. In contrast to IRBD, the risk for phenoconversion to a neurodegenerative disease is unknown in parasomnia overlap disorder. This condition is rare, and only few cases have been confirmed by video-PSG. We reported video-PSG documentation of a patient with NREM parasomnia and normal REM sleep that after several years of follow-up developed RBD with NREM parasomnia persistence.[57]

ANTI-IgLON5 DISEASE

The recently described anti-IgLON5 disease is a novel neurologic condition initially described in 8 unrelated adults in whom subacute (2 cases) and chronic (6 cases) presentations were noted.[58] Patients presented clinically with witnessed apneic events, abnormal sleep behaviors, and additional waking neurologic symptoms such as gait instability, dysarthria, dysphagia, and mild dysautonomia. Patients had no previous history of disorders of arousal and were unaware of their sleep behaviors that were only noted by the bed partner. Video-PSG showed a very complex and novel sleep pattern characterized by 1) normal occipital alpha rhythm during wakefulness, 2) slightly reduction of total sleep time and sleep efficiency, 3) a distinctive temporal sequence of sleep stages and behaviors taking place, from most abnormal at the beginning of the night to normalization at the end, 4) infrequent normal N1 sleep and infrequent normal N2 sleep, 5) normal N3 sleep with delta waves only in the second half of the night, 6) initiation of sleep and reentering of sleep after awakenings characterized by theta activity and rapid repetitive leg movements that do not fit criteria of periodic leg movements in sleep, 7) periods of diffuse delta activity, typical of normal N3 sleep, mixed with spindles, 8) poorly structured stage N2 sleep characterized by clear spindles and K complexes with frequent vocalizations (eg, talking, laughing, crying) simple motor activity (eg, raising the arm, punching) and finalistic behaviors (eg, goal directed behaviors like sucking the thumbs while apparently eating, manipulating wires), 9) RBD, and 10) obstructive sleep apnea and inspiratory stridor secondary to vocal cord palsy. Longitudinal follow-up by V-PSG showed no dramatic deterioration of these sleep features with time. Autoantibodies against IgLON5, a neuronal cell adhesion protein, were identified in all patients. The haplotypes DQB1*0501 and DRB1*1001 were detected in all 4 patients tested. Most of the patients deceased after sudden death during wakefulness or at sleep. Neuropathology performed in 2 patients showed a tauopathy mainly involving the tegmentum of the brainstem and the hypothalamus.

After this initial presentation, other patients were reported and neuropathological criteria were established for this new entity.[59–66] A recent review of 22 patients revealed that the median age was 64 years (range: 46–83 years).[67] At the initial visit, 15 (68%) patients already complained of sleep symptoms. By the time of the diagnosis of the disorder (median delay from symptom onset: 2.5 years, range: 2 months to 18 years), 4 clinical presentations were identified: 1) a predominant sleep disorder with non-REM parasomnia and sleep breathing symptoms; 2) bulbar syndrome characterized by dysphagia, dysarthria, sialorrhea, and acute respiratory insufficiency; 3) a syndrome resembling progressive supranuclear palsy, and 4) cognitive impairment resembling Huntington disease. Reasons for referral were sleep disturbances in 8 patients, gait dysfunction in 8, and other symptoms in 6 (3 bulbar, 2 chorea, 1 cognitive decline). Thirteen of 15 (86.6%) patients had the HLA-DRB1*10:01 and HLA-DQB1*05:01 alleles. The risk ratio calculation indicated that DRB1*10:01 was 36 times more frequent in these patients than in the general population. Thirteen patients had IgLON5 antibodies in serum and CSF, and 2 only in serum. The disease was refractory to immunotherapy by the time of diagnosis, and postmortem findings are consistent with a novel neuronal tauopathy mainly involving the hypothalamus and tegmentum of the brainstem. It is still unclear if we are facing a neurodegenerative or an autoimmune disease.

RESTLESS LEGS SYNDROME

Restless legs syndrome (RLS) is a chronic sensorimotor entity characterized by an urge to move the legs, usually accompanied by unpleasant or uncomfortable sensations in the legs that begins or worsens during periods of rest or inactivity such as lying or sitting. Typically, RLS starts in the evening or at night and is partially or totally relieved by movement such as walking, stretching, or stamping.[68] The unpleasant sensations are habitually felt deep inside the legs and most patients define them as creeping and crawling. Some patients, however, have difficulties to find a precise word or term to describe their abnormal sensations in the legs. Only a few patients describe their sensations in the legs as painful. RLS may involve one or both lower limbs, and in some cases, the symptoms spread to the upper limbs and, in severe cases, to the trunk, neck, and face. In the lower limbs, the legs are almost always affected, but it is not rare that the uncomfortable sensations reach the tights and hips. Involvement of the feet is unusual but it may occur. In the upper limbs, shoulders, arms, elbows, and forearms are more frequently affected than wrists and hands. In a few cases, RLS symptoms may occur exclusively in the abdomen or in other body parts. RLS peak intensity is between 23:00 and 3:00, and nadir is in the morning between 6:00 and 10:00. Neurologic examination is usually normal except in those cases where RLS is secondary to varicose veins and polyneuropathy.

The clinical spectrum of RLS is wide, ranging from mild to severe forms. Severity of RLS depends on the frequency and intensity of both the urge to move and unpleasant sensations in the legs. Some patients have a progressive course, others have a stable course, and others present unpredictable long fluctuations and remissions. In some individuals, RLS may be precipitated or aggravated by some specific circumstances including pregnancy, iron deficiency anemia, and the introduction of some medications such as antidepressants and antidopaminergics. Patients with mild RLS usually do not seek medical attention because symptoms are mild, sporadic, and not bothersome. Severe cases usually seen in medical practice may be associated with impaired general quality of life linked either to insomnia, sleep fragmentation, daytime sleepiness, depression, anxiety, fatigue, inability to concentrate, or social limitations (eg, inability to enjoy quiet activities at night that require sitting such as driving for a long time, traveling by plane, dinning in a restaurant, and watching a movie at the theater).[68]

RLS may be sporadic, familial, or secondary to several conditions including end-stage renal disease, iron deficiency, pregnancy, some forms of peripheral neuropathy, and the use of antidopaminergic medications. RLS affects both sexes and all ages.[69] For unknown reasons, it is more frequent in women than in men. Prevalence of RLS increases with age in both genders reaching a plateau in the sixth decade. One study reported that experiencing RLS more than 4 nights per month occurred in 3% of participants aged 18 to 29 years, 10% of those aged 30 to 79 years, and 19% of those 80 years and older. About 20% of adults with RLS report onset of the symptoms between the ages of 10 and 20 years. A positive family history occurs in approximately 30% to 50% of the cases. In some cases, an autosomal dominant mode of inheritance may be present. RLS is linked to some genetic variants in the BTBD9, MEIS1, and MAP2K5-LBXCOR1 genes.[70–72]

There is a growing body of literature that indicates that the pathophysiology of RLS is linked to decrease dopaminergic tone in the spinal cord and iron insufficiency in the brain.[73,74] Dopaminergic agonists (pramipexole, ropinirole, and rotigotine) are considered the first line therapy for RLS.[75] However, in RLS, long-term therapy with dopaminergic agents may be related to a change in symptomatology termed augmentation.[76,77] The augmentation phenomenon is a complication, which consists in 1) an overall increase of RLS symptoms severity, 2) earlier onset of symptoms in the afternoon, 3) extension of the symptoms to previously unaffected body parts including the upper limbs, and 4) a shorter therapeutic effect of the dopaminergic medication. Management of the augmentation phenomenon includes decreasing the dose or withdrawal the dopaminergic agent.

Dopamine agonists may also induce control impulsive disorders.

Nondopaminergic medications such as gabapentin, pregabalin, and oxycodone are also effective in the treatment of RLS. Iron replacement is necessary in cases with iron deficiency or when iron is normal, but serum ferritin levels are low or in the lower normal range.[75,76]

PERIODIC LIMB MOVEMENTS IN SLEEP

Periodic limb movements in sleep (PLMS) are stereotyped repetitive movements characterized by dorsal flexion of the foot and sometimes flexion of the knee and even the hip in severe cases. The period length between 2 consecutive leg movements is 5 to 90 seconds. Each movement lasts between 0.5 and 10 seconds. PLMS appear in series of at least 4 movements. They may occur in one or both legs.[78] PLMS occur in about 80% to 90% of the patients with RLS. PLMS are also found in other disorders and in healthy individuals without motor, sensory, or sleep complains. In healthy subjects, the prevalence of PLMS increases with age. In healthy people older than 60 years without sleep complains, the mean number of PLMS is 25 per hour.[79] Thus, the absence of PLMS does not exclude RLS, and the presence of PLMS is not specific for RLS.

PLMS may be asymptomatic or may fragment sleep continuity leading to a nonrestorative sleep. PLMD refers to the situation where PLMS induce clinically significant sleep disturbance such as insomnia or hypersomnia.[1] We recently reported a new form of PLMD that is associated with vigorous limb and body movements and unpleasant dreams mimicking IRBD.[80] They were 15 men and 2 women with a median age of 66 years who consulted because of abnormal sleep behaviors and nightmares resembling RBD, but video-PSG ruled out this REM sleep parasomnia and showed frequent and vigorous PLMS in NREM sleep involving the 4 limbs and trunk and associated with semipurposeful behaviors and vocalizations occurring during arousals that followed these prominent PLMS. After treatment with dopaminergic agonists, PLMS were less frequent and vigorous, and unpleasant dreams and behaviors during sleep were dramatically improved. This form of severe PLMS should be considered as another condition that may simulate RBD symptoms and part of the PLMD spectrum. Sleep specialists and neurologists should be aware of this entity in the differential diagnosis of RBD and consider video-PSG as the instrument able to distinguish RBD from this extreme form of PLMS or other entities that can mimic RBD symptoms such as obstructive sleep apnea.[81]

DISCLOSURE

The author has no disclosures regarding the topic covered in this article.

REFERENCES

1. American Academy of Sleep Medicine. International classification of sleep disorders. 3rd edition. Darien, IL: American Academy of Sleep Medicine; 2014.
2. Lecendreux M, Bassetti C, Dauvilliers Y, et al. HLA and genetic susceptibility to sleepwalking. Mol Psychiatry 2003;8:114–7.
3. Heidbreder A, Frauscher B, Mitterling, et al. Not only sleepwalking but NREM parasomnia irrespective of the type is associated with HLA DQB1*05:01. J Clin Sleep Med 2016;12:565–70.
4. Oudiette D, Leu S, Pottier M, et al. Dreamlike mentations during sleepwalking and sleep terrors in adults. Sleep 2009;32:1621–7.
5. Zadra, Desautels A, Petit D, et al. Somnambulism: clinical aspects and pathophysiological hypothesis. Lancet Neurol 2013;12:185–294.
6. Iranzo A, Santamaria J, Tolosa E. Idiopathic rapid eye movement sleep behaviour disorder: diagnosis, management, and the need for neuroprotective interventions. Lancet Neurol 2016;15:405–19.
7. Boeve B. REM sleep behaviour disorder. Updated review of the core features, the REM sleep behaviour disorder-neurodegenerative disease association, evolving concepts, controversies, and future directions. Ann N.Y Acad Sci 2010;1184:15–54.
8. Iranzo A, Lomeña F, Stockner H, et al. For the Sleep Innsbruck Barcelona (SINBAR) group. Decreased striatal dopamine transporter uptake and substantia nigra hyperechogenicity as risk markers of synucleinopathy in patients with idiopathic rapid-eye-movement sleep behaviour disorder: a prospective study. Lancet Neurol 2010;9:1070–7.
9. Postuma RB, Gagnon JF, Vendette M, et al. Olfaction and color vision identify impending neurodegeneration in rapid eye movement sleep behavior disorder. Ann Neurol 2011;69:811–8.
10. Iranzo A, Stockner H, Serradell M, et al. Five year follow-up of substantia nigra echogenicity in idiopathic REM sleep behavior disorder. Mov Disord 2014;29:1774–80.
11. Postuma RB, Gagnon JF, Vendette M, et al. Markers of neurodegeneration in idiopathic rapid eye movement sleep behavior disorder and Parkinson's disease. Brain 2009;13:3298–307.
12. Iranzo A, Valldeoriola F, Lomeña F, et al. Serial dopamine transporter imaging of nigrostriatal function in patients with idiopathic rapid-eye-movement sleep

behaviour disorder: a prospective study. Lancet Neurol 2011;10:797–805.
13. Fantini ML, Farini E, Ortelli P. Longitudinal study of cognitive function in idiopathic REM sleep behavior disorder. Sleep 2011;34:619–25.
14. Schenck CH, Bundlie SR, Mahowald MW. Delayed emergence of a parkinsonian disorder in 38% of 29 older men initially diagnosed with idiopathic rapid eye movement sleep behavior disorder. Neurology 1996;46:388–92.
15. Schenck CH, Boeve BF, Mahowald MW. Delayed emergence of a parkinsonian disorder or dementia in 81% of older males initially diagnosed with idiopathic REM sleep behavior disorder (IRBD): 16 year update on a previously reported series. Sleep Med 2013;14:744–8.
16. Iranzo A, Molinuevo JL, Santamaria J, et al. Rapid-eye-movement sleep behaviour disorder as an early marker for a neurodegenerative disease: a descriptive study. Lancet Neurol 2006;5:572–7.
17. Iranzo A, Tolosa E, Gelpi E, et al. Neurodegenerative status and post-mortem pathology in idiopathic rapid-eye-movement disorder: an observational cohort study. Lancet Neurol 2013;12:443–53.
18. Iranzo A, Fernández-Arcos A, Tolosa E, et al. Neurodegenerative disorder risk in idiopathic REM sleep behavior disorder: study in 174 patients. PLoS One 2014;9(2):e89741.
19. Postuma RB, Gagnon JF, Bertrand JA, et al. Parkinson risk in idiopathic REM sleep behavior disorder: preparing for neuroprotective trials. Neurology 2015;84:1104–13.
20. Wing YK, Li SX, Mok V, et al. Prospective outcome of rapid eye movement sleep behaviour disorder: psychiatric disorders as a potential early marker of Parkinson's disease. J Neurol Neurosurg Psychiatry 2012;83:470–2.
21. Youn S, Kim T, Yoon IY, et al. Progression of cognitive impairments in idiopathic REM sleep behavior disorder. J Neurol Neurosurg Psychiatry 2015. https://doi.org/10.1136/jnnp-2015-311437.
22. Postuma RB, Iranzo A, Hogl B, et al. Risk factors for neurodegeneration in idiopathic rapid eye movement sleep behavior disorder: a multicenter study. Ann Neurol 2015;77:830–9.
23. Sprenger FS, Stefanova N, Gelpi E, et al. Enteric nervous system α-synuclein immunoreactivity in idiopathic REM sleep behavior disorder. Neurology 2015;85:1761–8.
24. Vilas D, Iranzo A, Tolosa E, et al. Assessment of α-synuclein in submandibular glands of patients with idiopathic rapid-eye-movement sleep behaviour disorder: a case-control study. Lancet Neurol 2016;15:708–18.
25. Tolosa E, Pont-Sunyer C. Progress in defining the premotor phase of Parkinson's disease. J Neurol Sci 2011;310:4–8.

26. Iranzo A, Gelpi E, Tolosa E, et al. Neuropathology of prodromal Lewy body disease. Mov Disord 2014;29: 410–5.

27. Postuma RN, Lang AE, Gagnon JF, et al. How does parkinsonism start? Prodromal parkinsonism motor changes in idiopathic REM sleep behaviour disorder. Brain 2012;27:617–26.

28. Iranzo A, Rye DB, Santamaria J, et al. Characteristics of idiopathic REM sleep behavior disorder and that associated with MSA and PD. Neurology 2005; 65:247–52.

29. Wetter TC, Trenkwalder C, Gershanik O, et al. Polysomnographic measures in Parkinson's disease: a comparison between patients with and without REM sleep disturbances. Wien Klin Wochenschr 2001;113:249–53.

30. Gagnon JF, Vendette M, Postuma R, et al. Mild cognitive impairment in rapid eye movement sleep behaviour disorder and Parkinson disease. Ann Neurol 2009;66:39–47.

31. De Cock VC, Vidailhet M, Leu S, et al. Restoration of normal muscle control in Parkinson's disease during REM sleep. Brain 2007;130:450–6.

32. Sixel-Doring F, Trautmann E, Mollenhauer B, et al. Associated factors for REM sleep behaviour disorder in Parkinson disease. Neurology 2011;77: 1048–54.

33. Pont-Sunyer C, Iranzo A, Gaig C, et al. Sleep diosrders in parkinsonian and nonparkinsonian LRRK2 mutation carriers. PLoS One 2015;10(7):e0132368.

34. Wallace DM, Shafazand S, Carvalho DZ, et al. Sleep-related falling out of bed in Parkinson's disease. J Clin Neurol 2012;8:51–7.

35. De Cock VC, Vidailhet M, Leu S, et al. Restoration of normal motor control in Parkinson's disease during REM sleep. Brain 2007;130:450–6.

36. Plazzi G, Corsini R, Provini F, et al. REM sleep behavior disorders in multiple system atrophy. Neurology 1997;48:1094–7.

37. De Cock V, Debs R, Oudiette D, et al. The improvement of movement of speech during rapid eye movement sleep behavior disorder in multiple system atrophy. Brain 2011;134:856–62.

38. Palma JA, Fernandez-Cordon C, Coon EA, et al. Prevalence of REM sleep behavior disorder in multiple system atrophy: a multicenter study and meta-analysis. Clin Auton Res 2015;25:69–75.

39. Gaig C, Iranzo A, Tolosa E, et al. Pathologically description of a non-motor variant of multiple system atrophy. J Neurol Neurosurg Psychiatry 2008;79: 1399–400.

40. Tachibana N, Kimura K, Kitajama K, et al. REM sleep motor dysfunction in multiple system atrophy: with special emphasis on sleep talk as its early clinical manifestation. J Neurol Neurosurg Psychiatry 1997; 63:678–81.

41. McKeith IG, Dickson DW, Lowe J, et al. Diagnosis and management of dementia with Lewy bodies. Third report of the DLB consortium. Neurology 2005;65:1863–72.

42. Boeve BF, Silber MH, Ferman TJ, et al. REM sleep behavior disorder and degenerative dementia. An association likely reflecting Lewy body disease. Neurology 1998;51:363–70.

43. Boeve BF, Silber MH, Parisi JE. Synucleinopathy pathology and REM sleep behavior disorder plus dementia or parkinsonism. Neurology 2003;61:40–5.

44. Ferman TJ, Boeve BF, Smith GE, et al. Inclusion of RBD improves the diagnostic classification of dementia with Lewy bodies. Neurology 2011;77: 875–82.

45. Dugger BN, Boeve BF, Murray ME, et al. Rapid eye movement sleep behavior disorder and subtypes in autopsy-confirmed dementia with Lewy bodies. Mov Disord 2012;27:72–8.

46. Pao WC, Boeve BF, Ferman TJ, et al. Polysomnographc findings in dementia with Lewy bodies. Neurologist 2013;19:1–6.

47. Terzaghi M, Arnaldi D, Rizzetti MC, et al. Analysis of video-polysomnographic sleep findings in dementia with Lewy bodies. Mov Disord 2013;28:1416–23.

48. Ferman TJ, Smith GE, Dickson DW, et al. Abnormal daytime sleepiness in dementia with Lewy bodies compared to Alzheimer's disease using the Multiple Sleep latency Test. Alzheimers Res Ther 2014;6(9):76.

49. Ratti PL, Terzaghi M, Minafra A, et al. REM and NREM sleep enactment behaviors in Parkinson's disease, Parkinson's disease dementia and dementia with Lewy bodies. Sleep Med 2012;13:926–32.

50. Dumitrascu O, Schenck CH, Applebee G, et al. Parasomnia overlap disorder: a distinct pathophysiological entity or a variant of rapid eye movement sleep behavior disorder? A case series. Sleep Med 2013;14:1217–20.

51. Matos N, Iranzo A, Gaig C, et al. Video-polysomnographic documentation of non-rapid eye movement sleep parasomnia followed by rapid eye movement sleep behavior disorder: a parasomnia overlap disorder? Sleep Med 2016;23:46–8.

52. Sabater L, Gaig C, Gelpi E, et al. A novel non-rapid-eye movement and rapid-eye-movement parasomnia with sleep breathing disorder associated with antibodies to IgLON5: a case series, characterisation of the antigen, and post-mortem study. Lancet Neurol 2014;13:575–86.

53. Gelpi E, Höftberger R, Graus F, et al. Neuropathological criteria of anti-IgLON5-related tauopathy. Acta Neuropathol 2016;132:531–43.

54. Högl B, Heidbreder A, Santamaria J, et al. IgLON5 autoimmunity and abnormal behaviours during sleep. Lancet 2015;385:1590.

55. Simabukuro MM, Sabater L, Adoni T, et al. Sleep disorder, chorea, and dementia associated with

IgLON5 antibodies. Neurol Neuroimmunol Neuroinflamm 2015;2:e136.

56. Montojo MT, Piren V, Benkhadra F, et al. Mimicking progressive supranuclear palsy and causing Tako-Tsubo syndrome: a case report on IgLON5 encephalopathy [abstract]. Mov Disord 2015;30(Suppl 1): 710.

57. Brüggemann N, Wandinger KP, Gaig C, et al. Dystonia, lower limb stiffness, and upward gaze palsy in a patient with IgLON5 antibodies. Mov Disord 2016; 31:762–4.

58. Schröder JB, Melzer N, Ruck T, et al. Isolated dysphagia as initial sign of anti-IgLON5 syndrome. Neurol Neuroimmunol Neuroinflamm 2016;4(1): e302.

59. Haitao R, Yingmai Y, Yan H, et al. Chorea and parkinsonism associated with autoantibodies to IgLON5 and responsive to immunotherapy. J Neuroimmunol 2016;300:9–10.

60. Zhang W, Niu N, Cui R. Serial 18F-FDG PET/CT findings in a patient with IgLON5 encephalopathy. Clin Nucl Med 2016;41:787–8.

61. Gaig C, Graus F, Compta Y, et al. Clinical manifestations of the anti-IgLON5 disease. Neurology 2017; 88(18):1736–43.

62. Allen RP, Picchietti DL, Garcia-Borreguero D, et al. Restless legs syndrome/Willis-Ekbom disease diagnostic criteria: updated International Restless Legs Syndrome Study Group (IRLSSG) consensus criteria–history, rationale, description, and significance. Sleep Med 2014;15:860–73.

63. Garcia-Borreguero D, Egatz R, Winkelmann J. Epidemiology of restless legs syndrome: the current status. Sleep Med Rev 2006;10:153–67.

64. Stefansson H, Rye D, Hicks A, et al. A genetic risk factor for periodic limb movements in sleep. N Engl J Med 2007;357:703–5.

65. Winkelmann J, Schormair P, Lichtner P, et al. Genome-wide association study of restless legs syndrome identifies common variants in three genomic regions. Nat Gen 2007;39:1000–6.

66. Winkelmann J, Schormair B, Xiong L, et al. Genetics of restless legs syndrome. Sleep Med 2016;(16): 30255–6. pii: S1389-9457.

67. Rye DB. Parkinson's disease and RLS: the dopaminergic bridge. Sleep Med 2004;5:317–28.

68. Paulus W, Trenkwalder C. Less is more: pathophysiology of dopaminergic-therapy-related augmentation in restless legs syndrome. Lancet Neurol 2006; 10:878–86.

69. Winkelman JW, Armstrong MJ, Allen RP, et al. Practice guideline summary: treatment of restless legs syndrome in adults: report of the guideline development, dissemination, and implementation subcommittee of the American academy of neurology. Neurology 2016;87:2585–93.

70. Garcia-Borreguero D, Silber MH, Winkelman JW, et al. Guidelines for the first-line treatment of restless legs syndrome/Willis-Ekbom disease, prevention and treatment of dopaminergic augmentation: a combined task force of the IRLSSG, EURLSSG, and the RLS-foundation. Sleep Med 2016;21:1–11.

71. García-Borreguero D. Dopaminergic augmentation in restless legs syndrome/Willis-Ekbom Disease: identification and Management. Sleep Med Clin 2015;10:287–92.

72. Iber C, Ancoli-Israel S, Chesson A, et al, for the American Academy of Sleep Medicine. The AASM manual for the scoring of sleep and associated events: rules, terminology and technical specifications. 1st edition. Westchester, IL: American Academy of Sleep Medicine; 2007.

73. Pennestri MH, Whittom S, Adam B, et al. PLMS and PLMW in healthy subjects as a function of age: prevalence and interval distribution. Sleep 2006;29: 1183–7.

74. Gaig C, Iranzo A, Pujo M, et al. Periodic limb movements during sleep mimicking REM sleep behavior disorder. Sleep 2016. pii: sp-00337-16. [Epub ahead of print].

75. Iranzo A, Santamaría J. Severe obstructive sleep apnea mimicking REM sleep behavior disorder. Sleep 2005;28:203–6.

76. Iranzo A, Borrego S, Vilaseca I, et al. a-Synuclein aggregates in labial salivary glands of idiopathic rapid eye movement sleep behavior disorder. Sleep 2018;41(8).

77. Fernández-Arcos A, Vilaseca I, Aldecoa I, et al. Alpha-synuclein aggregates in the parotid gland of idiopathic REM sleep behavior disorder. Sleep Med 2018;52:14–7.

78. Antelmi E, Donadio V, Incensi A, et al. Skin nerve phosphorylated a-synuclein deposits in idiopathic REM sleep behavior disorder. Neurology 2017;88: 2128–31.

79. Doppler K, Jentschke HM, Schulmeyer L, et al. Dermal phospho-alpha-synuclein deposits confirm REM sleep behaviour disorder as prodromal Parkinson's disease. Acta Neuropathol 2017;133:535–45.

80. Stefani A, Iranzo A, Holzknecht E, et al. Alpha-synuclein seeds in olfactory mucosa of patients with isolated rapid-eye-movement sleep behaviour disorder. Brain 2021;144:1118–26.

81. Iranzo A, Fairfoul G, Ayudhay N, et al. Cerebrospinal fluid alpha-synuclein detection by RT-QuIC in patients with isolated REM sleep behavior disorder. Lancet Neurol 2021;20:203–12.

Neurodegenerative Disorders and Sleep

Raman K. Malhotra, MD

KEYWORDS

• Parkinson disease • Alzheimer disease • Dementia • Rapid eye movement sleep behavior disorder
• Sleep apnea • Insomnia • Circadian rhythm disorder • Restless legs syndrome

KEY POINTS

• Sleep disorders are common in neurodegenerative conditions.
• Certain sleep disorders are more common in specific neurodegenerative conditions. REM sleep behavior disorder is more commonly seen in Parkinson disease than in Alzheimer disease.
• Common sleep disorders that may occur in most neurodegenerative conditions include insomnia, sleep apnea, restless legs syndrome, and circadian rhythm disorders.

INTRODUCTION

Cerebral neurodegenerative disorders, such as Parkinson disease (PD) and dementia, are increasing in prevalence as the population ages. These disorders are characterized by neuronal cell loss and abnormal accumulation of protein in cells of the brain. Symptoms, such as tremor, muscle rigidity, imbalance, and impaired cognition, progressively worsen with time. Not only are there challenges in managing the primary symptoms of these conditions, but many of these patients also suffer from sleep complaints, such as insomnia or hypersomnia. Others may suffer from abnormal movements during sleep, known as rapid eye movement (REM) sleep behavior disorder (RBD). This disorder may be dangerous and disruptive to sleep, and can sometimes precede the development of other symptoms of neurodegenerative disorders by years or even decades. High rates of sleep disorders, such as insomnia, hypersomnia, sleep apnea, restless legs syndrome (RLS), and circadian rhythm disorders, in older adults with neurodegenerative disorders are likely caused by the underlying symptoms of the disease along with damage to sleep-controlling regions of the brain. It is important to recognize and properly manage these sleep disorders because treatment may improve symptoms of the neurodegenerative condition and improve quality of life.

PARKINSON DISEASE AND OTHER SYNUCLEINOPATHIES

PD is a progressive neurodegenerative condition that causes motor symptoms of bradykinesia, shuffling gait, tremor, and rigidity. It is the second most common neurodegenerative condition affecting more than 1% of the population older than 60 years of age.[1] Patients commonly present with postural instability and falls. The pathologic hallmark of PD is Lewy bodies, which are intraneuronal a-synuclein inclusions. Lewy bodies first involve lower brainstem areas before spreading next to the substantia nigra and eventually areas throughout the brain. Motor symptoms of PD typically respond well to dopamine therapy early in the course of the disease. There are a variety of nonmotor symptoms of PD, including autonomic, olfactory, and mood dysfunction, and poor sleep. Sleep disorders are seen in most patients with PD.[2] The most common sleep disorders are insomnia, periodic limb movement disorder, sleep-disordered breathing, and RBD. In addition to PD, other synucleinopathies (which are central nervous system degenerative conditions caused by abnormal a-synuclein accumulation) include Lewy body dementia and multiple system atrophy, which are also associated with high rates of the same sleep disorders typically seen in patients with PD.

Washington University Sleep Medicine Center, Department of Neurology, Washington University in St. Louis School of Medicine, 1600 S. Brentwood Boulevard, #600, St. Louis, MO 63144, USA
E-mail address: raman.malhotra@wustl.edu

Sleep Med Clin 17 (2022) 307–314
https://doi.org/10.1016/j.jsmc.2022.02.009
1556-407X/22/© 2022 Elsevier Inc. All rights reserved.

sleep.theclinics.com

Sleep is disrupted in PD and other synucleinopathies for numerous reasons. The motor and nonmotor symptoms described previously can lead to poor sleep at night. Many medications used for PD can have side effects of sleepiness and poor sleep. In addition, the sleep-controlling centers of the brain are also affected by the underlying neurodegenerative process in the brain. Involvement of the pedunculopontine nucleus, locus ceruleus, pontine ceruleus alpha nucleus, and raphe nuclei are implicated in disorders of REM sleep and slow wave sleep, and have been directly localized as areas of involvement in some animal models of PD.[3]

Insomnia

Insomnia is defined by a complaint of repeated difficulties with initiating sleep, maintaining sleep, or waking up earlier than desired that occurs despite adequate time and opportunity for sleep. The symptoms should result in some form of daytime impairment to meet criteria for this disorder.[4] Patients suffering from synucleinopathies, such as PD, commonly complain of insomnia. Patients with PD more commonly suffer from sleep maintenance insomnia as compared with sleep-onset insomnia. One study cites sleep problems in 60% of patients with PD, with 76% complaining of poor sleep.[2] Insomnia may occur from a variety of issues (**Box 1**). The motor symptoms of PD can cause issues with muscle cramps, stiffness, and difficulties with turning or rolling in bed. Nonmotor symptoms, such as autonomic dysfunction (which can lead to frequent nocturia) or mood disorders, also contribute to sleep disruption. Many medications used for PD can cause disrupted sleep at night or sleepiness during the daytime (causing less sleepiness overnight). Sleep-controlling areas of the brain may be damaged leading to insomnia. As the PD and nervous system degeneration

progresses, insomnia also worsens in incidence and severity. Underlying mood disorders and worsening motor and nonmotor PD symptoms also contribute to worse insomnia later in the course of the disease. Polysomnography in patients with PD demonstrates prolonged sleep latency and fragmented sleep with reduced slow wave sleep and REM sleep. Insomnia may often result in subjective complaints of daytime fatigue, irritability, mood changes, poor attention, trouble with motor skills, and may result in decreased ability to function at baseline during waking hours.

Diagnosis and evaluation of insomnia typically involves a good history of sleep habits, bedtimes, wake times, naps, and awakenings at night. Directed questions in regards to causes or exacerbating factors of insomnia, such as RLS, medications, motor symptoms of PD, sleep apnea, and circadian rhythm disorders, should be performed. Sleep logs, diaries, and sleep trackers, such as actigraphy or wearable devices, are helpful. Polysomnography may be necessary if insomnia is thought to be secondary to sleep apnea, periodic limb movement disorder, or parasomnias.

Management of insomnia includes identifying and addressing any underlying primary sleep disorders. In addition, good sleep habits and hygiene should be encouraged. Medications and their timing should be scrutinized and possibly altered. If motor symptoms of PD are keeping the patient up at night, dopamine therapy at night may be necessary to alleviate the symptoms to help induce and maintain sleep. Short-acting carbidopa/levodopa, long-acting carbidopa/levodopa, dopamine agonists, and transdermal dopamine (ie, rotigotine patch) have shown small benefits in motor symptoms during the night in small trials.[5] Sometimes the dopamine agent itself may be causing insomnia. A decrease in dose or change in timing of the doses may improve sleep.

Primary sleep disorders, such as RLS and circadian rhythm disturbances, need to be correctly identified as a cause of insomnia in patients with PD. RLS is seen in 15% to 20% of patients with PD.[6] RLS is difficult to distinguish from other causes of leg pain in this population, such as muscle spasms and arthritis. Serum ferritin and iron studies should be evaluated in these patients and replaced if low (ie, ferritin <50). Other treatments for RLS include dopamine agonists, gabapentin, pregabalin, and opioids. Some patients who present with sleep maintenance insomnia or early morning awakenings may have a circadian rhythm disorder, such as advanced sleep-wake phase disorder. This condition is seen more commonly in the older population and in patients with neurodegenerative disorders.

Box 1
Common causes of insomnia in Parkinson disease

Motor symptoms (cramps, stiffness, impaired turning in bed)

Nocturia

Depression and/or anxiety

Medication side effect

Inadequate sleep hygiene

Restless legs syndrome

Sleep apnea

Circadian rhythm disorders

Delayed sleep-wake phase disorder is also seen in this population and may present with sleep-onset insomnia or difficulties awakening in the morning. Circadian rhythm disturbances have been described in patients with PD, including disruption of circadian markers, such as cortisol and melatonin levels.[7,8] Diagnosis should include a detailed history, sleep logs, and actigraphy. Patients with advanced sleep-wake phase disorder demonstrate evening sleepiness with difficulties in staying asleep. A prolonged sleep latency and later wake times are commonly reported in delayed sleep-wake phase disorder. Treatment of advanced sleep-wake phase disorder involves evening bright light therapy. Treatment of delayed sleep-wake phase disorder involves bright light on awakening in the morning along with evening melatonin several hours before desired bedtime.

Hypnotic medications should be used judiciously in this population because of concerns of causing falls, worsened balance, and impaired cognition. Potential benefits of therapies should be weighed against their risks. Hypnotics used in the general adult populations are the same agents typically used in patients with PD. There are limited studies evaluating use in this specific population. Studies have demonstrated effectiveness of eszopiclone and another with doxepin in improving subjective impression of sleep in patients with PD, but not objective measurements.[9,10] Sedating antidepressants have been used, but there should be caution because they may worsen RLS or periodic limb movements of sleep. As in the general population, cognitive behavioral therapy for insomnia is strongly suggested as first-line therapy for treatment of insomnia, although again evidence is scarce in relation to its effectiveness specifically in patients with PD.

Hypersomnia

Excessive daytime sleepiness is a common symptom in patients with PD. Because hypersomnia is a side effect of dopamine therapy, this may present early on in the disease process when dopamine therapy is initiated for motor symptoms.[11] However, this is not the only reason that excessive daytime sleepiness may present in this population (**Box 2**). Many wake-promoting regions in the brain are affected in PD, including the locus coeruleus, raphe nucleus, and hypocretin neurons, among other areas. One study suggests that hypersomnia precedes the development of other motor symptoms in PD, demonstrating sleepy adults had a three times higher risk of developing PD than nonsleepy adults.[12] Sleepiness may present with sleep attacks, or sudden onset sleep, which are more

---

Box 2
Common causes of hypersomnia in Parkinson disease

Sleep apnea

Medication side effect

Loss of hypocretin neurons (central nervous system hypersomnia)

Insufficient sleep

Circadian rhythm disorder

REM sleep behavior disorder

Sleep-disordered breathing

---

commonly reported in patients with PD (up to 14%) than age-matched control subjects.[13] Sleep attacks are dangerous if they occur during driving, work, or other activities where a sudden change in alertness may be dangerous. Sleep attacks can also be a side effect of dopamine agonists commonly used as treatment in patients with PD. In PD and multiple system atrophy, there has been evidence of damage to hypocretin neurons in the hypothalamus, leading to a narcolepsy-like condition with related symptoms.[14] Low hypocretin levels have been measured in patients with PD with these symptoms.[15]

A careful interview and evaluation for primary sleep disorders (eg, sleep apnea, restless legs, insomnia) is an important first step. Sleepiness as a possible side effect of dopamine therapy must also be recognized in patients with PD presenting with hypersomnia. If these factors and other causes of hypersomnia have been addressed, then use of a wake-promoting agent is considered. Agents used to treat hypersomnia and narcolepsy in the general population are the same ones used in patients with PD with hypersomnia. Caffeine, modafinil, and methylphenidate have all been shown to improve sleepiness in patients with PD.[16,17] One trial used sodium oxybate and demonstrated improvement in symptoms.[18] Given the age of the population, caution must be used when starting wake-promoting agents in patients with comorbid cardiac or psychiatric disorders, and adverse effects, such as hypertension, confusion, and agitation, should be monitored.

Sleep-disordered breathing in the form of central and obstructive sleep apnea is seen in a greater proportion of patients with PD than in age-matched control subjects, although some studies dispute this finding.[19] Polysomnography is the proper diagnostic test in this population, because typically there is also concern for RBD and periodic limb movement disorder, both of which are not able to be identified with home sleep apnea testing. A randomized placebo-controlled crossover study of patients with PD showed improvements in sleep architecture and objective measures in sleepiness in the patients treated with continuous positive airway pressure (CPAP).[20] As in the general population, positive airway pressure is typically effective in treating obstructive sleep apnea, but adherence remains a glaring challenge. Use of CPAP in patients with multiple system atrophy demonstrated that more than 66% discontinued CPAP after a year in one study.[21] In addition to typical obstructive sleep apnea symptoms, patients with multiple system atrophy may present with stridor and laryngeal dysfunction, which is a poor prognostic factor and requires treatment with positive airway pressure or other forms of nocturnal ventilation.[22]

Parasomnias

Patients with PD may complain of abnormal movements during sleep. This may be from a variety of conditions including sleep myoclonus, periodic limb movements of sleep, tremor, dystonia, or parasomnias. RBD is the most common parasomnia seen in patients with PD, seen in up to 60% of patients with PD. RBD is even more common in multiple-system atrophy and Lewy body dementia (75% or higher).[23] RBD involves repeated episodes of sleep-related vocalization and/or complex motor behaviors that occur during REM sleep. Motor activity is reaching, grabbing, kicking, or other vigorous motor activity that could lead to injury of the patient or bed partner.[4] Nonviolent behaviors, such as smiling, laughing, or shouting, can also occur. The patient does not typically ambulate, with almost all motor activity occurring in or next to the bed. Eyes are typically closed and the patient does not interact with the environment. If awoken from the event, the patient returns to normal levels of consciousness, but may remember dream content related to the motor activity. Patients with PD with RBD have fewer tremors, more falls, more autonomic dysfunction, and more cognitive dysfunction than patients with PD who do not have RBD.[24] RBD has been shown to be a prodromal stage for PD and other synucleinopathies. Studies following patients with idiopathic RBD have demonstrated high rates of conversion to PD and other synucleinopathies, with a 45% rate of conversion at 5 years, 76% rate at 10 years, and more than 90% rate at 14 years.[25] These patients with RBD at high risk for central nervous degenerative disorders will likely be ideal candidates for neuroprotective therapy when they become available, although at this time no proven therapies of this kind exist. Patients with idiopathic RBD need to be counseled in regards to this risk and followed for early signs of cerebral neurodegenerative conditions, namely synucleinopathies. This follow-up may include questioning in regards to symptoms; serial neurologic examinations to look for early signs of disease; or more formal testing, such as neuropsychological testing or imaging of the brain.

RBD diagnosis requires not only a clinical history of dream enactment behavior, but also in the sleep laboratory, attended polysomnography demonstrating REM sleep without atonia.[4] In addition to standard chin and lower extremity surface electromyogram recording leads, additional upper extremity electromyogram leads in the arms or shoulders are used to increase sensitivity in identifying REM sleep without atonia.[26] Polysomnography is also useful in ensuring there are no other causes of abnormal movements during sleep, such as periodic limb movements of sleep or sleep-disordered breathing triggering increased muscle tone during REM sleep (pseudo-RBD).

Initial therapy for RBD includes securing the sleep environment and avoiding injury to the patient or bed partner. This includes removing sharp objects and weapons from the bedroom, possibly sleeping in separate beds, moving the bed away from windows, or placing the mattress on the floor. It is also necessary to educate the patient on possible triggers for RBD including medications and sleep deprivation. Treating any underlying primary sleep disorders, such as RLS or sleep-disordered breathing, should also be emphasized. Pharmacologic treatment of RBD includes two major therapies: clonazepam and melatonin.[27] Clonazepam was the first medication shown to be effective in treating RBD. The mechanism of action is unclear. Clonazepam is effective in improving RBD motor activity, but there are significant concerns in older adults in regards to possible side effects of cognitive impairments, sleepiness, and increased risk for falls. Melatonin at high doses has also been shown to improve RBD symptoms, with less potential for side effects.[28] For refractory cases, combination of melatonin and clonazepam has been used along with a customized bed alarm. Cases series and other small studies demonstrate possible effectiveness of rivastigmine, dopamine agonists, desipramine, clozapine, and carbamazepine.[27]

ALZHEIMER DEMENTIA AND OTHER TAUOPATHIES

Dementia is defined as progressive memory decline and diminished cognition in at least one additional domain: aphasia, apraxia, agnosia, or executive dysfunction. These impairments impact social or occupational functioning. There were an estimated 24 million people in the world with dementia in 2001, with the number expected to double in the next 20 years because of the increase in life expectancy of the population.[29]

Alzheimer disease (AD) is a neurodegenerative condition that causes progressive memory decline and other cognitive deficits. AD is the most common cause of dementia worldwide, and represents approximately 50% to 70% of cases. The neuropathologic hallmark of AD is neuronal loss with cerebral atrophy, b-amyloid plaques, and neurofibrillary tangles composed of tau. There are other neurodegenerative disorders associated with abnormal buildup of tau, including progressive supranuclear palsy (PSP) and corticobasal degeneration. All of these tauopathies are commonly associated with sleep disorders. The same processes that damage areas of the brain causing dementia also cause dysfunction in control of sleep, alertness, and the circadian rhythm. Degeneration of neurons in brain areas, such as nucleus basalis of Meynert, pedunculopontine tegmental and later-odorsal tegmental nuclei, and noradrenergic neurons of the brainstem, can lead to reduced REM sleep in AD. Unlike in PD (and other synucleinopathies), RBD is rarely seen in AD.

Degeneration of neurons of the suprachiasmatic nucleus and reduction in melatonin levels in patients with AD has been demonstrated.[30] Further reports suggest that this decrease in melatonin level and disruption of the circadian rhythm may appear early in the course of the disease, and may be potentially responsible for progression of the disease.[31] An interesting association has been reported between sleep disruption or deprivation and b-amyloid levels in normal control subjects, suggesting sleep disruption as an accelerating factor in the progression to AD.[32] One hypothesis is that sleep plays an important role in clearing toxic protein accumulation, such as b-amyloid, in the central nervous system.[33] Sleep changes are also prominent in patients with mild cognitive impairment (MCI), which is a prodromal phase of AD. Studies have shown that up to 60% of patients with MCI have sleep complaints.[34] Patients with MCI were found to have more arousals during slow wave sleep, prolonged REM sleep latency, and increased wake after sleep onset.[35]

Sleep disturbances in AD may also be caused by underlying psychiatric, medical, and primary sleep disturbances; medication-related effects; and insufficient light during the day or excessive light at night before bedtime. Polysomnography studies in patients with AD demonstrate decreased sleep efficiency, percentage slow wave sleep, and REM sleep, and prolonged REM sleep latency.[36] Although some of these may be age-related changes, the findings in AD are more prominent than in age-matched control subjects. Sleep spindles and K-complexes become poorly formed as the condition progresses, making distinction between stage N1 and N2 sleep more difficult in electroencephalography.[37]

Insomnia

Even early in the course of disease, patients with AD complain of disrupted sleep, insomnia, and frequent nighttime awakenings. The insomnia is multifactorial, likely caused by comorbid medical conditions and medication side effects, and damage to areas in the brain that control sleep, wakefulness, and the circadian rhythm. A different hypothesis suggests altered orexin levels in cerebrospinal fluid resulting in sleep dysregulation.[38] Circadian rhythm disorders are seen at higher rates in patients with dementia, because there have been studies demonstrating altered levels of melatonin in these patients and damage to the suprachiasmatic nucleus.[30] Patients generally present clinically with prolonged wakefulness during the night along with excessive sleepiness during the daytime in the forms of naps. This disrupted sleep pattern can cause worsening behavior, confusion, and agitation in the evening and nighttime, which has been called "sundowning." Environmental factors also play a role in exacerbating these symptoms, such as decreased physical exercise and decreased bright light exposure.[39] In patients with dementia in skilled nursing facilities, nocturnal awakenings are exacerbated by roommates, ambient noise, or bed-checks. In addition, exacerbation of any underlying medical issue (ie, infection, metabolic abnormality) can trigger sundowning or worsen sleep. This insomnia and sleep disruption can affect not only the patient, but also the caregiver's sleep and may lead to a visit to an emergency department or placement into a facility if the disruption persists.

Management of insomnia includes educating the patient and caregivers about good sleep hygiene and habits (**Box 3**). Circadian rhythm disorders in patients with AD are treated with properly timed bright light therapy and exogenous melatonin to reset the intrinsic clock to their desired bedtime and wake times. Both nighttime melatonin and morning light exposure for 1 hour improved daytime alertness and reduced sleep disruption in patients with AD.[40] Evidence demonstrates that melatonin at night in this population

Box 3
Sleep hygiene recommendations
Keep a regular bedtime and wake time throughout the week
Engage in relaxing activities (winding down) before bedtime
Limit liquids before bedtime
Avoid caffeine, tobacco, and alcohol in the evening time
Avoid long naps (>30 minutes) during the day
Limit exposure to light before bedtime (including light from electronic devices)
Make sure sleep environment is quiet and comfortable

may improve sleep quality and daytime functioning.[41]

Hypnotics in patients with dementia should be used cautiously. Careful consideration of the benefits versus risks of the pharmacotherapy needs to be assessed. Possible side effects of hypnotics in this age group with dementia include risks of falls and worsened cognition. There are limited studies of hypnotics in patients with dementia, although in practice, many of the same hypnotics used in the general population are used in this specific patient population. These include zolpidem, eszopiclone, zaleplon, ramelteon, and triazolam. Trazodone in low doses is also commonly used and was shown to improve sleep in one small randomized, placebo-controlled study.[42] Melatonin (prolonged release) helped improve sleep in patients with mild to moderate AD in one randomized, placebo-controlled multicenter study.[43]

Obstructive Sleep Apnea

It is unclear if there is a higher incidence of sleep-disordered breathing in patients with AD as compared with age-matched control subjects, although there are numerous studies suggesting a higher risk.[44] The incidence of sleep-disordered breathing in older patients is higher than the general population. There is some evidence to suggest that obstructive sleep apnea may lead to a higher risk or earlier onset of dementia or MCI.[45,46] Diagnosis should be confirmed with objective testing in the form of an in-laboratory attended polysomnography or home sleep apnea test in appropriate patients. Treatment options remain the same as in the general population, including positive airway pressure, weight loss, positional therapy, and oral appliances. CPAP has been shown to reduce

subjective daytime sleepiness in AD[47] and decrease arousals and increase stage N3 sleep.[48] CPAP as treatment in patients with AD with sleep apnea has demonstrated improved cognition and slowing of cognitive decline.[49,50] Adherence with CPAP therapy, which is already challenging in the general population, may be even more challenging in patients with dementia given their cognitive deficits and possibly worsening confusion at bedtime.

PROGRESSIVE SUPRANUCLEAR PALSY

Patients suffering from PSP also have numerous sleep complaints. PSP is a neurodegenerative condition caused by abnormal accumulation of tau in the central nervous system. Symptoms include axial rigidity, postural instability, and a supranuclear gaze palsy. Patients with PSP commonly suffer from insomnia for similar reasons as other patients with dementia and neurodegenerative conditions mentioned previously (eg, damage to sleep-controlling areas of the brain, muscle spasms, medication side effects, mood disorder). Sleep studies in patients with PSP have demonstrated reduced REM sleep and spindle formation[51] and frequent arousals.[52] Patients with PSP also have more RLS, which may contribute to insomnia.[53] RBD is noted at high rates in PSP, but not as high as PD or other synucleinopathies.[54]

CLINICS CARE POINTS

- Sleep disorders are commonly seen in patients with neurodegeneratives conditions, but remain unrecognized and untreated.
- Treating underlying sleep disorders and improving sleep in these patients may result in improvement in underlying symptoms related to the neurodegenerative condition as well as slow progression.

DISCLOSURE

The author has no relevant disclosures, nor any financial or commercial conflicts of interest.

REFERENCES

1. de Lau LM, Breteler MM. Epidemiology of Parkinson's disease. Lancet Neurol 2006;5(6):525–35.
2. Tandberg E, Larsen JP, Karlsen K. A community-based study of sleep disorders in patients with Parkinson's disease. Mov Disord 1998;13(6):895–9.

3. Takakusaki K, Saitoh K, Harada H, et al. Evidence for a role of basal ganglia in the regulation of rapid eye movement sleep by electrical and chemical stimulation for the pedunculopontine tegmental nucleus and the substantia nigra pars reticulata in decerebrate cats. Neuroscience 2004;124(1):207–20.

4. American Academy of Seep Medicine. International classification of sleep disorders. In: Diagnostic and coding manual. 3rd edition. Westchester (IL): American Academy of Sleep Medicine; 2014.

5. Pierantozzi M, Placidi F, Liguori C, et al. Rotigotine may improve sleep architecture in Parkinson's disease: a double-blind, randomized, placebo-controlled polysomnographic study. Sleep Med 2016;21:140–4.

6. Ondo W, Vuong K, Jankovic J. Exploring the relationship between Parkinson disease and restless legs syndrome. Arch Neurol 2002;59:421–4.

7. Breen DP, Vuono R, Nawarathna U, et al. Sleep and circadian rhythm regulation in early Parkinson disease. JAMA Neurol 2014;71(5):589–95.

8. Videnovic A, Noble C, Reid KJ, et al. Circadian melatonin rhythm and excessive daytime sleepiness in Parkinson disease. JAMA Neurol 2014;71(4):463–9.

9. Menza M, Dobkin RD, Marin H, et al. Treatment of insomnia in Parkinson's disease: a controlled trial of eszopiclone and placebo. Mov Disord 2010;25(11):1708–14.

10. Rios Romenets S, Creti L, Fichten C, et al. Doxepin and cognitive behavioural therapy for insomnia in patients with Parkinson's disease: a randomized study. Parkinsonism Relat Disord 2013;19(7):670–5.

11. Frucht S, Rogers JD, Greene PE, et al. Falling asleep at the wheel: motor vehicle mishaps in persons taking pramipexole and ropinirole. Neurology 1999;52:1908–10.

12. Abbott RD, Ross GW, White LR, et al. Excessive daytime sleepiness and subsequent development of Parkinson disease. Neurology 2005;65:1442–6.

13. Hobson D, Lang A, Wayne Martin W, et al. Excessive daytime sleepiness and sudden-onset sleep in Parkinson disease. A survey by the Canadian movement disorder group. JAMA 2002;287:455–63.

14. Arnulf I. Excessive daytime sleepiness and parkinsonism. Sleep Med Rev 2005;9:185–200.

15. Wienecke M, Werth E, Poryazova R, et al. Progressive dopamine and hypocretin deficiencies in Parkinson's disease: is there an impact on sleep and wakefulness? J Sleep Res 2012;21(6):710–7.

16. Postuma RB, Lang AE, Munhoz RP, et al. Caffeine for treatment of Parkinson disease: a randomized controlled trial. Neurology 2012;79:651–8.

17. Ondo WG, Fayle R, Atassi F, et al. Modafinil for daytime somnolence in Parkinson's disease: double

blind, placebo controlled parallel trial. J Neurol Neurosurg Psychiatry 2005;76:1636–9.

18. Ondo WG, Perkins T, Swick T, et al. Sodium oxybate for excessive daytime sleepiness in Parkinson disease: an open-label polysomnographic study. Arch Neurol 2008;65(10):1337–40.

19. Trotti LM, Bliwise DL. No increased risk of obstructive sleep apnea in Parkinson's disease. Mov Disord 2010;25(13):2246–9.

20. Neikrug AB, Liu L, Avanzino JA, et al. Continuous positive airway pressure improves sleep and daytime sleepiness in patients with Parkinson disease and sleep apnea. Sleep 2014;37(1):177–85.

21. Shimohata T, Nakayama H, Aizawa N, et al. Discontinuation of continuous positive airway pressure treatment in multiple system atrophy. Sleep Med 2014;15(9):1147–9.

22. Silber MH, Levine S. Stridor and death in multiple system atrophy. Mov Disord 2000;15(4):699–704.

23. Palma JA, Fernandez-Cordon C, Coon EA, et al. Prevalence of REM sleep behavior disorder in multiple system atrophy: a multicenter study and meta-analysis. Clin Auton Res 2015;25(1):69–75.

24. Sixel-Doring F, Trautmann F, Mollenhauer B, et al. Associated factors for REM sleep behavior disorder in Parkinson disease. Neurology 2011;77:1048–54.

25. Iranzo A, Fernandez-Arcos A, Tolosa E, et al. Neurodegenerative disorder risk in idiopathic REM sleep behavior disorder: study in 174 patients. PLoS One 2014;9:e89741.

26. Frauscher B, Iranzo A, Hogl B, et al. Quantification of electromyographic activity during REM sleep in multiple muscles in REM sleep behavior disorder. Sleep 2008;31:724–31.

27. Aurora RN, Zak RS, Maganti RK, et al. Best practice guide for the treatment of REM sleep behavior disorder (RBD). J Clin Sleep Med 2010;6:85–95.

28. Kunz D, Mahlberg R. A two-part, double-blind, placebo-controlled trial of exogenous melatonin in REM sleep behaviour disorder. J Sleep Res 2010;19:591–6.

29. Plassman BL, Langa KM, Fisher GG, et al. Prevalence of dementia in the United States: the aging, demographics, and memory study. Neuroepidemiology 2007;29(1–2):125–32.

30. Mishima K, Tozawa T, Satoh K, et al. Melatonin secretion rhythm disorders in patients with senile dementia of Alzheimer's type with disturbed sleep-waking. Biol Psychiatry 1999;45(4):417–21.

31. Bedrosian TA, Nelson RJ. Pro: Alzheimer's disease and circadian dysfunction: chicken or egg? Alzheimers Res Ther 2012;4(4):25.

32. Spira AP, Gamaldo AA, An Y, et al. Self-reported sleep and beta-amyloid deposition in community-dwelling older adults. JAMA Neurol 2013;70(12):1537–43.

33. Xie L, Kang H, Xu Q, et al. Sleep drives metabolite clearance from the adult brain. Science 2013;342:373–7.

34. Beaulieu-Bonneau S, Hudon C. Sleep disturbances in older adults with mild cognitive impairment. Int Psychogeriatr 2009;21:654–66.

35. Westerberg CE, Mander BA, Florczak SM, et al. Concurrent impairments in sleep and memory in amnestic mild cognitive impairment. J Int Neuropsychol Soc 2012;18:490–500.

36. Bliwise DL. Sleep in normal aging and dementia. Sleep 1993;16(1):40–81.

37. Ktonas PY, Golemati S, Xanthopoulos P, et al. Potential dementia biomarkers based on the time-varying microstructure of sleep EEG spindles. Conf Proc IEEE Eng Med Biol Soc 2007;2007:2464–7.

38. Liquori C, Romigi A, Nuccetelli M, et al. Orexinergic system dysregulation, sleep impairment, and cognitive decline in Alzheimer disease. JAMA Neurol 2014;71(12):1498–505.

39. Sullivan SC, Richards KC. Predictors of circadian sleep-wake rhythm maintenance in elders with dementia. Aging Ment Health 2004;8(2):143–52.

40. Dowling GA, Burr RL, Van Someren EJ, et al. Melatonin and bright-light treatment for rest-activity disruption in institutionalized patients with Alzheimer's disease. J Am Geriatr Soc 2008;56(2):239–46.

41. de Jonghe A, Korevaar JC, van Munster BC, et al. Effectiveness of melatonin treatment on circadian rhythm disturbances in dementia. Are there implications for delirium? A systematic review. Int J Geriatr Psychiatry 2010;25(12):1201–8.

42. Camargos EF, Louzada LL, Quintas JL, et al. Trazadone improves sleep parameters in Alzheimer disease patients: a randomized, double-blind, and placebo controlled study. Am J Geriatr Psychiatry 2014;22(12):1565–74.

43. Wade AG, Farmer M, Harari G, et al. Add-on prolonged release melatonin for cognitive function and sleep in mild to moderate Alzheimer's disease: a 6 month randomized, placebo-controlled, multicenter trial. Clin Interv Aging 2014;9:947–61.

44. Ancoli-Israel S, Klauber MR, Butters N, et al. Dementia in institutionalized elderly: relation to sleep apnea. J Am Geriatr Soc 1991;39(3):258–63.

45. Yaffe K, Laffan AM, Harrison SL, et al. Sleep-disordered breathing, hypoxia, and risk of mild cognitive impairment and dementia in older women. JAMA 2011;306(6):613–9.

46. Osorio RS, Gumb T, Pirraglia E, et al. Sleep-disordered breathing advances cognitive decline in the elderly. Neurology 2015;84(19):1964–71.

47. Chong MS, Ayalon L, Marler M, et al. Continuous positive airway pressure reduces subjective daytime sleepiness in patients with mild to moderate Alzheimer's disease with sleep disordered breathing. J Am Geriatr Soc 2006;54(5):777–81.

48. Cooke JR, Ancoli-Israel S, Liu L, et al. Continuous positive airway pressure deepens sleep in patients with Alzheimer's disease and obstructive sleep apnea. Sleep Med 2009;10(10):1101–6.

49. Troussiere AC, Monaca CC, Salleron J, et al. Treatment of sleep apnea syndrome decreases cognitive decline in patients with Alzheimer's disease. J Neurol Neurosurg Psychiatry 2014;85(12):1405–8.

50. Ancoli-Israel S, Palmer BW, Cooke JR, et al. Cognitive effects of treating obstructive sleep apnea in Alzheimer's disease: a randomized controlled study. J Am Geriatr Soc 2008;56(11):2076–81.

51. Petit D, Gagnon JF, Fantini ML, et al. Sleep and quantitative EEG in neurodegenerative disorders. J Psychosom Res 2004;56(5):487–96.

52. Aldrich MS, Foster NL, White RF, et al. Sleep abnormalities in progressive supranuclear palsy. Ann Neurol 1989;25(6):577–81.

53. Gama RL, Tavora DG, Bomfim RC, et al. Sleep disturbances and brain MRI morphometry in Parkinson's disease, multiple system atrophy and progressive supranuclear palsy: a comparative study. Parkinsonism Relat Disord 2010;16:275–9.

54. Sixel-Doring F, Schweitzer M, Mollenhauer B, et al. Polysomnographic findings, video-based sleep analysis and sleep perception in progressive supranuclear palsy. Sleep Med 2009;10(4):407–15.

Moving?

Make sure your subscription moves with you!

To notify us of your new address, find your **Clinics Account Number** (located on your mailing label above your name), and contact customer service at:

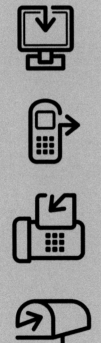

Email: journalscustomerservice-usa@elsevier.com

800-654-2452 (subscribers in the U.S. & Canada)
314-447-8871 (subscribers outside of the U.S. & Canada)

Fax number: 314-447-8029

**Elsevier Health Sciences Division
Subscription Customer Service
3251 Riverport Lane
Maryland Heights, MO 63043**

ELSEVIER